Western Biomedicine
and
Eastern Therapeutics

An Integrative Strategy for
Personalized and Preventive Healthcare

Western Biomedicine and Eastern Therapeutics

An Integrative Strategy for Personalized and Preventive Healthcare

Sun-Chong Wang
National Central University, Taiwan

World Scientific
NEW JERSEY • LONDON • SINGAPORE • BEIJING • SHANGHAI • HONG KONG • TAIPEI • CHENNAI

Published by

World Scientific Publishing Co. Pte. Ltd.
5 Toh Tuck Link, Singapore 596224
USA office: 27 Warren Street, Suite 401-402, Hackensack, NJ 07601
UK office: 57 Shelton Street, Covent Garden, London WC2H 9HE

Library of Congress Cataloging-in-Publication Data
Wang, Sun-Chong, 1963–
Western biomedicine and Eastern therapeutics : an integrative strategy for personalized and preventive healthcare / by Sun-Chong Wang.
p. ; cm.
Includes bibliographical references and index.
ISBN 978-9814412872 (hardcover : alk. paper)
I. Title.
[DNLM: 1. Integrative Medicine. 2. Medicine, Ayurvedic. 3. Medicine, Chinese Traditional. WB 113]
616--dc23

2012046513

British Library Cataloguing-in-Publication Data
A catalogue record for this book is available from the British Library.

Typeset by Stallion Press
Email: enquiries@stallionpress.com

Printed by FuIsland Offset Printing (S) Pte Ltd Singapore

To my mother, Gao-Yue Wang,
for her love and patience

Contents

Preface

Medicine has made great strides since the late 19th century, with advances in chemistry, pharmacology, surgery, molecular biology and laboratory technologies. Together with education and accreditation systems, modern medicine, which originated in the West, has penetrated and dominated the healthcare of the world. Life expectancy at birth has more than doubled in a century, with decreased mortalities among infants and patients with infectious, cardiovascular or endocrine diseases. Modern western medicine (MWM) has, however, been less successful in treating chronic and degenerative conditions, such as sleep disturbance, dysmenorrhea, diabetes, cancer and dementia, which are increasingly recognized as multifactorial complex disorders. Multitarget holistic approaches to complex diseases, termed "systems pharmacology," have recently been called for toward personalized and preventive medicine.

None of the holistic, individualized and preventive modes of therapy is new to ancient eastern medicines such as traditional Indian medicine (Ayurveda) and traditional Chinese medicine (TCM). Ayurveda deduced three fundamental forces, called *doshas*, for all living organisms. An individual's phenotype, including psychophysiological traits, disease susceptibility, prognosis and treatment, are determined by his or her predominant dosha(s). Ayurveda and Yoga prescribe a package of interventions including lifestyle, diet, detoxification, purification, herbal mixtures and meditation. TCM's model of human physiology focuses on functional interactions among the body subsystems, called *zang–fu*. Imbalance in the functions, due to emotional or environmental disturbances, causes disease. TCM treatment for the patient's pattern of functional imbalance, called *zheng*, includes multi-ingredient herbal formulas and acupuncture. Both Ayurveda and TCM prescribe lifestyle and dietary regimens for disease prevention.

MWM and Ayurveda/TCM can be considered two radical paradigms of complex systems. The microscopic and reductionist approach of the West prevails in acute and single-gene conditions such as infection and Mendelian disorders. The macroscopic and holistic approach of the East potentially fares well in subclinical, chronic and complex conditions such as lumbago, obesity and ageing. This book serves three purposes: (1) to help MWM, Ayurveda and TCM professionals get acquainted with one another; (2) to help identify common grounds for MWM, Ayurveda and TCM, rather than blindly westernizing eastern medicines or vice versa; and (3) to help translate the complementarity of MWM and Ayurveda/TCM into integrated, multicomponent, evidence-based healthcare. To this end, we introduce theories and tenets of the three medicines. We use bioenergetics to reconcile West and East, as ATP generation, *prana* and *qi* are central to MWM, Ayurveda and TCM, respectively. We discuss clinical trials of varying experimental rigor for the assessment of the scientific evidence for treatment effectiveness. We hold that a federal unity of therapies consisting of MWM, Ayurveda and TCM better serves the wellbeing of humankind.

Chapter 1 shows how evidence for effectiveness is evaluated in MWM. Chapters 2 and 3 introduce the fundamental principles of MWM, Ayurveda and TCM. Chapter 4 illustrates how western and eastern therapies can be integrated. Examples in this chapter serve to inspire design of holistic therapies with the core principles outlined in Chapters 2 and 3. Taiwan is one of the few areas in the world that practice both modern and traditional medicine.

Moreover, pharmacoepidemiology (including pharmacovigilance) of TCM is facilitated by the single-payer, national health insurance system covering all residents patronizing either medicine. Chapters 6–9 emanate from results of 35 million TCM prescriptions, stored in the (deidentified) reimbursement database, which were made by about 4800 licensed TCM doctors in Taiwan in a year. Chapter 6 covers benign and malignant cancers. Chapter 7 includes the top 10 causes of death across the globe according to the World Health Organization. Chapter 8 contains the top 20 frequent conditions for which TCM is sought after. Chapter 9 involves reproductive system disorders. In Part II, known disease mechanisms are presented together with the herbal medicines, which typically serve as being complementary or alternative to conventional remedies. For example, some side effects of cancer chemotherapy have been shown to be alleviated by herbal medicine. Low-fat diet or exercise can be combined with oral hypoglycemics for efficient diabetic management. Ovulation-inducing drugs together with *yin*-nourishing herbs improve fertility. Ayurvedic/TCM holism offers insights into longevity. To reap the rich harvest of holistic concepts, Chapter 10 reviews modern as well as traditional theories of aging. Chapters 11 and 12 present individualized lifestyles and diets for healthy aging.

This book is for advanced students, academics, researchers and professionals, including physicians, pharmacists, nurses and regulators, in conventional as well as unconventional healthcare. It is also beneficial to a general audience interested in evidence-based holistic self-care. I am indebted to Lan-Ying Huang, Pei-Hsun Chiu and Jie-Ping Lin for insightful discussion and clerical assistance.

Sun-Chong Wang
Zhongli Taoyuan, Taiwan
September 2012

Part I

Basics

1

Evidence-Based Practice

Medicine is the knowledge of healing. Clinical practice of the knowledge by medical doctors seeks to resolve or prevent health problems of individuals. Reliability of the knowledge therefore matters to patients and to society at large. Reliable knowledge is believed to be most efficiently accumulated by scientific methods where hypotheses or models for a phenomenon are tested in well-defined and -designed experiments. The assertion of the experimenter will have to be reproduced by other, independent investigators. Evidence that supports the hypothesis and assertion is then considered substantial. Modern medicine, which is based on scientific evidence, is in sharp contrast to ancient medicines, which are based on personal experience and anecdotal evidence, such as intuition, rules of thumb, folklore and custom. As healthcare absorbs a sizable chunk of public and private spending, evidence-based medicine helps keep quack medicine from wasting healthcare resources. To illustrate the role of evidence-based approaches in the decision-making of healthcare providers, we outline the process of new drug development and approval in the United States, which is one of the largest drug markets in the world. We elaborate on evidence bases and echo innovative development of translational research beyond health services.

1.1 The FDA Drug Approval Process

In the United States, as in other jurisdictions, promotion and production of drugs are regulated. The agency that receives and approves new drug applications is the Food and Drug Administration (FDA). The focuses of the FDA review are the safety, effectiveness, labeling and manufacturing of the candidate drug. The FDA itself does not conduct tests for the effectiveness of the new drug. It is the responsibility of the drug sponsor, usually a pharmaceutical company, to provide evidence for the benefits of the new drug.

Before formal application, the sponsor most likely has spent years on the biology and synthesis of the new drug, usually a chemical compound. The safety and dosage of the compound have also been assessed in laboratory animals. After consulting with the FDA about the potential benefits of the new drug, the sponsor files an investigational new drug application to test the new drug in humans. If the safety and ethics of the proposed clinical study can be assured, the drug enters a phase I clinical trial.

In a phase I clinical trial, 20–80 healthy volunteers are enrolled to evaluate any acute adverse effects of the drug. Pharmacokinetics, including dosage, metabolism and excretion of the drug, is also studied. A phase II clinical trial involves dozens to 300 patient volunteers. Efficacy and short-term side effects of the drug are evaluated via placebo-controlled studies. If the drug looks promising after phase II, it enters phase III for verification of the effectiveness of the drug in randomized controlled trials with hundreds to 3000 patient volunteers across clinics and hospitals. With a larger sample size, effects due to different population/dosage and drug–drug interaction can be studied. Long-term side effects will also be monitored. The main objective of phase III is extrapolation of the result to the general population. As the scale of the study increases with the phase, the time and costs increase too. It usually takes one, two and three years for phase I, II and III clinical trials, respectively. It was estimated that a phase III clinical trial devoured two-thirds of the costs.

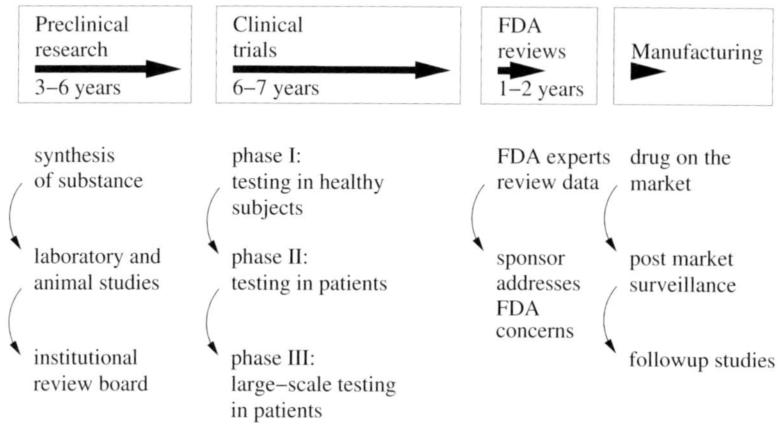

FIGURE 1.1
The process and timetable for a new drug to obtain FDA approval.

With results of the clinical and animal studies, the drug sponsor submits to the FDA a new drug application. The Center for Drug Evaluation and Research of the FDA then assigns a panel of scientists, consisting of physicians, statisticians, chemists, pharmacologists, microbiologists and other experts, to review the application. The issues of concern range from the manufacturing, bioavailability, stability, pharmacodynamics, benefits and risks to the proposed labeling of the drug. If the benefits are demonstrated to outweigh the risks, the drug is approved to be marketed under the labeling in the United States. The FDA is required to respond within 10 months of the submission of the new drug application. In a survey of the new drug applications made by the 50 largest pharmaceutical companies in the period of 1993–2004, the average success rate of clinical approval through June 2009 was 19% [DiMasi *et al.*, 2010].

1.2 Randomized Controlled Trial

Clinical trials allow information on the safety and effectiveness of the health intervention in human subjects to be collected. Well designed clinical trials provide compelling evidence for the benefits of the drug. The FDA normally considers at least two randomized controlled trials (RCTs) as mandatory for the qualification of the evidence. As such, most phase III clinical trials and some phase II clinical trials are randomized controlled trials.

The first RCT was run by England's Medical Research Council in 1946. Since then, RCTs have become gold standard in modern evidence-based medicine. Three elements are essential in the design of RCTs:

(1) Randomization randomly assigns the subjects to one of two groups. One group receives the new drug; the other receives a fake treatment, such as an inert pill, called a placebo.
(2) Blinding refers to unawareness of the actual treatment which the subject receives. If only the subjects are unaware, it is called single-blind. If both the subjects and the clinicians are unaware, it is called double-blind. If none of the subjects, clinicians and assessors of the data are aware, the design is called triple-blind.
(3) Controlling provides a reference for the comparison. Sometimes, the controls receive, instead of a placebo, the best available or standard-of-care treatment. The trials are then called active-controlled.

Randomization prevents biases due to confounding factors that are unknown at the time of the trial. For example, if aging plays a role in the disease, random assignment of the subjects would in principle result in two groups of similar age distributions, avoiding the comparison of a young treated group with an old untreated group. Blinding prevents potential biases due to differential care which the clinicians provide for the subjects. For example, physicians may display sympathy toward the placebo-receiving patients for the fake treatment. Patients may show improvement in the symptom because of their subjective perception of the treatment effect. This phenomenon is called the placebo effect. The placebo-controlled design aims to isolate the effect in the sense that the medical improvement of the drug has to better than that of the placebo.

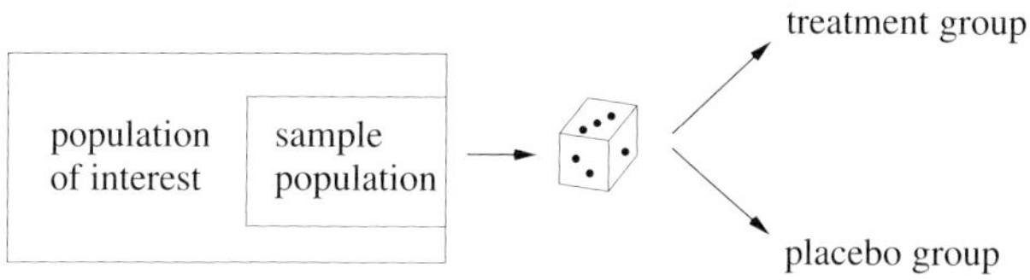

FIGURE 1.2
In a randomized controlled trial, recruited patients are randomly divided into two groups. One group receive treatment which is under investigation. The other group receive inert treatment or standard treatment, serving as control. The inert treatment patients are called the placebo control group, and the standard treatment patients the active control group.

Note that the condition of the placebo-receiving patients may deteriorate after the trial. Patients have to be informed that they are receiving either treatment or placebo in the trial, and written consent has to be obtained from the participating patients.

1.3 Level of Evidence

In situations where placebos are not acceptable or alternate therapies are not available for the controls, the trials then involve only one group, i.e. the treatment group. These are called single-arm studies. Although randomized, double-blind, placebo-controlled trials are the design of choice, the FDA has accepted single-arm design in the clinical trials for new drugs for such indications as metastasizing cancers. It is therefore useful to have in mind the quality of evidence generated from diverse medical research.

An evidence scale also helps healthcare professionals determine the best practice for the patients. The rating is based on the benefits and risks of the treatment or diagnosis. A ranking of the evidence by the Preventive Services Task Force of the United States is the following:

(i) Randomized controlled trials
(ii) Controlled trials
(iii) Cohort or case control studies

(iv) Multiple time series
(v) Opinions of authorities and experts

On the other hand, the National Health Services of the United Kingdom also ranks the evidence from different studies:

(i) Consistent randomized controlled trials and cohort studies
(ii) Consistent cohort and case control studies
(iii) Case series
(iv) Expert opinions, physiology, laboratory research and first principles

Both cohort and case control studies are observational studies commonly seen in epidemiology. In a cohort study, a group of people sharing a common characteristic, such as nurses, are interviewed on a regular basis for a period of time. The conditions and other factors of the subjects are examined and recorded in the

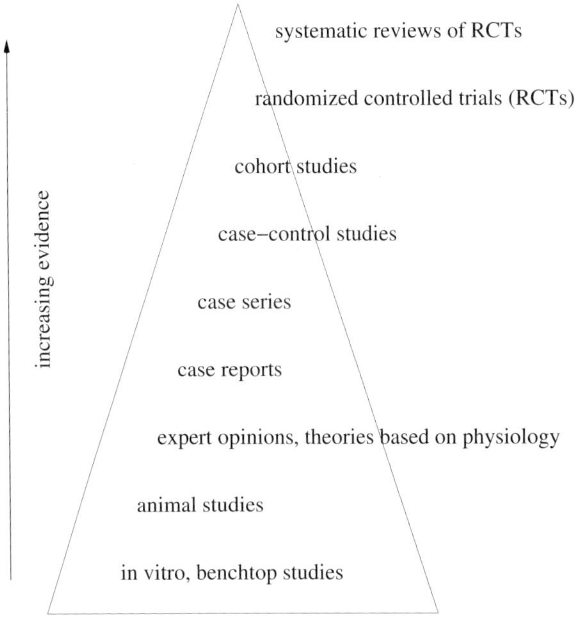

FIGURE 1.3
The hierarchy of scientific evidence from various studies.

interview throughout the study. A condition, such as the body mass index (BMI), is then correlated with factors like levels of physical activity and calorie intake. A statistically significant correlation between calorie intake and BMI may then suggest calorie intake as an effective intervention for the obese condition. In a case control study, two groups of subjects are similar in all but one respect. For example, a group of old prostate cancer patients are compared to a group of old healthy men for the identification of differences in the prostate genomes. Identified sequence mutations are then considered risk factors for the disease. Case series and multiple time series are small-scale descriptive cohort studies. They are thought to be prone to selection bias because of the small sample size.

Clinical studies infer the effect of treatment or intervention on the subjects from the correlation between treatment and outcome. In observational studies such as cohort and case-control studies, assignment of subjects to treatment or reference groups is outside the control of the investigators. In contrast, in controlled studies, including randomized controlled studies, investigators separate the subjects to account for potential confounding factors. Within a design, studies can give different and sometimes conflicting results due for example to the stochastic nature of disease processes or the varying degree of experimental quality. An undertaking that systematically consolidates the study findings is needed.

1.4 Cochrane Review

It is not uncommon that results from different biomedical laboratories are at odds. Different techniques, methodologies, subpopulations, inpatient settings and analyses can contribute to the variance. A journal of a field of inquiry may publish narrative reviews, usually by invited authors, from time to time. A systematic review, however, aims to appraise and synthesize the evidence in the published literature in an objective and transparent way. Among the systematic reviews, Cochrane Reviews are unique in that they are

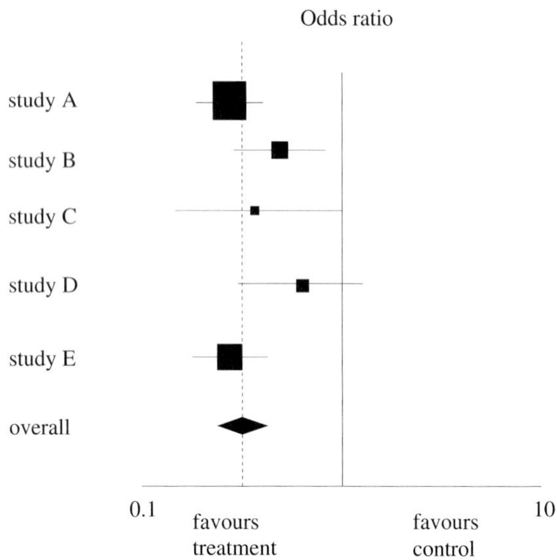

FIGURE 1.4
In the meta-analysis of a systematic review, treatment effects — odds ratios in this example — from eligible studies are summarized into an overall effect. The size of the solid square indicates the weight in the summarization.

prepared by the Cochrane Collaboration (www.cochrane.org), which, having been an independent and not-for-profit organization since 1993, advocates evidence-based healthcare for healthcare providers, policy-makers and patients through a network of 28,000 volunteering contributors from 100 countries around the world. Cochrane Reviews, with stringent and explicit guidelines for unbiased selection and rigorous assessment of primary research, address diverse healthcare interventions, including treatment, prevention, rehabilitation and diagnosis, for a wide range of medical conditions.

A systematic review starts with a comprehensive search of the public databases such as MEDLINE for the original studies on a specific healthcare topic. Most of the studies included in a Cochrane Review are controlled trials and observational studies. Clear criteria for the incorporation of studies are specified during the search. For example, only randomized, double-blind, placebo-controlled trials are incorporated. Data are then independently extracted from the eligible studies by two of the review authors. The effect of the intervention, which is usually in terms of the effect size if the intervention outcome is continuous or the odds ratio if the outcome is dichotomous, varies from one study to another, owing to differing sample sizes and/or the probabilistic nature of underlying biochemical reactions. An important component of the systematic review is then to output, in a procedure called meta-analysis, an overall effect by the weighted average of the effects from the individual studies. The weighting in the average can be the inverse of the variance of the effect in each incorporated study. Combining individual studies is believed to enhance the statistical power of detecting or rejecting an effect. The Cochrane Collaboration has so far published over 4600 systematic reviews available online in the database of Cochrane Reviews in the Cochrane Library.

Meta-analysis can be considered an observational study of evidence [Egger *et al.*, 1997]. New studies are published as technologies advance. Systematic reviews have to be updated too. In addition, since published results are predominantly positive with negative results piling up file drawers, the so-called publication bias needs to be addressed in a meta-analysis. For example, Chinese herbal medicine clinical trials published in Chinese journals seldom concluded negative results [Shang *et al.*, 2007]. An indication of publication bias is the observation of the trend of a decreasing effect size with an increasing sample size among the published results. In this case, many of the small sample size studies measured no effect and went unpublished and those that were published were just false positives. In meta-analysis, a step can be taken to test if the overall effect remains significant when the small sample size studies are excluded. Likewise, individual studies can be scored according to their experimental quality. The overall effect is then estimated to test if it is sensitive to exclusion of low-equality studies. Finally, conflicts of interest have to be stated in journal publication. A similar sensitivity test should be performed on the studies whose authors disclose financial ties to commercial sponsors. A systematic review provides healthcare

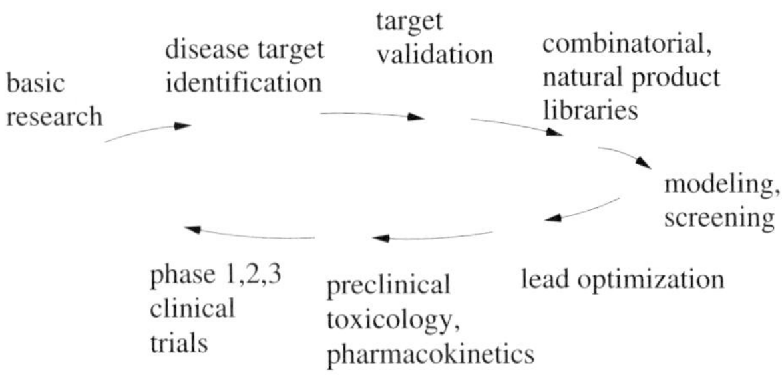

FIGURE 1.5
Steps of drug development leading to clinical trials.

providers, policy-makers and patients with the best available evidence for the effectiveness of an intervention. For example, in the United States, the Preventive Services Task Force, based on the evidence from up-to-date systematic reviews of well-controlled clinical trials, releases health intervention recommendations, which are then followed by most medical groups.

1.5 Drug Development

Biological macromolecules such as proteins and nucleic acids are involved in almost all essential biological processes in living organisms. They have served as targets in drug development in which a small compound is sought to modify, e.g. inhibit, the activity of the target when the compound is brought in contact with the target in cell cultures. Examples of established targets are G-protein-coupled receptors and protein kinases, which play important roles in signal transduction. Indeed, over 60% of the targets of FDA-approved drugs were found to be membrane proteins even though only under 40% of disease genes expressed in cell membrane [Yildirim *et al.*, 2007]. The international, 13-year endeavor of the Human Genome Project (HGP), which was completed in 2003, identified about 23,000 genes in human DNA. One of the great opportunities and also challenges in the post-HGP era is the identification of new functional targets for new drug discovery.

In combinatorial chemistry, with the help of robotics and information science, high-throughput screening (HTS) methods have been developed, allowing the performance of millions of biochemical tests in hours. HTS determines the potency and selectivity of chemical libraries, resulting in a series of lead compounds. Further screening on the grounds of drug likeness isolates one or two lead compounds for subsequent studies on animals. Despite advances in combinatorial chemistry, according to an updated review by researchers at the National Cancer Institute of the United States [Newman and Cragg, 2007], 63% of all the 974 FDA-approved small molecule chemical entities from January 1981 to June 2006 are derivatives or semiderivatives of natural products called natural product mimics. If the drug indications are limited to cancer, then the proportion is even higher, with 73% of the 155 anticancer small molecule chemical entities approved by the FDA during the period from the 1940s to June 2006 being natural product mimics [Newman and Cragg, 2007]. Since species in an ecosystem have evolved competitive, predatory or symbiotic relations among them through (co)evolution, bioactive compounds are believed to be abundant in nature. If this is the case, many of the botanic plants that have long been used in ethnopharmacy hold promise for new drug discovery.

A lead compound, either natural or synthetic, while showing its stability and mass-manufacturability, undergoes toxicity tests in two — e.g. murine and canine — animals. The results help determine the dose and schedule for human clinical trials. It was estimated that 1 out of 5000 candidate compounds in preclinical investigations entered clinical trials. Estimation of the average cost of a drug from benchtop to bedside varied, ranging from 500 million to 2 billion U.S. dollars [Adams and Brantner, 2006]. The time spent was about 10 years.

1.6 Translational Medicine

The spending by large pharmaceutical companies on research and development continues to rise, having tripled since 1995. However,

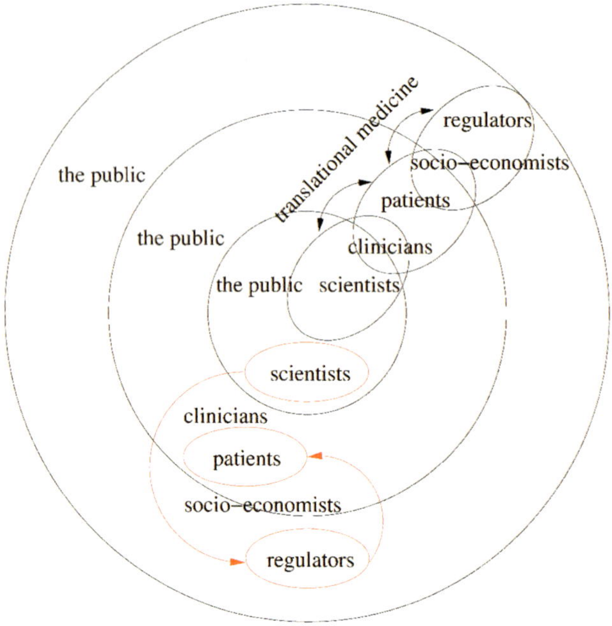

FIGURE 1.6
Translational medicine aims to shorten the pathway from laboratory discovery to clinical application by aligning biomedical scientists, clinicians, biotechnologists, health economists and policy–makers. Each of the professions is part of the public. Note that the interactions (arrows) between those involved in translational medicine are bidirectional.

the number of FDA-approved new drugs had fallen from an average of 37 per year between 1995 and 1999 to an average of 21 per year between 2000 and 2010. A call was made to speed up the translation of research findings into health and economic benefits [Coller and Califf, 2009; Bornstein and Licinio, 2011]. Toward this goal, the infrastructure of the whole healthcare system, including clinical research, will have to be overhauled. Such a change will definitely involve academia, industry and government, which are driven by such different factors as individual success, shareholders' interests and public mandate.

An approach to translational medicine is a bidirectional transfer of knowledge between laboratory researchers and clinical practitioners. In particular, "-omics" and cross-disciplinary researches can help identify new drug targets, raising the confidence in drug discoveries. For example, the crystal structure of a retroviral protease that had baffled scientists for a decade was solved to a sufficient quality by online players of a protein folding game in just three weeks [Khatib *et al.*, 2011]. Furthermore, creative designs of clinical trials that do not sacrifice efficacy for safety reduce not only costs but also time. This approach of translational medicine concerns basic science.

The other layer of translational medicine focuses on patient-driven healthcare development. On this layer, the acceptability and cost-effectiveness of the intervention are assessed via such tools as consumer research and health economics. Clinical decisions may be modified based on demographic factors and competing priorities. For example, chronic illness patients should be provided with cheaper or alternative interventions which, although having lower levels of scientific evidence for the effectiveness, do not compromise their quality of life. This layer engages socioeconomic science.

An ongoing projection of translational medicine is evidence-based public policies for sustainable solutions in healthcare. For example, promotion and implementation of preventive measures against obesity through education of the public and tax on fattening foods should be part of an integrative intervention against the epidemic. This front of translational medicine touches political science.

2

Modern Western Biomedicine

The word "biology", meaning "the study of life and living organisms," first appeared in German as "*biologie*" in the 18th century. The invention of optical microscopes in the 17th century contributed greatly to the development and identification of the basic building block of life: the cell. Studies of the chemical processes and energy flow for the homeostasis of cellular functions began in the late 19th century. It was not until the discovery of the double-helical structure of DNA in the mid-20th century that biologists started to unravel the complex interactions between biological molecules responsible for the inheritance of organismal traits including human pathologies. Applications of biological principles to the functions and forms of organs/systems help advance clinical diagnosis and therapy of human disease. This chapter covers biochemistry, molecular biology and genetics, which are the three pillars of modern biology.

2.1 ATP Hydrolysis

One of the characteristics of living organisms that distinguish them from inanimate objects is the quality or ability of motion. In animals, motion is carried out by muscle contraction, which consumes energy. Growth and reproduction of an organism involve transportation and reorganization of biomolecules, which demands energy too. Energy transformation therefore accompanies most living processes. In chemistry, energy is stored in the electrons in chemical bonds, rearrangement of which can release energy. For example, in the hydrolytic reaction, ATP + $H_2O \rightarrow$ ADP + H_3PO_4 (= Pi) + energy, energy is liberated because the high-energy electrons in the phosphanhydridic bonds of adenosine triphosphate (ATP) subside in the new bonds in adenosine diphosphate (ADP) and inorganic phosphate (Pi).

In under the standard condition, the released energy is 30.5 kJ/mol or 7.3 kcal/mol, which is equal to the energy released by 1.3 g of peanuts. The energy-rich content of ATP makes it appealing to reactions that require energy. That is to say, reactions that do not occur without energy proceed fast once they are coupled to ATP hydrolysis. ATP is therefore considered a battery for the energy-consuming processes, including motility by motor proteins, synthesis and transportation of biological macromolecules (DNA, RNA, proteins), and signal transduction in intra- and extracellular signaling.

2.2 Oxidative Phosphorylation, the Electron Transport Chain, the Krebs Cycle

ATP, the molecular unit of energy transfer in biology, is synthesized in aerobic organisms by the so-called oxidative phosphorylation (OXPHOS), ADP + Pi + ATP synthase $\rightarrow$ ATP + ATP synthase, in mitochondria, which are a double-membraned organelle. OXPHOS requires input of energy as it is the reverse of the energy-releasing ATP hydrolysis. The energy comes from downhilling of protons, i.e. H^+ ions, through the proton gradient from the mitochondrial intermembrane space to the mitochondrial matrix. Moving down of the protons through the gradient drives rotation and reconformation of ATP synthase, yielding ATP. Before the proton gradient is utilized by ATP synthases, it, in brown fat tissue, can be dissipated by enzymes, called thermogenins, in the inner membrane. The dissipation generates heat for the maintenance of thermal homeostasis in hibernating mammals and human infants. The mechanical work by the proton-motive force also lashes flagella back and forth to propel cells.

The proton gradient is established by three proton pumping enzymes, i.e. complexes I, III, IV, on the mitochondrial inner membrane through a series of redox reactions called the electron transport chain (ETC). A redox reaction consists of paired reactions called reduction and oxidation. An example of redox reaction is corrosion of iron, $4\ Fe + 3\ O_2 \rightarrow 2\ Fe_2O_3$, where the electrons lost by iron are gained by oxygen in the formation of rust. In a redox reaction, if the electrons bind more weakly to the electron donor than to the electron acceptor, the transfer of electrons from the donor to the acceptor is thermodynamically favored with release of energy. Electron donors, called reductants or reducing agents, lose electrons and are oxidized; electron acceptors, called oxidants, gain electrons and are reduced. In the ETC, oxidation of nicotinamide adenine dinucleotide (NADH) and ubiquinol (QH_2) by O_2 drives the pumping of protons from the mitochondrial matrix to the mitochondrial intermembrane space, creating a proton gradient.

NADH, QH_2 and other energy-rich electron carriers are produced in mitochondria by cyclical steps of biochemical reactions called the Krebs cycle: acetyl-CoA + 3 NAD^+ + Q + GDP + Pi + 2 $H_2O \rightarrow$ CoA-SH + 3 NADH + 3 H^+ + QH_2 + GTP + 2 CO_2. The molecule acetyl-CoA is derived from oxidation of glucose, fatty acids and some amino acids. Other amino acids enter the cycle in its intermediate steps. Furthermore, intermediary compounds of the Krebs cycle also serve as precursors for the synthesis of other molecules. The Krebs cycle therefore plays a dual role in the breakdown and buildup of biological macromolecules.

2.3 Glycolysis, Aerobic Respiration, the Warburg Effect

In cellular respiration, chemical energy in nutrients is extracted in the form of ATP with the release of waste products. An immediate precursor of acetyl-CoA is pyruvate, which is produced by glucose in cytosol via a 10-step enzymatic reaction called glycolysis. In aerobic organisms, acetyl-CoA together with oxygen is then fed into mitochondria for efficient ATP production. In addition to pyruvate, fatty acids are also converted to acetyl-CoA in the mitochondrial matrix of heart tissue via a process called beta oxidation. The carbon skeletons of some amino acids are readily transformed into pyruvate and acetyl-CoA. Other amino acids enter the Krebs cycle directly. Glucose, fatty acids and amino acids are, respectively, the basic units of carbohydrates, fats and proteins, which constitute the three primary sources of calories in our diet.

Glycolysis gives a net yield of 2 ATPs per glucose in cytosol: glucose + 2 NAD^+ + 2 ADP + 2 Pi $\rightarrow$ 2 pyruvate + 2 NADH + 2 H^+ + 2 ATP + 2 H_2O. To continue glycolysis, NAD^+ is replenished via oxidation of NADH with pyruvate as the electron acceptor, i.e. pyruvate + NADH + H^+ $\rightarrow$ lactate + NAD^+, in a process called lactic acid fermentation. On the other hand, the theoretical net yield per glucose via the aerobic route of the Krebs cycle, ETC and OXPHOS in mitochondria is 36 ATPs. Aerobic respiration is more efficient than anaerobic respiration. Nevertheless, anaerobic respiration is seen in anaerobic microbes, overworked muscles and proliferating tissues.

Moreover, cancer cells — cells that proliferate uncontrollably — were observed to predominantly utilize glycolytic fermentation over oxidative phosphorylation even in the presence of sufficient oxygen to support oxidative phosphorylation [Warburg, 1956]. An explanation for the phenomenon, called aerobic glycolysis or the Warburg effect, is a mis-crosstalk between proliferating signal transduction pathways and metabolic pathways, leading to a proliferating phenotype of cancer cells.

2.4 Reactive Oxygen Species, Oxidative Stress, Redox Signaling

In mitochondrial ETC, electrons pass down the chain from electron donors to acceptors while protons are translocated across the inner membrane. Oxygen is the final electron acceptor and gets reduced to water. During the passing down, electrons may escape and prematurely leak to oxygen, forming superoxide (O_2^-). Atoms and molecules are stable when they are in the ground state with paired electrons filling the outermost or valence shell. Superoxide, lacking only one electron, is unstable and reactive, in that it tries to steal one electron from the molecules in its surroundings in order to fill its shell. The surrounding molecules, such as DNA, proteins and lipids, can be damaged as a result of lost electrons. Superoxides are one example of reactive oxygen species (ROS), which are chemically reactive molecules containing oxygen.

It has been estimated that the fraction of electron leakage in the mitochondrial ETC is about 1%. Organisms have evolved a defense system that scavenges and detoxifies ROS. The system also includes mechanisms that repair damaged DNA and proteins. Irreparable components can trigger programmed cell death. However, imbalance in the oxidative damage over organismal responses leads to a challenge called oxidative stress. Oxidative stress has been implicated in many age-associated diseases, including Alzheimer's disease, Parkinson's disease, atherosclerosis, stroke, heart attack and chronic fatigue syndrome.

Despite the downside, ROS have their usefulness. Because of the nonspecificity of ROS to their targets, superoxides are utilized by phagocytes, a type of white blood cells of our immune system, as toxin to kill harmful objects, including dying cells and invading microbes. As the level of ROS has to be maintained within tolerance, variations in the ROS level and redox status (i.e. the ratio of the interconvertible reduced to the oxidized form of a molecule such as NAD^+/NADH) have to be precisely sensed and closely monitored. Thus, ROS, through posttranslationally modifying regulatory proteins, function as signaling molecules. The processes that are responsive to redox status include the mitogen-activated protein kinase (MAPK) pathway, embryogenesis, DNA methylation and histone modifications.

2.5 Cell Metabolism

The majority of biomass is made up of four classes of basic macromolecules: carbohydrates, amino acids, lipids and nucleotides. Examples of carbohydrates are sugar and cellulose. Strings of amino acids fold into proteins and enzymes. Lipids form membranes and steroids. Sequences of nucleotides form genes and mRNA. Other organic and inorganic compounds are also abundant and essential. They encompass coenzymes such as ATP, vitamins such as NAD^+/NADH, minerals such as sodium (Na^+), potassium (K^+), calcium (Ca^{2+}), magnesium (Mg^{2+}), chloride (Cl^-), phosphate (PO_4^{3-}) and bicarbonate (HCO_3^-), and metals such as iron (Fe) and zinc (Zn). All these materials exist as foods in the ecosystem. However, they are not in the forms and compositions that are readily useful to the consuming organisms. For example, chicken proteins are not functional in human cells. Mechanisms have evolved that efficiently break down the digested foods allowing for the extraction of nutrients (including ATP), from which mass of the right composition and form to the consumer is built up. Cell metabolism concerns the intertransforming processes of breaking down and building up biomass in cells.

ATP turnover and biomass transformation are two sides of the same coin. Carbohydrates, proteins and lipids represent the three main sources of energy for all living organisms. They are broken down into sugars, amino acids and fatty acids/glycerol via hydrolysis by extracellular digestive enzymes in the gut before being absorbed and oxidized in cells. The resulting acetyl-CoA is an important intermediate that goes on to aerobic respiration for efficient ATP production in mitochondria. When nutrients are plentiful, the surplus, in the form of acetyl-CoA, is converted to and stored as lipids via lipogenesis in the cytoplasms of liver and fat cells. An alternative to fat for long-term energy storage is glycogen, which is synthesized from glucose via glycogenesis in the liver and muscle. When the blood glucose concentration is low, glycogen polymers are broken down via glycogenolysis and fed to glycolysis. If the levels of blood glucose remain unmet, for example in the brain, a reversible glycolysis called gluconeogenesis takes place in the liver with glycerol and the Krebs cycle intermediates, including many amino acids, as substrates.

Not all glucose that enters glycolysis exits as pyruvate and glycogen. Instead, a diversion is the pentose phosphate pathway (PPP), which utilizes and transforms the six-carbon sugars as precursors for reductive biosynthesis of a variety of macromolecules, including fatty acids, steroids, amino acids and nucleic acids. Rapidly proliferating cells therefore express high levels of PPP enzymes. Macromolecular synthesis through glycolytic intermediates may underlie the Warburg effect.

Synthesis and degradation of biomolecules are, respectively, called anabolism and catabolism. Together, they are called metabolism. Control of metabolism in a cell can be regulated at two levels: intrinsic and extrinsic. An example of intrinsic regulation is in the multisteps of the Krebs cycle, where substrates initiate the reaction and products inhibit it. At the extrinsic level, cells sense and respond to extracellular signals such as hormones and growth factors from other organs. Hormones that induce catabolism (anabolism) are called catabolic (anabolic) hormones. Catabolic hormones include cortisol and adrenaline, secreted by the adrenal glands; glucagon, from the pancreas; and cytokines, from the immune and nervous systems. Anabolic steroids include growth hormone, from the anterior pituitary gland; insulin, from the pancreas; IGF-1, from the liver; estrogen, from the ovaries; and testosterone, from the testes.

2.6 The Central Dogma of Molecular Biology, the Genome

Much has been reviewed about energy flow among the entities in the biochemical world. Transformation of energy allows things to come alive. However, it is information flow that keeps living things alive. Moreover, accumulation of information across generations increases the complexity of organisms in evolution. Information in all known forms of life on Earth is encoded in double-helical chains of nucleotides called DNA. A nucleotide contains one of four types of nucleobases, abbreviated to A, C, G and T. A and T preferentially bind to each other; so do C and G. As a result of the base-pairing, double-helical DNA is structurally stable, making it suitable for information storage. Base-pairing also makes the double strands complementary: knowing one strand of DNA means knowing the other as well.

To decode the information, the sequence of a DNA segment or gene is copied into a single-stranded nucleotide-based molecule called messenger RNA (mRNA). The sequence of mRNA is the same as that of DNA except that T in DNA is replaced by U in mRNA. The copying is facilitated by enzymes called RNA polymerases and the process is known as transcription. Because of the single strand characteristic, mRNA molecules are short-lived.

Next, the mRNA is transported to the vicinity of a ribosome where the RNA sequence is translated into an amino acid sequence. During the translation, a triplet of nucleotides called the RNA codon specifies one amino acid. For example, a 9-nucleotide sequence translates into a 3-amino-acid sequence. Since there are only 20 amino acids while there are $4^3 = 64$ codons, 3-letter codons unequivocally specify an amino acid sequence. The amino acid chain then folds into a three-dimensional structure called protein. Different amino acid sequences fold into different structures. Protein functions are dictated by the structure. Information of the DNA sequence thus manifests in protein functions. The process of gene transcription and mRNA translation into functional proteins is called gene expression. The faithful, deterministic and irreversible flow of biological information from DNA to RNA and from RNA to protein is universal for all life and is called the central dogma of molecular biology.

The entirety of the hereditary information of an organism is called the genome. The human genome has about 23,000 genes. The size of a gene varies and is on average about a few kilobases. Gene expression is energy-consuming. Therefore, only the genes that are needed by the cell at that moment are expressed. Still, about 40% of the genes in a human cell are constitutively expressed to a high level across all conditions. They participate in the maintenance of the cell and are called housekeeping genes. To no surprise, many of the housekeeping genes are metabolism-related. Other genes are facultative and their expression is condition-specific. Among them are a type of genes whose expression products return and bind to DNA. The bound regions are usually upstream of genes called promoter regions. The effect of protein-promoter binding is that transcription of the gene downstream of the promoter is induced or suppressed. The DNA-binding proteins are called transcription factors (TFs). TFs bind only to the target DNA sequences that they recognize. Extracellular signals, through signal transduction, activate the expression of TFs, which in turn regulate the expression of their target genes. Target genes can be a TF, and the interactions among the TFs and targets form a transcriptional regulatory network. The response of the cell or organism is coded in the genome, which is passed from one cell generation to the next.

The linear DNA molecules wrap around proteins called histones into structures called chromosomes. The number of chromosomes making up a genome varies from species to species.

2.7 Eukaryotic Cell Division Cycle

Eukaryotes, including animals, plants, fungi and algae, are organisms whose cells have nuclei. A nucleus, as one of the organelles of a cell, envelops DNA and histones. Organelles, or specialized parts, are to a cell what organs are to the body. Other important organelles of a eukaryotic cell include mitochondria, ribosomes and the Golgi apparatus. Mitochondria are cellular power plants which respire aerobically. RNA is transcribed in the nucleus. Ribosomes, with the help of other molecules, synthesize proteins. Posttranslational modifications of proteins such as phosphorylation and glycosylation occur in the Golgi apparatus. All the components are held in position by a structure called the cytoskeleton and enclosed in a lipid bilayer called plasma membrane. Cell membrane, through channels or pumps, is permeable to some substances. In addition, the cell surface has receptors that bind and sense signaling molecules. A typical eukaryotic cell measures 10 microns and weighs 1 ng.

Living organisms maintain homeostasis by metabolism. They express genes in response to stimuli. Also, living organisms reproduce, and through natural selection adapt to changing and new environments. The process of cell growth and DNA replication leading to two identical cells is called the cell division cycle or cell cycle. Progression of the cell cycle is regulated like falling dominoes, where a stage begins only when the preceding stage is completed. Cells reproduce when circumstances allow; for example, when nutrients abound. The cell cycle is therefore usually triggered by growth factors.

Four distinct phases compose a cycle: G1, S, G2 and M. Each phase readies cells for the next phase. For example, in the G1 phase, enzymes for DNA replication are produced. In the S phase, DNA molecules and associated histone proteins are replicated and synthesized in the nucleus. In the G2 phase, microtubules, a cytoskeleton structure, are produced. Finally, in the M phase, replicated DNA divides and the cell separates into two cells. Regulation of the cell cycle involves the evolutionarily conserved cyclins, cyclin-dependent kinases (CDKs), and the target genes of the cyclin–CDK complexes, representing an example of the transcriptional regulatory network. In particular, mechanisms have evolved that detect and repair DNA damages at the points of G1/S and

G2/M phase transitions, ensuring that incomplete DNA is not passed to daughter cells.

Cells spend only 10% of the cycling time in phase M or mitosis. The rest is spent in the G1, S and G2 phases, altogether called the interphase. However, some types of cells, e.g. nerve and heart cells, do not or seldom divide once they reach maturity. Such quiescent cells express little cyclins and CDKs, and stay in the G1 phase indefinitely or extendedly. Other cells lose the ability to divide because of senescence-associated DNA attrition and stay arrested in G1. The senescent phase can be thought of as a cellular alternative to apoptosis, by which cells die before the organism dies. Because of the role of cyclin–CDK complexes in cell cycle progression, inhibitors of the complexes are targets of drugs for neoplasms, which are characterized by uncontrolled cell proliferation.

2.8 Meiosis, Mendelian Inheritance, Genetic Disorder

Cell population grows through cycles of cell division, as seen in the enlargement of muscles and bones of a juvenile and in the adipose tissue of an adult. Human population grows by sexual reproduction, through which the genetic material, i.e. the DNA, of the father combines with that of the mother in the creation of an offspring. Chromosomes serve as the convenient unit of DNA replication. Because of sexual reproduction, a human cell has one complete set of paternal chromosomes and one complete set of maternal chromosomes. The paired sets of homologous chromosomes are called diploid. The human genome comprises 23 chromosomes, and thus a diploid human cell has 46 chromosomes.

Each of the human sex cells, i.e. sperm and egg cells, contains half the number of chromosomes of a nonsex or somatic cell, and is called haploid. The way that a diploid germ cell gives rise to haploid sex cells is through meiosis. If we take one chromosome to illustrate, the process can be broken down into the following steps:

(1) (black, white)
(2) (black/black, white/white)
(3) (black/blate, whick/white)
(4) (black/blate), (whick/white)
(5) (black), (blate), (whick), (white)

where "black" stands for a chromosome from a parent and "white" the homologous chromosome from the other parent. Parentheses delimit a cell, so the process starts from a diploid germ cell in step 1. Step 2 replicates the chromosomes to get two black and two white chromosomes in the cell. In step 3, a black chromosome recombines with a white chromosome to get a black–white (i.e. blate) chromosome and a white–black (i.e. whick) chromosome. Step 4 separates the recombined chromosomes. Step 5 segregates further to get four haploid gametes, i.e. sex cells. The steps can be readily extended to cells with multiple chromosomes. A haploid sperm fertilizes a haploid egg to create a diploid zygote, which develops into an embryo. The human life cycle is a cycle of meiosis and fertilization.

Mitosis of somatic cells doubles and then divides the cells with identical chromosomes in the daughter cells. By contrast, meiosis not only halves the number of chromosomes by a second division, but also shuffles the DNA sequences in a chromosomal crossover, as illustrated in step 3. Note that the position where two homologous chromosomes recombine can in principle be anywhere in the chromosome. The chromosome number remains and yet the DNA sequence diverges from generation to generation. Fitter offspring survive to reproduce, creating fitter offspring. Sexual reproduction is considered a better solution for species perpetuation than asexual reproduction.

An individual inherits a copy of the gene from each of his or her parents. The two genes can differ in the sequence at one position due, for example, to mutation. The variant nucleotide is called a single nucleotide polymorphism (SNP). Because of the redundancy in RNA codons, an SNP may not change the sequence of the amino acids and the functions of the gene product. However, many SNPs in a gene increase the chance of modifying gene functions. Variants of a gene are called alleles, and the trait (or phenotype) is affected by the allele (or genotype). In the middle of the 19th century, Gregor Johann Mendel, through a series of hybridization experiments on pea plants, described the observed patterns of inherited traits and summarized them into two laws. His findings are the basis of the biological discipline of genetics, which studies the functions of genes and the links between genotype and phenotype at the individual and the population level.

Mendel's first law or law of segregation states that a pair of alleles determines a trait and that a parent passes to its offspring one or the other allele with equal probability. The first law can be understood by meiosis, even though meiosis was not known at that time. Mendel's second law or law of independent assortment states that separate genes for separate traits pass independently of each other to the offspring. The second law can be understood again by meiosis if the two genes are located at different chromosomes. The significance of Mendel's work is that he conceptualized the existence of a heredity unit ahead of the discovery of chromosomes/genes.

Aberration in steps 4 to 5 of meiosis can result in a missing or extra chromosome and give rise to unviable or birth defect babies. For example, Turner syndrome is caused by an absent X chromosome in the female, and Down syndrome by an additional, 21st chromosome. Adult women with Turner syndrome are short and infertile. Individuals with Down syndrome show signs of delayed mental and physical development. Abnormalities in a single gene can have pathological consequences which can be passed down to subsequent generations. These monogenic disorders show a Mendelian pattern of inheritance and are called Mendelian disorders. For example, if a single defective allele is enough to cause the disease, then an affected parent carrying a single defective allele and an unaffected parent have a 50% chance of having an affected baby. An example of such dominant disorder is Huntington's disease, caused by a defect in the Huntington gene. If two defective alleles are necessary for causing the disease, unaffected parents, each carrying a single defective allele, have a 25% chance of conceiving an affected baby. Examples of such recessive disorders are sickle-cell anemia, cystic fibrosis and Tay–Sachs disease, caused by defects in the hemoglobin gene, CFTR and HEXA, respectively.

Many other disorders that have genetic components do not show clear patterns of familial inheritance, because the disorders are caused by multiple defective genes or the genetic abnormalities are formed after birth. Examples of the polygenic disorders are cancers. Yet other genetic disorders show vulnerabilities under certain environmental conditions, including lifestyle. The non-Mendelian disorders, e.g. asthma and diabetes, are a result of genetic and environmental interactions. Online Mendelian Inheritance in Men (OMIM), www.ncbi.nlm.nih.gov/omim, is a comprehensive, authoritative and up-to-date database of genetic traits and disorders, containing over 7000 gene–phenotype descriptions.

2.9 Chromatin Modification, Complex Disorder

Environmental cues can elicit an immediate and transient cellular response by, for example, activating transcriptional regulatory networks. In many other circumstances, however, it is advantageous for the cell to remember the incidence of an event which took place many cellular (or even organismal) generations ago. For example, because of the seasonal climate of each year, plants direct their resources to roots and leaves when the weather is warm before winter and then to flowers and seeds after winter. A prolonged period of cold is required for many plants prior to flowering. The ability of plants' perception and memory of cold winter lies in modifications of chromatin.

A DNA sequence coils around histone proteins like a string around spools. The complex of DNA and histones is called chromatin. The structure of chromatin, i.e. spools of string, helps package

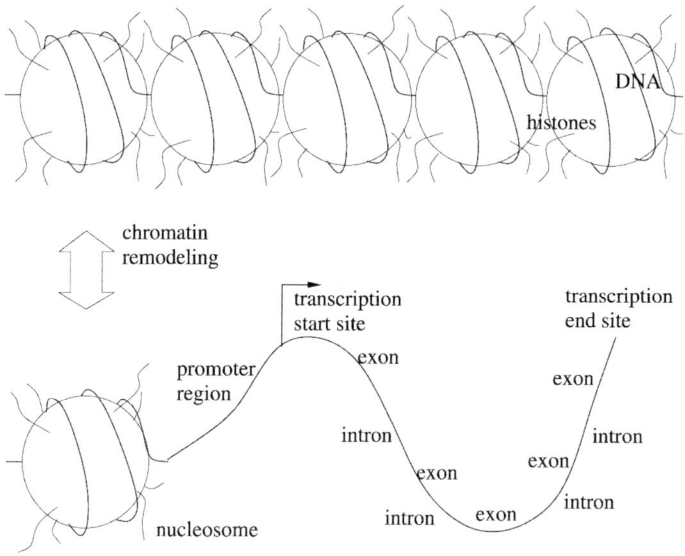

FIGURE 2.1

DNA wrapping around a histone octamer forms a nucleosome. Strings of nucleosomes constitute chromatin. Histones contain unstructured tails, covalent modifications of which are reversible and recognized by chromatin remodeling factors. Interactions between the chromatin remodelers compact or loosen chromatin structure. A sequence upstream of a transcription start site is called a promoter. Exon sequences encode protein peptides, whereas introns do not. Both promoters and introns are regulatory regions, protein binding or histone modifications of which regulate gene transcription. Chromatin is the relevant substrate for all genetic processes in eukaryotic nuclei.

DNA inside the nucleus. Moreover, amino acid residues on the unstructured histone tails can be posttranslationally modified, leading to a compact or loose chromatin structure. For example, acetylation of histone lysines loosens the coupling between DNA and the acetylated histones and between acetylated histones and neighboring acetylated histones, allowing access to the DNA sequence by the transcription machinery, such as transcription factors and RNA polymerases. Regions of loosened chromatin are thus associated with active transcription. On the other hand, histone deacetylation is associated with transcriptional silencing.

Other modifications such as methylation and phosphorylation at the same and/or other amino acid residues of the histone tail are found to enhance or counteract one another in remodeling the chromatin structure. Concurrent compacting and opening modifications at the gene body chromatin poise gene transcription, as found in undifferentiated stem cells. Histone modifications are reversible by enzymes. For example, histone acetyltransferases (HATs) and histone deacetylases (HDACs), respectively, acetylate and deacetylate histone lysines. Most importantly, once modified, the modifications are copied during mitosis and get passed down to daughter cells. The covalent modification profile of the histones and cytosines over the genome is called the epigenome.

If the genome is likened to a manual, then the epigenome can be thought of as paper clips that bind sheets of paper together. An adult human body has over 200 different cell types. The different somatic cell types have very different functions and morphologies, yet they share an identical DNA sequence in their nuclei. The epigenomes are found to be more different between cell types within an individual than they are between individuals within a cell type, indicating that chromatin remodeling plays an essential role in cell differentiation and organismal development. Epigenomes are more amenable to environmental perturbations than the DNA sequence. For example, in animal models, early-life stress was found to alter the brain epigenome to generate a gene expression change that persists to trigger a psychopathological phenotype later in life [Champagne and Curley, 2009]. Particles from traffic exhaust alter the leukocyte epigenome in humans [Baccarelli *et al.*, 2009]. Chronic sun exposure changes the skin epigenome in humans [Gronniger *et al.*, 2010]. Epigenomes serve as an integrator of environmental exposures and it is not surprising to find more and more reports of epigenomic aberrations in complex (i.e. non-Mendelian) disorders such as cancer, Alzheimer's disease and aging. Unlike DNA sequence mutation, many epigenomic modifications are reversible. The epigenomes thus emerge as a target for new drug development.

2.10 Immunity, Hematopoiesis

Organisms fight for limited resources for survival and reproduction against one another in the ecosystem. Jawed vertebrates, including humans, have developed sophisticated defense systems to ward off constant attacks from such infectious microorganisms as viruses, bacteria, fungi and parasites. The first layer of defense is skin, which creates a physical barrier against foreign matter. Tearing, sneezing and vomiting are also first-line mechanisms for expelling unwanted substances. Gastric acid in the stomach digests and gut flora in the intestines compete against invading bacteria.

Still, immediately after pathogens successfully breach the first line of defense, they are recognized by the innate immune system cells such as the resident macrophages and mast cells that are present in all tissues. Recognition is achieved by Toll-like receptors and other pathogen recognition receptors on the innate immune system cells that identify the conserved molecular motifs (e.g. bacterial carbohydrates, viral RNA and peptides) found in broad groups of microbes. The innate immune system cells (or infected cells) release cytokines (interferons) to recruit neutrophils (natural killer cells) to the site of the encounter (infection). The innate immune system cells also release short-lived inflammatory mediators that cause the classical inflammatory symptoms of swelling, redness, heat and pain at the damaged tissue. Acute inflammation is a response of the innate immunity to remove harmful stimuli and to initiate healing processes.

Still, some foreign agents may evade or overwhelm the innate immune system and emerge in the tissue fluid. In jawed vertebrates, another layer of defense involving lymphocytes in the lymph and blood circulating systems comes into play side by side with the innate immune system. Pieces — (i.e. proteins and polysaccharides) — of a cell or tissue such as bacterium, virus, pollen, transplanted organ, and transfused blood, which bind to lymphocyte receptors, are called antigens. Receptors of the lymphocytes which include T and B cells distinguish self from nonself or missing-self antigens. The naïve T cells in the lymph nodes recognize specific nonself antigens presented to them in the lymph nodes. After activation, the naïve T cells proliferate to become effector T cells, which perforate and induce apoptosis of the nonself-antigen-containing cells. Effector T cells are short-lived but some effector T cells are retained to become long-lived memory T cells. Resolution of non/missing-self antigens is also reinforced by helper T cells, which also act, by cytokine secretion, to activate macrophages and B cells. B cells recognize non/missing-self antigens in uncomplexed form. Upon recognition, B cells differentiate into plasma cells which secrete antibodies, i.e. immunoglobulins, that are specific to the activating antigens. The antigen-specific antibodies then neutralize the pathogens or mark the pathogens for destruction by phagocytes. Plasma cells are short-lived but some enter the quiescent state to become memory B cells. Swollen lymph nodes are an indication of T and B cell activations.

A repertoire of diverse T and B receptors is essential for matching the antigens of evolving pathogenic and tumorigenic cells. When progenitor T cells mature in the thymus and B cells differentiate in the lymph nodes, the variable regions of the antigen receptor genes undergo somatic recombination and mutation. The random recombination and hypermutation of the genetic regions keep diversifying the receptor proteins. The system is therefore adaptable. When the same pathogens are encountered the second time, the memory T and B cells respond quickly by immediate reproduction. Furthermore, new naïve T cells and B cells can be activated, leaving new clones of memory T and B cells. The adaptive immune system is considered a specific and strong response to pathogens. Vaccination is a preventive or therapeutic measure which, by the use of a weakened form of pathogens called vaccine, provokes an adaptive immune reaction of the body. The adaptive immune system recognizes the vaccine as foreign, destroys it and remembers it. The next time the body encounters the wild pathogens, the antibodies, memory B and memory T cells can readily recognize and destroy them.

Red blood cells, platelets and all white blood cells, including T cells, B cells, natural killer cells, neutrophils, macrophage and mast cells, are derived from hematopoietic stem cells (HSCs). Stem cells are undifferentiated cells that are able to (1) differentiate into specialized cells and (2) self-renew. Neutrophils, lymphocytes and macrophages account for the majority of white blood cells. Their lifetimes range from hours to weeks. In an adult, HSCs reside in the interior of bones, including vertebrae, pelvis, cranium and sternum. Decrease in the number of white blood cells (mostly neutrophils) to below the normal level — due, for example, to a recent infection, folate deficiency, radiation therapy or chemotherapy — can increase the risk of infection. On the other hand, acute illness can cause proliferation and release of leukocytes (primarily neutrophils) from the bone marrow, raising the white blood cell count. Rapid growth of abnormal or immature white blood cells in the bone marrow, which interferes with the production of normal white blood cells, is a cancer of the white blood cells, called acute leukemia.

3

Traditional Oriental Ethnomedicine

India and China, two of the world's oldest civilizations, have developed their indigenous theories and practices of disease prevention, treatment and diagnosis. For example, Sushruta (*c.* 800 BCE), known as the father of surgery, performed hundreds of different surgical operations, including cataract and plastic surgery, in the Ganges region of north India about 3000 years ago. In addition, yoga, which originated in ancient India, aims for the relief of all suffering via an austere self-discipline including abstinence and meditation. On the other hand, in China, Zhongjing Zhang (150–219 CE) systematically characterized disease progressions and the corresponding herbal formulas, thrusting forward the development of ancient Chinese internal medicine. As part of multicomponent therapeutics, acupuncture has been prescribed alongside herbal regimens since ancient China. A feature of traditional Indian and Chinese medicines is that harmonious interactions among the body, mind and changing environment are key to disease prevention and health maintenance.

3.1 Ayurveda

The word "Ayurveda" comes from the Sanskrit "*ayur*" (meaning "life; living") and "*veda*" (meaning "science or knowledge"). Ayurveda therefore translates to "the science of life." It has been a traditional Indian medicine since the Vedic period of ancient India, i.e. about 1400 BCE. The earliest and authoritative texts on Ayurveda are *Charaka Samhita* (*c*. 250 BCE), *Susruta Samhita* (*c*. 350 CE) and *Ashtanga Hridaya of Vagbhata* (*c*. 700 CE). Ayurveda covers a wide range of specialties, including internal medicine, surgery, treatment of the head and neck, gynecology, obstetrics and pediatrics, toxicology, psychiatry, care of the elderly and rejuvenation, and sexual vitality.

It was believed in ancient India that five basic elements, namely space, air, fire, water and earth, made up all material creations, including living and nonliving things. Human living, which includes body, mind and behavior, is therefore interconnected with the environment. Ayurveda aims to integrate and balance body, mind and behavior with the environment in maintaining a healthy life. It is therefore considered a holistic medicine, in contrast to the reductionist approach of modern western biomedicine.

Specifically, Ayurveda considers health to be a state of balanced *doshas*, good appetite, functional *dhatus*, normal *malas* and blissful mind. *Malas* are the excretions, including sweat, urine and feces. *Dhatus* are the tissues, including plasma, blood, muscle, fat, bone, bone marrow and nervous system, and sperm and ovum. In the tissue hierarchy of Ayurveda, foods converts into plasma, which fuels blood, which in turn supports muscles, ..., and so on. *Doshas* refer to the three forces with the following elemental predominance and physiological effects:

- *Vata* (space, air): movement and communication, e.g. cell division, blood flow, nerve conduction, breathing, waste discharge
- *Pitta* (fire, water): metabolism and transformation, e.g. appetite, hormones, digestive system, endocrine system
- *Kapha* (water, earth): cohesion and structure, e.g. strength, immunity, stability, weight

In Ayurveda, an individual bears a unique combination of the three *doshas* at the moment when he or she is born. The unique combination then predisposes an individual's psychophysiological phenotype, in that *vata*-predominant individuals tend to be thin, light and dry-skinned. They act quickly and dislike cold weather. They are likely to be fearful and worried, sleep lightly, and are predisposed to constipation, heart disease, neurological conditions and rheumatoid arthritis. *Pitta*-predominant individuals have a moderate build and medium speed. They dislike hot weather and like cold foods/drinks. They are easily hungry, irritable, short-tempered, and are susceptible to hypertension, infectious diseases and digestive conditions. *Kapha*-predominant individuals have a solid build and oily and smooth skin. They are strong, enduring and slow. They sleep long and digest slowly. They are steady, tranquil, greedy, and are at risk of obesity, diabetes, cancer and respiratory conditions.

Not only plants and animals but also minerals, the time of the day and the season of the year through the predominant basic elements have their own predominant *doshas*. Thus, the *doshas* of a human being throughout his or her life are constantly being formed and reformed by foods, activities and the environment. Ayurveda holds that when the *doshas* are in harmony the body is impervious to disease and that imbalanced *doshas* incur disease. Ayurveda has developed strategies, throughout life from conception to death, for the prevention and treatment of disease.

One of the primary strategies is diet. Foods in Ayurveda have one of the following six tastes:

- Sweet (earth, water), e.g. sugar, milk, butter, rice, bread
- Sour (earth, fire), e.g. yogurt, lemon, cheese
- Salty (water, fire), e.g. salt
- Pungent (air, fire), e.g. spicy foods, peppers, ginger
- Bitter (air, space), e.g. spinach, green leafy vegetables
- Astringent (earth, air), e.g. beans, walnuts

The effects of the foods on *doshas* are, according to Ayurveda:

- Decreasing *vata* with sweet, sour and salty foods

- Decreasing *pitta* with sweet, bitter and astringent foods
- Decreasing *kapha* with pungent, bitter and astringent foods

So, a *kapha*-predominant individual would be recommended to more frequently consume pungent, bitter and astringent foods to decrease the *kapha*. Likewise, to increase *pitta*, one should consume pungent, sour and salty foods, avoiding sweet, bitter and astringent foods. Indian cuisine extensively utilizes a variety of spices, including turmeric, coriander, cumin, ginger, garlic and cinnamon, to help digestion.

In Ayurveda, *doshas* peak at times of the day in the following way:

- *Vata* peaks at 2 a.m. to 6 a.m. (i.e. sunrise) and 2 p.m. to 6 p.m.
- *Pitta* peaks at 10 a.m. to 2 p.m. and 10 p.m. to 2 a.m.
- *Kapha* peaks at 6 a.m. (i.e. sunrise) to 10 a.m. and 6 p.m. to 10 p.m.

Since *pitta* helps digestion, one would have one's main meal at noon and leave light meals to breakfast and dinner. Furthermore, since *vata* is associated with lightness and *kapha* with heaviness, one would get up by sunrise and go to bed by 10 p.m. Moreover, since the other peak of *pitta* starts at 10 p.m. and *pitta* drives metabolism, falling asleep by 10 p.m. fosters efficient biosyntheses, rejuvenating the body.

Seasons show their doshic trends:

- *Vata* (cold, dry, windy) peaks in late autumn and winter
- *Pitta* (hot) peaks in summer and early autumn
- *Kapha* (cold, wet) peaks in spring

Kapha-predominant individuals are therefore recommended to increase their physical activities in spring because of the aggravating *kapha* in spring. Likewise, *pitta*-predominant individuals are suggested to limit their outdoor exposure in summer. *Vata*-predominant individuals are advised to oil-massage their skin in winter. Ayurveda therefore prescribes a natural way of living, deviation from which leads to illness.

In addition to the diet and lifestyle strategies for maintaining *dosha* balance, Ayurveda also provides means of removing accumulated wastes from within the body. Ayurvedic detoxification therapy includes: fasting; sinus cleansing to strengthen the skull; emesis to expel excessive mucus and toxins from the stomach and the respiratory system; purgation to expel bile and *pitta* toxins from the small intestine and the liver; herbal enemas to purify the large intestine; and bloodletting to stimulate new blood production. Ayurvedic medicinals are mostly plant- and animal-based. The predominant basic elements in the habitats and foods of an animal determine the predominant basic elements of its flesh. The therapeutic effects are discussed in terms of the predominant basic elements in *Susruta Samhita*. For example, earth-, fire- and water-predominant medicinals allay *vata*; earth-, water- and air-predominant medicinals quell *pitta*; space-, fire- and air-predominant medicinals relieve *kapha*. On the other hand, space- and air-predominant medicinals increase *vata*; fire-predominant medicinals activates *pitta*; earth- and water-predominant medicinals promote *kapha*. Similarly, for better effectiveness, laxatives are made from earth- and water-predominant medicinals; emetics from air- and fire-predominant medicinals; tranquilizers from space-predominant medicinals; astringents from air-predominant medicinals; digestants from fire-predominant medicinals; lipolytics from air- and fire-predominant medicinals; roborants from earth- and water-predominant medicinals, and so on. The number of common medicinals in the three Ayurvedic classics was estimated to be 670. However, as use of the language declines, many of them have lost the identities and become unknown today. Ayurveda also has rejuvenation therapy with herbal preparations that are said to bring back youth.

3.2 Asana, Pranayama, Dhyana

Yoga, one of the six orthodox schools of classical Indian philosophy, encompasses a system of physical, mental and spiritual disciplines to help one clarify reality, remove suffering and achieve wellbeing.

The Sanskrit word "*yoga*" has a root, "*yuj*," which means "to yoke, to join or to unify." Health is considered a state of equilibrium of the body, mind and spirit. Yoga aims to still the restless mind and to join the body, mind and spirit in the search for self-awareness and health. Note that although the development of yoga has a Hindu element, the practice of yoga requires no spiritual beliefs or religious observances.

The *Yoga Sutras of Patanjali* (*c*. 200 BCE) is the earliest, most thorough and systematic description of the practice of the yoga philosophy. In it, eight limbs or steps are laid down for the adherents of yoga:

(1) *Yama*: to follow such behavioral norms as nonviolence, truthfulness, nonstealing, sexual abstinence and noncovetousness
(2) *Niyama*: to control emotions by body-cleaning, satisfaction, austerity, studying and devotion
(3) *Asana*: to sit in a physical posture and stay comfortable, relaxed and without effort
(4) *Pranayama*: to regulate the breathing by inhalation, exhalation and withholding of the breath
(5) *Pratyahara*: to withdraw the five senses (eyes, ears, nose, mouth, anus) so that awareness is far removed from the senses
(6) *Dharana*: to concentrate the awareness on a single object of thought
(7) *Dhyana*: to sustain awareness of only the object of thought with minimal self-consciousness
(8) *Samadhi*: to merge consciousness with the object of thought to achieve wholeness, i.e. no subject–object relationship

The first two limbs prescribe attitudes and values for the physical and mental practices of yoga. *Asanas* comprise a number of physical postures for improving the strength, flexibility and endurance of the body. For example, 84 main postures were developed to balance the left–right, front–back, internal–external, passive–active and overworked–underworked parts of the body. Stretching, compressing or twisting in the postures massages the internal organs

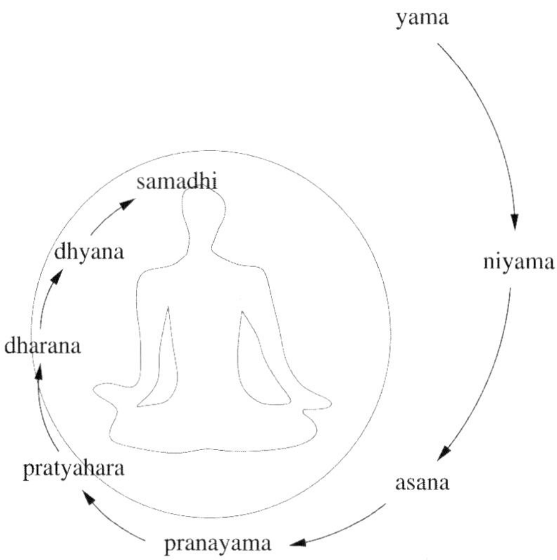

FIGURE 3.1

The first five external aids and the last three internal aids to yoga, a discipline of the mind and body.

and strengthens the muscles. In addition, joints and ligaments are lubricated. "*Prana*" in Sanskrit means "life force, vital energy or breath." *Pranayama* controls or extends *prana* by conscious prolongation of inhalation, retention and exhalation of the breath, strengthening the respiratory system. The first four limbs are to conquer an obsessed and addicted body to serve the search for a peaceful mind of the last four limbs.

Limb 5 promotes limb 6, which, by concentrating the mind on one point, region or object, helps *dhyana*. Yogic philosophy holds that the greatest suffering or stress comes from fluctuations of the mind as it oscillates constantly between future worries/obligations and past mistakes/frustrations. *Dhyana* aims to limit the drifting of the mind by, for example, directing the constant flow of attention to the same point, region or object of meditation. Meditation thus helps regulate impulses and decondition the mind. Finally, when the mind and the object are merged together, a quiescent state of nonegoism is reached and one is liberated from suffering. According to the yoga philosophy, the universe consists of two realities: consciousness and matter. Matter comprises inanimate and animate substances, while consciousness fuses with the mind and body of the animate. As a sentient being falsely identifies itself with the physical body, bondage and suffering arise. Realization of the misidentification and awareness of one's place in and relation with the universe are achieved in *samadhi*, which is the goal of yoga.

3.3 Traditional Chinese Medicine

Traditional Chinese medicine (TCM) is believed to have originated in the Shang Dynasty of ancient China (*c*. 1350 BCE) and is the major alternative medicine in East Asia, including China, Taiwan, Hong Kong and Singapore. The development of traditional Korean, Japanese, Vietnamese and Tibetan medicines was greatly influenced by TCM. The earliest, authoritative TCM texts are *The Yellow Emperor's Inner Canon* (*c*. 200 BCE), *Shennong's Materia Medica* (*c*. 100 BCE), *Treaties on Cold Damage Disorders and Miscellaneous Illnesses* (*c*. 200 CE) and *Canon of Difficult Questions* (*c*. 200 CE). Notably, shamanistic accounts of the cause and treatment of illness were excluded from *The Yellow Emperor's Inner Canon*. TCM is therefore said to have separated from shamanism since at least 2000 years ago.

In TCM, a human being is a microcosm of the macrocosm. The ultimate macrocosm, i.e. the universe, comprises *qi* (pronounced "chi") and five elements, and operates under the duality principle of *yin* and *yang*. *Qi* is considered a form of energy and the five elements are wood, fire, earth, metal and water. *Yin* and *yang* are seemingly opposite but actually complementary or alternating qualities or forces of the perennial nature. For example, light, in opposition to darkness, brightens darkness but loses this utility in bright space. A single-sex population, i.e. either female (*yin*) or male (*yang*), cannot continue without the opposite sex. Cold in winter is followed by heat in summer, which is in turn followed by a cold winter. A trough turns into a peak, and vice versa, in the wave motion of ripples. *Yin* and *yang* are thus interdependent, opposite aspects of an object or phenomenon in relation to the greater whole of a dynamic system. A *yin* object can further have *yin* and *yang* components, depending on the scale of investigation. Man, in TCM, is composed of *qi*, blood, bodily fluid, *zang–fu* organs and meridians. The components, having their functions and *yin–yang* qualities, work in harmony. Disturbance in the *yin–yang* balance due to external and/or internal factors gives rise to disorder. External factors are diet, lifestyle and environmental extremes, including wind, cold, fire, dampness, dryness and summer heat. Internal factors include joy, anger, anxiety, pensiveness, grief, fear and fright.

Qi in the body not only provides energy but also defense. Sources of *qi* are parents during conception, and air, foods and drinks after birth. Blood nourishes and moisturizes the body. Bodily fluids include those nonblood fluids such as tears, sputum, saliva, gastric juice, joint fluid, sweat and urine. *Zang* organs, including the *xin*, *pi*, *fei*, *shen* and *gan*, are responsible for the production and storage of *qi*, blood and other essence. Specifically,

- The *xin* (heart) governs mentality, blood and blood vessels. It opens at the tongue and is affected by joy.
- The *pi* (spleen) governs transformation, absorption and ascending pure essence. It connects flesh, extends to limbs and opens at the mouth. It is hurt by pensiveness.
- The *fei* (lung) governs respiration and disseminating, descending and liquefying *qi*. It vents airways and waterways, extends to skin and hair, and opens at the nose. It is susceptible to grief.
- The *shen* (kidney) governs growth, development, maturation, reproduction and water metabolism. It produces blood and maintains the brain, marrow and bones. It opens at the ears and is vulnerable to fear.
- The *gan* (liver) governs unclogging and spreading in the regulation of *qi*, emotions and enhancement of the digestive function of *pi*. It joins tendons and opens at the eyes. It is sensitive to anger.

Fu organs, including *xiaochang* (small intestine), *wei* (stomach), *dachang* (large intestine), *pangguang* (bladder), *dan* (gall bladder)

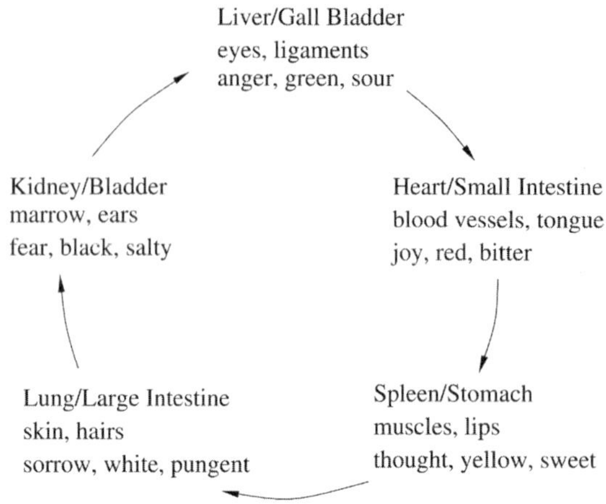

FIGURE 3.2

The five *zang* and the associated *fu*, peripheral tissues, emotions, colors and flavors in TCM. Arrows indicate the relationship of coactivation; so kidney problems can breed liver problems, etc. Green or sour foods are said to affect most the liver and its meridian. Sadness can hurt the lungs, etc.

and *sanjiao* further assist *zang* organs in the digestion of foods and transmission of wastes. Meridians extend *zang–fu* organs to form a web of pathways throughout the body for the distribution of *qi*, blood and bodily fluids. Note that the TCM model of the body and classification of organs are based on functions instead of anatomies. For example, TCM *shen* governs water metabolism, reproduction, growth, development, brain, marrow, bones and blood production. It is not merely the anatomical kidneys in modern physiology.

A disturbed *yin–yang* harmony of the body, by the external and/or internal factors, can manifest as a medical condition. TCM diagnostics therefore lies in identifying a "pattern of disharmony" or "pattern of functional disturbance" called *zheng* in TCM. Methods of *zheng* identification include inspection, smelling/listening, inquiring and palpation. Identified *zheng* is usually summarized by the so-called eight principles:

- Exterior: skin, hair, flesh, meridians
- Interior: *zang*, *fu*, bone marrow, *qi*, blood

- Cold: aversion to cold, cold limbs, pale, light color tongue with white coating
- Heat: aversion to warmth, fever, sweating, red color tongue with yellow coating
- Deficiency: weakness, fatigue, depression
- Excess: stagnation, acuteness or nondeficiency
- Yin: cold, deficient, interior, blood, hypoactivity
- Yang: heat, excess, exterior, *qi*, hyperactivity

Zheng can reflect the trend of syndrome development. For example, an exterior (or excessive) *zheng* is usually initiated by climatic variations in the environment. If there is unsuccessful intervention, an acute exterior (excessive) *zheng* can intrude and entrench the *zang/fu* organs, becoming a chronic interior (deficient) *zheng*. The eight-principle *zheng* differentiation is usually followed by further identification of the more subtle *zang*, *fu* or meridians that are out of balance.

Herbal remedies have been one of the major health interventions in TCM since *Shennong's Materia Medica* (*c*. 100 BCE), which lists 365 medicinals derived from mostly plants (69%) and also from animals (18%) and minerals (13%). This manual classified medicinals into three grades. Those of the top grade, a total of 120 medicinals, are tonic and nontoxic and can be consumed for long periods of time. Those of the medium grade number 120, and they are healing but can be toxic and should therefore be taken judiciously. For the bottom grade there are 125 medicinals, which are toxic but can be healing and should not be indefinitely consumed. Any medicinal has one of four natures — cold, cool, warm and hot — and one (or many) of the five flavors — sweet, bitter, acrid, sour, salty and bland. In TCM herbalism, acrid medicinals are dispersing, moving and moistening. Sweet medicinals are nourishing, mediating and slowing. Sour medicinals are absorbing and astringing. Bitter medicinals are dispersing, drying and hardening. Salty medicinals are softening. TCM herbal medicine is allopathic, as is modern western medicine. Identified cold TCM syndromes, i.e. *zheng*, will therefore be treated by warm or hot medicinals in order to rebalance *yin–yang* and restore *zang/fu* functions. The targeted body meridians of each medicinal were also indicated in the *materia medica*, and so were the parts, preparation and growing regions in China of the herbs. Further development of TCM herbalism in the successive dynasties of Chinese history by official and private TCM practitioners has, based on the paradigm of *Shennong's Materia Medica*, greatly expanded and improved the knowledge of TCM herbal remedies. The number of TCM medicinals has now reached 13,000.

TCM herbalism also combines single herbs into herbal formulas, as documented in *The Yellow Emperor's Inner Canon* and *Recipes for 52 Ailments*. The latter, containing 247 medicinals and 283 formulas, was excavated in 1973 from a tomb in south-central China, which was sealed in 168 BCE. According to TCM, prescribing herbs for a syndrome is likened to leading an army against an enemy. A TCM formula consists of monarch, minister, assistant and guide herbs. Monarch herbs are those that counteract the main syndrome. A formula can have up to two monarchs. Minister herbs are those that either enhance the effects of the monarch or counteract the secondary syndrome of the patient. There can be one or multiple ministers in a formula. Assistant herbs are those that counteract the secondary syndrome of the patient or neutralize the adverse effect of the monarch. There are usually one or two assistants. Guide herbs are those that harmonize the ingredients in the formula or guide the formula to the designated meridians. There are at most two guides in a formula. An example of a TCM formula is *ma huang* decoction for the wind–cold syndrome of influenza. The formula, first seen in *Treaties on Cold Damage Disorders and Miscellaneous Illnesses* (*c.* 200 CE), consists of four herbs: *Ephedra sinica*, *Cinnamomum cassia*, *Prunus armeniaca L.* and *Glycyrrhiza uralensis*. The first herb resolves the exterior symptom by causing sweating, it being the monarch. The second herb enhances the effect of the monarch and is minister. The third herb relieves the secondary symptom of coughing, serving as an assisant. The last herb harmonizes the formula and is a guide. The weights of the ingredient herbs in a formula usually decrease from monarch to minister to assistant to guide. TCM herbalism therefore concerns not only the herbs but also their relative weights in a formula. Classical TCM formulas were divided into 22 categories according to their therapeutic actions in *Collected Exegesis of Recipes*, by Ang Wang (1615–1694 CE). The categories, which are widely used today, are tonifying, fire-purging, dampness-eliminating, blood-regulating, exterior-relieving, exterior–interior, mediating, phlegm-dissolving, wind-expelling, *qi*-regulating, peptic, carbuncle-treating, gynecologic, cold-dispelling, dryness-treating, tranquilizing, heat-clearing, astringing, interior-warming, vomiting, parasite-killing and vision-improving.

3.4 Acupuncture

Another common therapeutic practice in TCM is acupuncture, which first appeared in *The Yellow Emperor's Inner Canon* (*c.* 200 BCE). The five *zang* and six *fu* organs together with *xinbao* (pericardium) constitute 12 organs in the interior of a TCM body. Each of the organs extends its functions through the left, right, front or back of the body to the terminal of the four limbs or the head via a meridian. The 12 main meridians and 8 or more minor meridians interconnect the internal organs and the peripheral of the body, forming a network of channels for the conduction of *qi* throughout the body. *Qi* in TCM is a form of energy for actuation, warming, defense, containment and transformation. Clogs in *qi*'s flow upset the *yin–yang* balance, leading to illness or pain in TCM. Acupuncture is a technique that unclogs the flow by insertion and manipulation of needles at certain positions along the meridians, called acupuncture points or acupoints.

Acupuncture points are the locations on the surface of the body where the flow of *qi* merges. Dysfunctions of the organ manifest in the acupoints of the corresponding meridian. Stimulation of the acupoints by needling aims to mobilize stagnant *qi* or redirect excessive *qi*, depending on the identified *zheng*. Reading of the radial pulses is an important method for detecting deficiency or excess of the troubled TCM organs/meridians. The position at the wrist crease where the radial artery passes is called *cun*. A finger's breadth from *cun* away from the palm is called *guan* and a finger's breadth from *guan* away from the palm is called *chi*. Pulses at the *cun–guan–chi* positions are felt by the tips of a TCM doctor's index, middle and ring fingers, respectively. Pulses at *cun–guan–chi* on the left hand are associated with the heart, liver and kidney, and those on the right hand with the lung, spleen and kidney. If pulses are felt with slight (heavy) pressing of the fingers, exterior (interior) *zhengs* are indicated. If pulses are strong (weak), excess (deficiency) *zhengs* are implied. If pulses are sparse (dense), cold (heat) *zhengs* are assumed. The first book to be devoted to pulsology, *The Pulse Classics*, by Shuhe Wang (201–280 CE), listed 24 pulse patterns and their associated *zhengs* and clinical significance.

Modern needles are stainless steel needles with round tips. The length ranges from 13 to 130 mm. The type of needles and the depth of insertion depend on the chosen acupoints. Once inserted, the needle can be twisted at the butt to enhance the acupunctural stimulation. A sensation of soreness, numbness, distention and heaviness felt by the patient at the insertion acupoint and along the meridian indicates the arrival of *qi* and the effectiveness of acupuncture. After the arrival of *qi*, the needle can remain inserted for 10–20 minutes for regular syndromes and up to hours for chronic and interior syndromes. For excess syndromes, insertion and twisting are usually fast and rough to drain the excessive *qi*. For deficiency syndromes, insertion is slow and twisting is gentle. There is no more twisting during needle retention. Acupuncture with sterile needles by well-trained acupuncturists is generally considered safe.

4

Integrative Medicine

The development of western medicine has been greatly aided by autopsy and biopsy. In a pathological autopsy, the body may be dissected for internal examination. In a clinical biopsy, part of a tissue is removed from the patient for microscopic (or histological) examination. Structural changes identified through autopsy and biopsy help determine causes of death and clarify progressions of disease. In the case of autopsy, the body is dead, not operating. In the case of biopsy, the sampled tissue is isolated, not interacting with the rest of the living body. By contrast, in Ayurveda and TCM, knowledge of illness and health has largely been learned from a living individual as a whole. Ayurveda and TCM are in principle better at functional disorders, in which bodily functions are impaired without discernible structural abnormities. Many functional disorders are chronic disorders and, if left untreated, can progress to become structural disorders. As Ayurveda and TCM are only concerned about living individuals, it is not surprising that both medicines have placed emphasis on the flow of energy within the body and between the body and the environment. While energy does not flow in dead bodies and isolated tissues, transformation of energy via anaerobic fermentation and aerobic respiration in single cells is well studied in biochemistry. Western modern biomedicine and eastern ancient therapeutics have the best chance of integration in the grand picture of a unified cell-level and organism-level bioenergetics.

A cell, while interacting with other cells in the organ, is regulated by the constraint imposed on the organ. Organs and tissues, such as the heart, liver and brain, interact with one another through the psychoneuroimmunological system and are constrained by the activities of the individual, which are in turn constrained by the physical and social environments he or she is in. The perceived environment can, through top-down processing, affect gene expression and thus bodily functions and symptoms. A therapy that integrates mind and body interventions is therefore considered more efficient. Furthermore, gene expression differences from cell line experiments, which culture cells isolated from diseased or normal tissue, do not account for the multiscale, hierarchical nature of gene regulation in living organisms. This explains the low success rates of laboratory-discovered drugs upon clinical trials. Innovative designs of clinical trials that include arms of flexible, multicomponent interventions will help identify effective integrative medicines.

4.1 Bioenergetics, Tridosha, Chronic Disorder

Survival and reproduction characterize life on Earth. Both characteristics demand energy from the environment. Living organisms are thus open systems through which energy constantly flows. Energy is consumed to generate and sustain the structure for survival and reproduction. Different structures confer on species different advantages at specific niches in the ecosystem. For example, reptiles in the swamp and primates in the jungle are evolved. Information on such anatomical structure is encoded in the form of a DNA sequence in the nucleus. Mutation and recombination of the nuclear DNA generate biodiversity, leading to subspecies or new species via natural selection.

Nuclear DNA mutations can be lethal, as they potentially alter anatomy and development. The rate of nuclear DNA mutation, set by variations in the energy reservoir of the environment over the geological timescale (10,000–100,000 years), is therefore low. On the other hand, mitochondrial DNA (mtDNA), being maternally inherited, has a higher mutation rate. The sequences of mtDNA from present-day people around the world were found to cluster into continents [Chen *et al.*, 1995]. Furthermore, the diversity of the mtDNA from a region decreases with the distance between the region and East Africa, supporting the recent single-origin hypothesis that anatomically modern humans migrated out of Africa between 60,000 and 125,000 years ago. mtDNA encodes some of the polypeptide genes for proton translocation, i.e. complexes I, III, IV and V, in the electron transport chain and oxidative phosphorylation of aerobic respiration. Mutation of the bioenergetic genes in mtDNA therefore helped human physiology adapt to the energy environments specific to the regions.

Within each region, people in their lifespan adapt to energy fluctuations across seasons and between day and night. Monthly reproductive cycles also require alteration in the bioenergetic physiology which cannot be achieved by irreversible genetic changes. High-energy intermediates in cells include acetyl-CoA, S-adenosylmethionine (SAM) and ATP. Acetyl-CoA and SAM are substrates for histone acetylation and methylation. ATP-dependent phosphorylation is involved in virtually all signal transductions. Adaptation to short-term cyclical energy fluctuations is therefore mediated by reversible chromatin modifications and signal transductions.

Bioenergetics plays a central role in Ayurveda, yoga and TCM, as manifested in Ayurvedic/yogic *prana* and TCM *qi*. In addition, in Ayurveda, the three energetic forces, or *doshas*, are required for life to happen. *Vata* is responsible for all movement in the body, *pitta* for all metabolism in the body, and *kapha* for all structure in the body. We can interpret *vata* as the mechanism that moves energy into and out of the living form. If energy simply passed though without dissipation, the living organism or structure would decay to randomness according to the second law of thermodynamics. *Pitta* is the mechanism that transforms the input energy into generation and maintenance of the structure. Finally, *kapha* is the mechanism that stores surplus energy in forms that facilitate adaptation to a variable environment. The tridoshic view of life applies to all living forms, from simple single cells to sophisticated multicellular organisms. TCM *zang/fu* organs' functions can readily be grouped into input–output, transformation and storage. For example, the heart and lung are *vata*-like, the liver and spleen are *pitta*-like, and the kidney and sanjiao is *kapha*-like. TCM *zang/fu* is, unlike *tridosha*, specific to humans.

Deleterious mtDNA mutations and/or aberrant epigenome modifications can disrupt coordinated expression of dispersed bioenergetic genes, leading to imbalance in *tridoshas*. The resulting disorders are the common complex diseases including metabolic and degenerative diseases. The development of molecular and cellular biology has identified the functions of many genes on nuclear DNA, contributing to great advances in the diagnosis of anatomical and developmental disorders [Wallace, 2010]. Capitalizing on the development, the pharmaceutical industry has also developed small chemical drugs, most of which target receptors of signal transductions. In the perspective of bioenergetics, modern western biomedicine has thus been successful in the diagnosis of developmental disorders and the treatment of acute medical conditions including microbial infections. On the other hand, Ayurvedic medicine through dietary and lifestyle interventions can be helpful in such chronic medical conditions as metabolic and degenerative disorders. This relevance to chronic disorders also applies to TCM, as the balance of *qi* in particular and the homeostasis of *yin–yang* in general are sought by TCM herbalism and acupuncture in the pursuit of health.

4.2 Complex Adaptive System, Yogic Cognitive-Behavioral Practice, Psychological Stress Management

The development of science has been greatly influenced by the paradigm of Newtonian reductionism, where a system's properties are studied by investigating the interactions between the components constituting the system. Advances have been made, especially in closed systems near thermodynamic equilibrium. However, many systems in nature are open, nonlinear and far-from-equilibrium. Their properties are not easily understood by reductionist approaches. They are called complex adaptive systems and often-cited examples are ecosystems and markets [Lansing, 2003]. Features of complex adaptive systems are:

- Large numbers of components
- Local interactions between components
- Positive and negative feedback loops
- A hierarchical organization
- Finite randomness

Local interactions can induce an aggregate pattern. For example, information on buying IBM stocks can trigger buying of the stocks of similar companies, such as companies in the industry of IT services and consulting. Positive feedbacks promote waves of buying when the prices are under target values. Negative feedbacks initiate selling to counteract further buying once the prices are above the targets. Individual industries, although autonomous, interact with other related industries, forming megaindustries or market sectors. Complex adaptive systems thus tend to have a hierarchical architecture. The performance of a sector constrains the performances of the industries in the sector, which in turn constrain the performances of the companies in individual industries. That is to say, the higher-level segment exerts influence downward to the lower-level segments. Constraints of an industry cannot be thoroughly understood by studying the companies in isolation. Complex adaptive systems have thus to be studied as a whole, not by the interactions between the freed parts. Random strategies of a few companies diversify and help the industry quickly respond or adapt to a changing market. An important property of a complex adaptive system is the absence of centralized control. The movement of a price can be initiated by any market player to meet the supply and demand of goods. Complex adaptive systems are efficient and robust.

The evolution of the genome made a quantum leap as the evolution of the genome for use as a medium of information storage and retrieval shifted to the evolution of the use of the genome to create a structure for information storage and retrieval. The resulting structure is the brain. The human brain, consisting of 100 billion neurons, each of which interacts with, approximately 1000 other neurons via synaptic transmissions, is considered a complex adaptive system. Connections of the neurons form three areas for the sensory, motor and association functions. Actively interacting neurons in the association area create models of the external environment. Each model fits differently with the environment. The choice of a particular model for the environment makes up one's mind.

Whenever one needs to adjust oneself to fit the environment, one is said to be under stress. If one chooses a model which indicates that one's survival or interests are at stake because one's coping resources cannot meet the environmental demands, one appraises the environment as threatening. On the other hand, if one's resources outweigh the demands in the chosen model, one appraises the environment as challenging. Threat appraisals result in negative emotions such as anxiety, fear and worry, in contrast to the eagerness, confidence and hope of positive emotions in challenge appraisals. Under stress, energy is mobilized from storage to muscle and brain via stress hormones including adrenaline and cortisol with such physiological changes as increased heart rate, blood pressure, breathing rate, pupil diameter, sweating and decreased digestion, growth, reproduction and immunity. Stress is not necessarily always damaging and detrimental. However, negative appraisals and emotions can be aggravated and prolonged by rumination on uncertainties/difficulties, leading to chronic stress. Pathophysiologies due to chronic stress include heart disease, rheumatoid arthritis, hypertension, Alzheimer's disease, atherosclerosis and aging. A balance between threat and challenge appraisals is therefore key to health.

Patanjali's eight limbs of yoga can be considered a whole system, i.e. a cognitive-behavioral approach to stress management. In particular, a technique called mindfulness meditation has been developed from yoga by Jon Kabat-Zinn; through control of attention, breathing and posture, it consciously regulates the mind, nerves and physiology for stress reduction. The recipe for mindfulness practice is:

(1) An upright sitting posture
(2) Attention to a predetermined object (such as the nose tip)
(3) Distraction of focused attention to thoughts
(4) Noticing the distractions without judgment
(5) Decentering as subject becomes object

The nonjudgmental attitude to any distractions in step 4 is essential, as our mind wanders around different thoughts, each of which is simply a model of the world created by the activating neurons in our brain. Thoughts come and go as the patterns of neuron connections drift and a thought does not necessarily represent the reality. With nonjudgmental awareness of the fleeting thoughts, a subjective perspective on mental content becomes objective in step 5. Mindfulness practice therefore reduces elaborate processing of past stimuli and future uncertainties and increases attentional resources for present-moment experience. As a result, an ambiguous behavior of e.g. a colleague is less likely to be interpreted as hostile intent and threat appraisals are shifted to being challenge appraisals. Note that TCM *tai chi* is a form of moving meditation that focuses on breath. It was shown that, through an eight-week mindfulness meditation program, the quality of life and overall stress symptoms were improved in breast and prostate cancer outpatients via reductions in the salivary cortisol level, blood proinflammatory cytokines and systolic blood pressure [Carlson *et al.*, 2007].

4.3 Placebo Effect, Acupuncture Analgesia, Chronic Pain

The brain, through direct innervation of the sympathetic and parasympathetic nervous systems and hormonal secretion of the hypothalamic–pituitary–adrenal axis, regulates physiology in a top-down manner. Regulated cellular and organic physiologies include antibodies, T cells, organ inflammation, glucose homeostasis by the liver and pancreas, thermogenesis of brown adipose tissue and kidney functions. Physiology can thus be changed by the mind, which is a chosen model of the world, actual or imagined. An example of the impact of imagination and expectation on physiology is the placebo response, where a measurable difference in effect, such as pain ratings, is observed between sham treatment and nontreatment [Klinger *et al.*, 2007; Colloca and Miller, 2011]. Differences have also been observed between overt and covert treatments, suggesting the effect of imagination, belief, expectation and emotion on clinical outcomes. Furthermore, once the association of an active agent with a neutral agent is established in the brain, application of the neutral agent alone can mimic the effect of the active agent. For example, when a drug is administered together with a drink, with experience of the pairing, the taste of the drink itself, through neural top-down control, creates the drug response. A therapy that maximizes the therapeutic efficacy by combining pharmacological effect and placebo response is beneficial to the patient.

Anatomically, portions of individual TCM meridians have been found to follow one or more successive connective tissue planes that separate muscles or are within muscles [Langevin and Yandow, 2002]. Acupuncture points were also found to coincide with the sites that allow access to more connective tissues at a depth of needle insertion, in comparison with nonacupoints. Connective tissue permeates the whole body, surrounding all organs and all nerves, blood vessels and lymphatics. The proposition that the continuous network of interstitial connective tissue planes form the anatomical basis of TCM meridians is therefore consistent with the TCM theory that meridians connect peripheral tissues and central viscera.

In the practice of acupuncture, after needle insertion the needle is rotated clockwise and counterclockwise or pistoned up and down. In response to the needle manipulation, the connective tissues beneath the acupoint, including subcutaneous tissue and deep fasciae, wind around the needle. The grasp of the needle is sought and felt by the acupuncturist, providing an indication of a working acupuncture therapy. The histological feature of acupoint-associated connective tissues lies in the abundance of sensory nerve endings, neurovascular bundles, neuromuscular attachments, capillary vessels, lymphocytes, fibroblasts and undifferentiated mesenchymal stem cells. These connective tissues, being part of the sensorineural and immune systems, are sensitive to mechanical signals. Acupuncture, through the mechanical coupling between needle and connective tissues, modifies the extracellular matrix composition, which in turn alters the neural and immune systems. Through connections of the network of connective tissue planes, the acupoints selected for needling need not be proximal to the area of affliction.

Acupuncture has been a relatively safe treatment for chronic pain, especially noninflammatory musculoskeletal pain, where modern western medicine is of little effectiveness [Audette and Ryan, 2004; Pyne and Shenker, 2008]. The sensation of skin penetration alone can elicit the placebo effect. However, some of the typical clinical features of acupuncture indicate that acupuncture analgesia is more than a placebo effect [Staud, 2007]. These clinical features include: (1) instead of immediate pain relief, the usual response is delayed for a few hours or days; (2) each subsequent acupuncture session improves or prolongs the pain relief; and (3) maximum effect is achieved after 3–6 treatment sessions. It is known that the nervous system reorganizes with or without structural changes. Structural change occurs with axonal and dentritic growth via stem cell neurogenesis, while nonstructural change happens with changes in synaptic membrane potential and NMDA receptor density. The central nervous system adapts its structure and function to the mechanical signals from the needle manipulation at acupoints. The adapted central nervous system raises pain tolerance or lowers pain sensitivity, achieving acupuncture analgesia. A most rigorous, detailed meta-analysis to date of 29 high-quality RCTs involving 17,922 patients, sponsored by the National Institutes of Health of the US, concludes that acupuncture is effective — compared to sham or nonacupuncture standard treatments — in reducing pains in chronic headache, neck and head pain, shoulder pain and osteoarthritis, and that the effect sizes are clinically relevant [Vickers *et al.*, 2012].

4.4 Periodontitis: An Example of Holistic Therapy

According to the NHS Evidence service of the UK (www.evidence.nhs.uk), the prevalence of plaque-induced inflammation of the gums, i.e. gingiva, in adults of the US and UK ranges from 50% to 90%, depending on the degree of infection. Untreated gingivitis spreads, developing into periodontitis. The prevalences of mild, moderate and severe periodontitis in UK adults are 54%, 43% and 8%, respectively. Risk factors for periodontitis include poor oral hygiene, ethnicity, socioeconomic status, smoking, decreased immunity and diabetes.

Oral bacteria feed on the food debris around the base of teeth. If the teeth are not cleaned thoroughly after a meal, a film of microflora grows around the gumline of the teeth, hardening into plaque. In response to the plaque-derived toxins, immune cells attack the plaque as well as the infected gums, causing inflammation. If the plaque and inflammation are not controlled, the gums recede and the infection progresses to ligaments. Dead tissue cells, white blood cells and bacteria form abscesses in the tooth-supporting tissue. Further inflammation leads to loss of the bone that supports the teeth, loosening them. Periodontitis is the major cause of tooth loss in adults.

Healthy gums are firm and pink. Soft, red–purple, swollen and bleeding gums mean inflamed gums. Visible deposits of plaque, receding gums and loose teeth are indications of periodontitis. Loss of supporting bones can be detected by dental X-rays. Modern western medical treatment of mild periodontitis is by antibiotics to control the inflammation. Daily tooth brushing and flossing are basic oral hygiene practices to control periodontitis. Professional tooth cleanings by e.g. ultrasonic scaling, at least twice a year, are suggested. In moderate-to-severe periodontitis, plaque deposits in the deep pockets between teeth and gums are removed. Gums are cut open to thoroughly clear off the abscesses and sutured back in place, with local anesthesia. Advanced tissue engineering techniques may be prescribed to regenerate lost tissue and bone. Loosened teeth are fixated to prevent loss of teeth. Note that antibiotics are effective only in the short term as oral bacteria quickly develop resistance to the drug.

In Ayurveda, descriptions of periodontal disease appeared in *Charaka Samhita* and *Ashtanga Hridaya* with the characteristics of swelling, bleeding gingiva and protruding teeth. Calculus was also noted and was called *Danta Shakkara* in Ayurveda. Periodontal disease is considered an imbalance of *pitta* in Ayurveda. To maintain oral hygiene and treat periodontal disease, Ayurveda has prescribed chewing sticks that are specific to the individual's doshic constitution (*prakriti*). Specifically, *vata*-predominant individuals should use bitter–sweet astringent chewing sticks, *pitta*-predominant individuals bitter chewing sticks, and *kapha*-predominant individuals pungent chewing sticks. Common chewing sticks are from twigs of arak, neem, mango, babul and guava plants. In usage, the bark of one end of the stick is peeled off; the wood is then chewed on until the fibers separate, and the fibers are used to rub the teeth as if they were a regular toothbrush. The action of chewing releases ingredients that were found to be antimicrobial, anti-inflammatory and/or antioxidant [Surathu and Kurumathur, 2011]. Ayurveda also prescribes oil gargling with sesame or

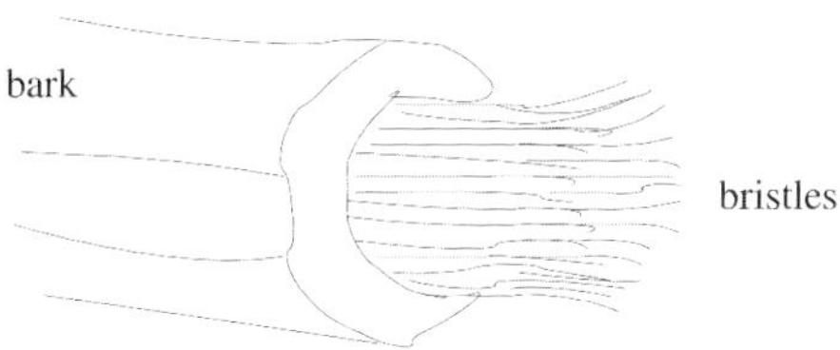

FIGURE 4.1

A chewing stick allows one to brush, floss, and chew on it. The juice in the stick, such as a miswak stick, is antibacterial. A chewing stick therefore functions like a toothbrush without the need for toothpaste.

sunflower oils as a detoxifying and purification therapy in the case of a mouth ulcer. Amla is a *rasayana* tonic for connective tissue regeneration in Ayurveda.

In TCM, periodontal disease is called *ya xuan*, which literally means "exposure of teeth." *The Yellow Emperor's Inner Canon* describes a feature of periodontal disease as long teeth with plaque. Plaque removal by a knife was described to cure periodontitis in *Wei Tai Mi Yao*, by Tao Wang (670–755 CE). The Chinese have manually cleaned teeth with salt since the Tang Dynasty (618–907 CE). Two toothbrush sticks made of bone material were unearthed in a tomb which had been sealed in 959 CE. Furthermore, descriptions of horse-tail toothbrushes and toothbrush-selling grocery stores appeared in various literature texts of the Song Dynasty (960–1279 CE). Periodontitis has two major subtypes in TCM. The first is stomach heat, which has such symptoms as swelling, dark-red gums and floating pulse. The second is kidney *yin* deficiency, characterized by receded, pale gums and weak pulse. The first corresponds to the acute and initial phase of periodontitis, and the second to the chronic and late phase of periodontitis. Stomach heat is believed to be caused by excessive intake of foods, digestion of which in the stomach heats up and "burns" the teeth. Teeth are bone residues in TCM. The kidney governs bone and bone marrow. As a consequence, when one is weak in the kidney due, for example, to old age, one's teeth loosen and come off. TCM herbal prescriptions for periodontitis therefore aim to cool stomach heat and enhance kidney *yin*. *Qing wei tang/san, yu nu jian, gan lu yin* and *gu chi wan/dan* are common herbal prescriptions. For example, *gu chi wan* was shown to inhibit osteoclast activity *in vivo* [Cao and Sun, 1998]. In addition, the stomach meridian passes through upper teeth and the large intestine meridian passes through lower teeth. As a consequence, acupuncture of stomach meridian and large intestine meridian acupoints usually accompanies TCM herbal prescriptions for the healing of upper and lower teeth, respectively. Tongue cleaning has been practiced in the two traditions, as both Ayurveda and TCM have relied on tongue inspection in diagnosis.

The topical intervention of periodontitis by modern western medicine effectively and acutely controls progression of the disease. By contrast, the systemic (or holistic) treatments of both Ayurveda and TCM, combining antibacterial/oxidant herbs and tissue-regenerative regimens, are likely to benefit the prognosis and even reversal of the disease. In addition, the *pitta* imbalance viewpoint of Ayurveda and stomach heat *zheng* of TCM converge on the role of dyshomeostatic metabolism in the disease. A thin and balanced diet is likely to prevent or control periodontal disease.

4.5 Practical Clinical Trial for the Effectiveness of Integrative Therapy

Randomized controlled trials (RCTs) have been the experimentally rigorous ways of establishing scientific evidence for the efficacy of a novel intervention. They have played a central role in translating laboratory biomedical discovery to FDA drug and labeling approval. In traditional RCTs, the eligibility criteria for participants are strict in order for the genotype of the clinical sample to match that of the cell lines on which the discovery was based. The experiments in RCTs are conducted under a highly controlled and specialized setting for the collection of dozens to hundreds of physiological variables per participant. The treatment in RCTs is fixed, following a predetermined protocol. Compliance of RCT participants is required and closely monitored. The design of traditional RCTs is therefore oriented toward substantiating mechanisms of action of the treatment.

In real-world situations, patients are of diverse genotypes and phenotypes. They differ in race, age, sex, environment and comorbidity. The intervention is often delivered in a community clinic, not a research-grade hospital. Based on clinical judgment, interventions can be changed, and thus are not fixed, along the course of the therapy. Patient compliance varies; some adhere while others may even quit. Traditional RCTs are considered to answer the question whether a treatment does more good than harm in an ideal circumstance. However, what matters to patients, clinicians and policy-makers is whether a treatment does more good than harm under (best-practice) clinical conditions.

The Cochrane Collaboration, an independent and not-for-profit organization, publishes up-to-date systematic reviews of healthcare therapies, including complementary and alternative medicine (CAM). A 2008 review of 68 Cochrane systematic reviews of TCM herbs and acupuncture found that 48% (20 out of 42) of the systematic reviews of TCM herbal medicine and 27% (7 out of 26) of the systematic reviews of acupuncture suggested benefits [Manheimer *et al.*, 2009]. The rest of the selected systematic reviews were found to be inconclusive on the evidence for the efficacy of the TCM intervention. Poor quality and quantity of the RCTs in the systematic reviews were attributed as a cause of the inconclusiveness. More studies were invariably called for in the conclusions of the systematic reviews.

RCT studies exercise the most experimental rigor. However, results of RCTs can suffer from clinical generalizability as the evidence is derived under ideal conditions. In the era of continuously escalating healthcare costs, limited resources, including time, should be allocated to meet the concerns of all the stakeholders. Design of clinical trials should therefore take into account such measures as quality of life, long-term effect, care-giving burden and use of health services. Specifically, the patient should live longer, feel better and spend less with the adopted clinical intervention. To this end, clinical trials can have three arms, comparing among conventional intervention, CAM intervention and integrative intervention combining conventional and CAM intervention. Intervention should be flexible, allowing individualized treatment. Assignment of participants to each arm should be random to avoid selection and unknown biases. The assessed clinical outcomes should also include self-report on improvements, long-term effect, quality of life and cost. Participating patients and clinics of the trial should be diverse and heterogeneous, reflective of the patients and practice in the real world. Results of such practical clinical trials are readily translatable to patients, healthcare providers and policy-makers. Ayurveda and TCM interventions tailored to patient *prakriti* and *zheng* are individualized. An Ayurveda intervention includes diet and detoxification therapy. TCM can prescribe herbal formulas and acupuncture. The interventions are multicomponent. RCTs, with their experimental rigor, help identify the active component and its optimal dose in the whole package of the CAM or integrative intervention.

Part II

Herbal Medicine

5

Safety and Regulation of Herbal Products

The use of herbal medicines has substantially increased in developed and developing countries in recent years. The surge is expected to continue in the future. Herbal medicines are considered complementary or alternative to conventional medicine. In Cochrane Summaries (summaries.cochrane.org), among the total of 526 systematic reviews within the CAM topic, we find 83 (16%), 74 (14%), 20 (4%) and 7 (1%) systematic reviews of the treatment effectiveness of "acupuncture," "Chinese herbal" medicine, "yoga" and "ayurvedic" medicine, respectively. Chinese herbal medicine can therefore be considered one of the most-investigated modes of therapies in traditional CAMs. A misconception about herbal remedies is that they are safe because they are natural. Plants interact with herbivores and pollinators through a plethora of released phytochemicals, some of which have been demonstrated to interfere with human physiology and medication. Surveys showed that 15% of adults in the US concomitantly consumed herbal medicines and conventional drugs. The concomitant rates went up to 39% and 49% for those in Taiwan and Israel, respectively. Potential adverse herb–drug interactions should not be overlooked. Herbal medicines should also be free from contaminations of pesticides, heavy metals and microbes. The safety, quality and efficacy of herbal products should therefore be regulated as strictly as for conventional drugs. The website nccam.nih.gov/news/alerts, by the National Center for Complementary and Alternative Medicine of the US government, maintains up-to-date information on the safety of particular botanical supplements.

5.1 Plant Secondary Metabolites

Plants cover a great proportion of the terrestrial surface. They also account for the majority of the biomass on Earth. However, they are stationary, self-feeding organisms. A rich set of secondary biochemical pathways is believed to have evolved in plants in order for them to respond to the specific environmental stimuli in their ecological niche. Examples of the stimuli are pollination, seed dispersal, nutrient fluctuations, herbivore attacks, pathogen infections and allelopathy. The chemicals in the secondary biochemical pathways which are not required for immediate survival but are essential for long-term fitness are called secondary metabolites. Plant secondary metabolites are responsible for the toxins, bitterness, scents and colors in deterring herbivores and attracting pollinators. Some plants are known to release secondary metabolites to attract predators of the herbivores upon herbivore attacks. Furthermore, some plants produce structural analogs of hormones endogenous to the herbivore in an effort to change the life course and behavior of the herbivorous insects. Other functions of plant secondary metabolites include: antioxidant, UV-light-absorbing, antibacterial, antifungal and antiviral.

The most abundant plant-derived secondary metabolites are alkaloids, terpenes and phenolics in regard to the chemical nature. Examples of alkaloids are caffeine and nicotine. Ginkgolides (from *Ginkgo biloba* leaves) and ginsenosides (from *Panax ginseng* roots) are examples of biologically active terpenes. Curcumin (from the Indian spice turmeric), resveratrol (from grape skins) and genistein (from soybeans) are well-known examples of phenolics. Toxicity of the phytochemicals tends to correlate with their ecological roles

[Kennedy and Wightman, 2011]. For example, alkaloids are neurotoxic based on the roles they play in deterring insects and other herbivores. Terpenes can be antimicrobial or prosymbiotic or both from their roles in pollination and seed dispersal. Phenolics are antioxidant through their roles in UV light protection and nontoxic deterrence of insects. A complication of secondary metabolite studies is that many of the secondary metabolites are induced upon environmental stress such as insect attacks. The chemical defense profiles of the same plant species from different geographical regions were also found to be specific to the types of local bugs. Naturally occurring combinations of herpenes were found to outweigh the combined activity of the constituent chemicals in terms of repellent and deterrent properties on insects [Nerio *et al.*, 2010; Gonzalez-Coloma *et al.*, 2006]. Synergies within and between chemical groups in a plant can therefore complicate the elucidation of the bioactive effects of phytochemicals. Recent sequencing of fungal genomes identified clusters of secondary metabolite genes. Furthermore, activation of the gene clusters and thus synthesis of secondary metabolites are regulated at the chromatin level [Strauss and Reyes-Dominguez, 2011]. It is plausible that plant-derived secondary metabolites interact with human cells through chromatin-modifying mechanisms [Hsieh *et al.*, 2011].

5.2 Pharmacodynamic and Pharmacokinetic Herb–Drug Interactions

Plant, insect and human cells share many of the biochemical pathways, including carbohydrate, lipid, protein and nucleic acid metabolisms. Other evolutionarily conserved cellular mechanisms include NO signaling, redox signaling, glutathione and cytochrome P450 (CYP) metabolisms. Neuropeptides, hormones and neurotransmitters in insects and mammals (including humans) are also highly conserved. Phytochemicals in herbal products, most of which are secondary metabolites, are pharmacologically active. Interactions between herbs and drugs therefore pose a risk for patients who concomitantly consume herbal medicines and conventional medications. For example, caffeine is psychoactive through adenosine receptor antagonism and can be contraindicated in insomniac patients taking sedatives. On the other hand, additive effects of herbs with drugs can result from their binding to the common receptor sites. Herb–drug interactions can thus either neutralize or precipitate the pharmacological effects of conventional drugs.

Most of the drugs and herbal products are orally administered. Xenobiotic substances, including drugs and toxins, are modified by the CYP isoenzymes in the liver and intestines in humans. Modified products are then pumped out of the intestinal cells by the p-glycoproteins (P-gp), one of the ABC transporters, in the intestines before entering the circulation in humans. Transporter proteins are also expressed in the kidneys and brain. If the coadministered herbal products induce (or inhibit) the intestinal and hepatic CYP and P-gp activities, the blood levels of the affected drugs are reduced (elevated). Oral bioavailability and systemic disposition of the conventional drugs can therefore be influenced by the coadministered herbal medicines. Examples of herbal products that contain CYP or P-gp inducers are garlic bulb, germander leaves, ginseng root and St John's wort. Examples of herbal products that contain CYP or P-gp inhibitors are cranberry fruit extract, ginseng root, grape seed, kava root, liquorice root and St John's wort [Fasinu *et al.*, 2012]. Fibers in some herbal medicines can increase gastrointestinal motility. The gastrointestinal transit time of the coadministered drug is decreased, and so is its absorption as a result. Phytochemicals are metabolized extensively by intestinal microbiota. Metabolites of the microbiota transformation may modulate the bioactivity of the drug in some way. Herbal medicines that increase the rate of urination can increase the renal elimination of other drugs. As a notable example of herbal nephropathy, aristolochic acid in *Aristolochia fangchi* causes end-stage kidney failure and urinary tract cancer in humans [Nortier *et al.*, 2000]. Use of *Aristolochia* species has ever since been heavily scrutinized. In addition to the issue of herb–drug interactions, other clinical concerns include contamination and adulteration of herbs. Regulation of herbal medicines regarding safety, quality and efficacy is therefore imperative for the health of consumers.

5.3 Regulation of TCM and Other Natural Herbal Products in China

In China, drugs, governed by the State Food and Drug Administration (SFDA), are defined to be the substances that are used for prevention, treatment and diagnosis of human diseases via regulation of the physiological functions of human beings. Drugs thus include not only chemical drug substances but also Chinese crude drugs, prepared slices of Chinese crude drugs and TCM preparations. In registration with the SFDA, medicinal substances and their preparations that follow the guidance of TCM theory are classified as traditional Chinese medicines, whereas natural medicinal substances and their preparations that follow modern medical theory are classified as natural medicinal products. The specifications and processing of TCM *materia medica* and natural medicinal products are required to meet the national and provincial standards. In addition, to support the study and development of TCM and the medicines of Chinese minorities, the SFDA issued a supplementary requirement for TCM registration in 2008. Under the supplementary requirement, partial exemption of the application data may be allowed, depending on the formulation, composition, indication and manufacture, for the marketing of TCM combination preparations which originated from historic, classic and well-known recipes. Also, herbal formulation registration may submit only nonclinical safety data and phase III clinical trial data if the herbal formulation is assessed by the SFDA to be reasonable in accordance with TCM theory. Supervision of herbal medicines in China is as strict as that of chemical drugs. Safety data are compulsory in herbal medicine registration although partial exemption in the application data is not impossible for demonstrably historic TCM formulations [Fan *et al.*, 2012].

5.4 *Kampo* Medicine in Japan

Traditional Japanese medicine, called *kampo*, was derived from the TCM which was introduced into Japan in the fourth century. Since then, substantial adaptation, refinement and improvement have been made by the Japanese practitioners. In particular, many of the original formulas have been validated through clinical experience since the 17th century, laying the foundation of *kampo* medicine. Approval of herbal medicine, including *kampo*, is regulated by the Ministry of Health, Labor and Welfare, and is subject to the same safety, quality and efficacy requirements as for conventional pharmaceuticals. A *kampo* formula can be approved as a prescription drug or over-the-counter (OTC) drug, depending on the medical claims. Some *kampo* formulas are both prescription drugs and OTC drugs in the Japanese market. *Kampo* preparations are mainly available in the form of ready-made powders or tablets from dry extracts which are manufactured by the process of decoction, condensation and spray-drying. Over 70% of Japanese licensed physicians prescribe *kampo*. Japanese national health insurance has covered *kampo* formulas since 1967. To date, 148 *kampo* formulas are reimbursed by the Japanese national health insurance program.

5.5 Regulation of TCM Medicine in Taiwan

The national health insurance of Taiwan has covered western medicine, TCM and dentistry since 1995. TCM herbs or formulas from the classical TCM literature recognized by the Committee on Chinese Medicine and Pharmacy, Department of Health, can be registered without clinical efficacy and safety data. Registered formulas and herbs in the form of concentrated extract granules and powders are reimbursable. TCM processing and manufacturing have to meet the Good Manufacturing Practice (GMP) standards required by the government. In particular, the total heavy metals have to be below 30 ppm, the total microbe number below

105 cfu/g and *Escherichia coli* and *Salmonella* spp. undetected in all concentrated Chinese medicinal preparations. To date, over 300 formulas and over 400 single herbs manufactured by over 100 GMP-compliant TCM pharmaceutical manufacturers in Taiwan are reimbursed. Chinese medicines listed in the classical Chinese literature used for new medical indications or by new administration routes have to apply for approval with clinical efficacy data. Chinese medicines unlisted in the classical Chinese literature have to provide clinical safety, efficacy and quality control data in the application.

5.6 Regulation of Natural Health Products in Canada

In Canada, herbs, plant-based remedies and traditional medicines (including TCM and ayurvedic medicine) are classified as natural health products (NHPs). Other examples of NHPs are vitamin/mineral supplements, omega-3, essential fatty acids, probiotics and homeopathic medicines. Commercial sales of NHPs in Canada require the NHP manufacturers, packagers, labelers or importers to apply to Health Canada for licenses. In the application, proper evidence for the safety and efficacy of the NHP and the health claims have to be provided. Depending on the health claims and overall risks, supporting evidence can come from clinical trial data or from references to published studies, journals, pharmacopoeias and traditional resources. Notably, the NHP licensing requirement does not apply to retailers of NHPs or to healthcare practitioners who compound products for their patients on an individual basis.

5.7 Botanical Products as Dietary Supplements in the United States

In the US, the FDA regulated product categories are: (1) cosmetic, (2) device, (3) dietary supplement, (4) drug, (5) food, (6) food additive. Botanical products or herbal medicines are not in the above categories. If a botanical product is intended for production and sale for general wellness, it is subject to FDA food regulation. If the botanical product is marketed as part of a regimen for the treatment of a disease, it is regulated by the FDA as a drug. If the botanical product is to become a new drug, it needs to provide safety, efficacy and quality data with well-designed clinical trials through the investigational new drug application and new drug application processes. Since 2000, for the new drug application of botanical mixtures such as TCM and other herbal medicines, purification and identification of the active compounds in the botanical mixtures have not been required. To further speed up the preclinical studies of TCM products, animal toxicology data are not required if the previous human use of the TCM products is deemed safe. Currently, most TCM products (including TCM raw herbs) are marketed and used as dietary supplements by acupuncturists and herbalists based on a one-to-one practitioner–client consultation in the US. In the labeling of dietary supplements, the manufacturer can make claims about the effect of the product on the structure or function of the body. A disclaimer reading "This statement has not been evaluated by the FDA. This product is not intended to diagnose, treat, cure, or prevent any disease." has to follow the claim.

5.8 Regulation of Traditional Herbal Medicinal Products in the European Union

Herbal medicines are required to have appropriate licenses for sales in the EU under the European Directive 2004/24/EC, which took effect on April 30, 2011. The typical route of registration for herbal medicines, including TCM but excluding animal materials and chemical compounds, is registration as traditional herbal medicinal products (THMPs). The "traditional" in THMPs is defined for herbal medicine products that have been in traditional medicinal use for 30 years preceding the date of application for the intended indications. In the 30-year usage, 15 years must have been within the EU. Traditional use also means that it is a herbal product (1) which is for use in minor, self-limiting conditions, such as the common cold and cough, suitable for self-management without the requirement for the intervention of a medical practitioner; (2) which is taken orally, of external use or inhalation; and (3) whose efficacy is plausible on the basis of longstanding use. The bibliographical evidence for traditional use from such sources as pharmacopoeia and official expert reports then replaces the usual requirements of toxicological and clinical studies on safety and efficacy. The quality of the herbal product, such as to meet the standards of Good Agricultural and Collection Practice, and Good Manufacturing Practice, has also to be demonstrated in the application. Labeling of the herbal product should contain the following statement: "Product X is a traditional herbal medicinal product for use in specified indications exclusively based on longstanding use."

6

Cancer

In TCM development, multiple herbs were combined, with specific weights, into a formula. Thousands of formulas have been devised. Those that have survived the test of time and are still in popular use today are called classical formulas. A classical formula may not suit every patient, because of idiosyncrasy. In tailoring, ingredient herbs are added to or subtracted from the standard classical formula. A TCM prescription can therefore consist of a classical formula together with a couple of herbs. The heavier an ingredient, the more prominent the role it plays in the prescription. In recent large-scale, nationwide pharmacoepidemiological studies of TCM use, we find that TCM doctors in Taiwan prescribe on average two or three formulas and two to four herbs per prescription for the diseases defined by modern western medicine. Formulas are found to be in general heavier than herbs in the prescription. A western drug comes with its labeling. Similarly, a classical TCM formula is designated its corresponding TCM *zheng* in TCM texts. TCM *zhengs*, i.e. sets of signs and symptoms, are summarized as cold/warm, exterior/interior, excess/deficiency, *yin/yang* and TCM viscera/meridians following TCM diagnostics; they do not readily find counterparts in modern western diagnostics. A combination of TCM *zhengs* may be required to describe an X-ray (Pap smear)-diagnosed lung (cervical) cancer. Differences between TCM holistic and western molecular diagnostics are thought to explain the multiplicity of formulas in a TCM prescription for a disease defined by modern western medicine. A compilation of TCM prescriptions for western diseases is the first step toward integrative medicine. This chapter results from analysis of over 100,000 TCM prescriptions for neoplasms. To avoid potential herb–drug interactions, administration of TCM prescriptions and conventional drugs should be staggered in time, following the doctor's advice. All the TCM formulas and herbs in the book have been standardized and are available from GMP-certified herbal product manufacturers.

6.1 Six Core and Two Emerging Hallmarks of Cancer

A tumor is not just an insular mass of proliferating cells. It is a complex tissue consisting of multiple distinct cell types interacting with one another and with the rest of the body. The interacting cells collude to enable the multistep process of tumorigenesis, starting from neoplastic formation and growth, continuing with invasion of adjacent tissues and ending with metastatic dissemination throughout the body. Four decades of intensive cancer research has helped recapitulate eight distinctive yet interrelated hallmark capabilities that allow cancer cells to survive, proliferate and disseminate [Hanahan and Weinberg, 2011].

The most fundamental capability of cancer cells involves their chronically unlimited proliferation. Normal cells operate a highly temporally and spatially regulated program of the cell division cycle to maintain cell number homeostasis within the tissue. Cancer cells upset the balance by overproduction of growth factors and/or growth factor receptors. Binding of growth factors to the cognate receptors activates intracellular signaling pathways, resulting in cell cycle initiation and progression. Such growth factors and growth factor receptors are called oncogenes. Notable examples are RAS, MYC and EGFR. MYC regulates not only target genes but also chromatin by recruitment of histone acetyltransferases. Growth signaling pathways generally come with negative feedback loops to damp the activation of proliferation. Normal growth is therefore transitory. Cancer cells, however, exhibit defects in the negative feedback loops. Prominent defects are Ras GTPase and PTEN phosphatase inactivities in the negative feedback loops; the former is by DNA mutation and the latter by promoter methylation. Sustained proliferative signaling, via constitutive growth factor (receptor) activation and/or negative feedback loop disruption, is the first hallmark of cancer.

In addition to growth-stimulatory signaling, normal cells are equipped with growth-suppressing signaling to maintain an adequate cell number. Tumor suppressors sense cellular physiology and trigger negative growth signaling, which governs the decision of whether the cell enters into the cell cycle, stays in senescence or goes through apoptosis. TP53 and RB are two of the dozens of known tumor suppressor genes. For example, TP53 will signal a halt to cell cycle progression when the glucose level is suboptimal or cause apoptosis when the genome damage is irreparable. Another example is NF2, whose product inhibits cell growth, by sequestering growth factor receptors, when the cell population becomes too dense. Evasion of growth suppressors, by loss of function of the tumor suppressor genes, represents the second hallmark of cancer.

In multicellular organisms, cells and cellular parts are recycled by apoptosis and autophagy, respectively. In apoptosis, cells with damaged DNA, sensed by TP53, are first disassembled through a cascade of proteolysis and then engulfed by neighboring cells and phagocytes (a type of white blood cells). In autophagy, organelles in cells under stress, such as nutrient deficiency, are broken down, by lysosomes, into low-molecular-weight metabolites. By contrast, necrosis is a form of acute cell death caused by extracellular factors such as infection, toxins and trauma. Necrotic cells release proinflammatory signals which recruit immune inflammatory cells to the site of injury. Immune inflammatory cells, assessing the degree of tissue damage and removing the necrotic debris, are able to foster angiogenesis and are thus tumor-promoting. Resistance to cell death, by attenuating apoptosis and/or by tolerating necrosis, constitutes the third hallmark of cancer.

As cells go through repeated cell cycles, the tips of the chromosomes, called telomeres, erode. Telomeres function to protect the genome from chromosomal end-to-end fusions. Telomere length therefore serves to count down the remaining cell generations. Cells with subcritically shortened telomeres enter into a nonproliferative but viable state called senescence. Cells of advanced senescence trigger a crisis and die via apoptosis. Few of the senescent cells, however, survive the crisis, becoming immortal. Telomerase is an enzyme able to elongate the lost telomeres. Its level of expression is almost zero in nonimmortalized cells but is significantly elevated in a majority of immortalized cells, including human cancer cells. Enabled replicative immortality, by telomerase activation to delay replicative senescence, gives the fourth hallmark of cancer cells.

Vasculature is a system for passing nutrients including oxygen, and wastes including carbon dioxide into and out of cells. Vasculature development, including vasculogenesis and angiogenesis, is switched on during embryogenesis and becomes quiescent after morphogenesis. In adults, angiogenesis is transient, occurring in wound healing or female reproductive cycling. VEGF-A, which binds to the cell surface receptors of vascular endothelial cells, is a well-known angiogenesis inducer. VEGF expression is upregulated directly by oncogene signaling in some tumors and produced indirectly by peritumoral inflammatory cells in others. Angiogenesis has been observed in a surprisingly early stage of tumorigenesis: the microscopic premalignant phase of neoplastic progression. Induction of angiogenesis for tumor neovasculature defines the fifth hallmark of cancer.

Invasion of cancer cells to local tissues and metastasis to distant tissues reflect the increased pathological grade of malignancy. For example, in invasive carcinoma cells are observed downregulation of molecules associated with cell-to-cell and cell-to-extracellular-matrix (ECM) adhesion and upregulation of molecules associated with cell migration. Six discrete steps have been used to schematize the sequence of cell-biologic changes of the cancer cells throughout invasions and metastasis: (1) local invasion; (2) intravasation into nearby blood and lymphatic vessels; (3) transit through the hematogenous and lymphatic systems; (4) extravasation into parenchyma of distant tissues; (5) formation of small aggregations called micrometastases; and (6) colonization via growth of micrometastatic lesions into macroscopic tumors. The ability of malignant cells to invade and disseminate is thought to be acquired by co-opting the processes involved in embryonic morphogenesis and wound healing. Transcription factors, which were initially identified by developmental geneticists in the migratory processes of embryogenesis, were found to be expressed in various combinations in a number of different malignant tumors. Notably, evidence from developmental genetics indicates that contextual signals from neighboring cells choreograph embryogenesis. Tumor-associated stromal cells must play an integral role in the induction of the invasive phenotype. On the other hand, the microenvironment of the distant tissues may not be hospitable to the micrometastases of the primary tumor. Disseminated micrometastases therefore do not necessarily result in successful colonization. These micrometastases appear dormant until they overcome, with much trial and error, the tough problem of tissue colonization decades after a primary tumor was surgically removed or pharmacologically contained. Invasion and metastasis activation sums up the sixth hallmark of cancer.

Normal cells consume glucose through anaerobic glycolysis in cytoplasm coupled with aerobic respiration (oxidative phosphorylation) in mitochondria. It has been observed by Otto Warburg in 1930 that cancer cells produce their energy largely by glycolysis even in the presence of oxygen. The phenomenon is called aerobic glycolysis. To compensate for the lower ATP production efficiency of glycolysis, cancer cells upregulate the expression of glucose transporter genes such as GLUT1. Glucose uptake and utilization are increased in many tumors, as a result. Since glycolytic intermediates can be redirected to various biosynthetic pathways for nucleoside and amino acid production, it is thought that upregulated glycolysis supports the large-scale biosynthesis required by continuously proliferating cancer cells. In addition, glycolytic fueling is associated with oncogene activation and the hypoxic condition, both of which operate within tumors. Reprogrammed energy metabolism is the first emerging hallmark of cancer.

Mice deficient in adaptive immunity such as cytotoxic T cells and/or in innate immunity such as natural killer (NK) cells have been demonstrated to show an increased incidence of tumors relative to immunocompetent controls. The results suggest that the immune system keeps recognizing and then eliminating incipient cancer cells, at least in some experimental models. However, human epidemiological studies of chronically immunosuppressed patients such as HIV patients did not show significantly increased rates of nonviral cancer. One explanation is that HIV patients are usually immunodeficient in T and B but not in cytotoxic T and NK cells; the other is that cancer cells may recruit immunosuppressive inflammatory cells to suppress the actions of cytotoxic T cells. Evasion of immune destruction, by evading surveillance or limiting killing of the immune system, represents the second emerging hallmark of cancer.

6.2 Mechanisms of Hallmark Acquisition: Genomic and Epigenomic Instability, Inflammation; Microenvironment

The hallmark capabilities for tumorigenesis which have been enumerated are acquired through a sequence of genome alterations and/or epigenome modifications, each of which confers selective advantage on subclones of the cells. As the mutant cells outgrow and dominate their normal counterparts, a succession of clonal expansions portrays the multistep development and progression of cancer. Rates of chance mutation have been kept very low in adaptive evolution by means of natural selection. To acquire the required combinations of mutant genotypes, cancer cells increase the rates by (1) increased sensitivity to mutagenic agents such as reactive oxygen species (ROS) and/or by (2) breakdown of the components of the genome maintenance and repair machinery.

Examples of the DNA maintenance machinery components are TP53 and telomerase; they behave like tumor suppressor genes. Loss of function of tumor suppressor genes also results from gene promoter methylation, which, like DNA mutation, is inherited from cell generation to cell generation. The latest high-resolution, next-generation DNA sequencing studies have revealed recurring defects in the genome maintenance and repair in a variety of human tumors. Genome instability is demonstrably one of the enabling mechanisms of cancer.

In virtually every neoplastic lesion, there have been detected varying grades of inflammation, ranging from subtle infiltrations of adaptive and innate immune cells detectable by cell-type-specific antibodies, to gross inflammations apparent by standard histochemical techniques. Inflammation in some cases is observed in the earliest stages of neoplastic progression. The observation reflects the antitumoral effects of the immune system. On the other hand, evidence also demonstrates that tumor-associated inflammation promotes neoplastic progression by supplying the tumor microenvironment with bioactive molecules including growth factors, survival factors, proangiogenic factors, transdifferentiating factors and mutagenic factors. Tumor-promoting inflammation is the other enabling mechanism for the acquisition of core hallmark capabilities.

A tumor is not a collection of homogeneous cancer cells that can be described by the cell autonomous properties studied by reductionist approaches. A tumor, instead, contains individual specialized cell types and the microenvironment it builds during the multistep tumorigenesis. The clonal heterogeneity of cancer cells also manifests in the histopathological diversity of human tumors. One of the specialized cell types in tumors is cancer stem cells (CSCs), which show enhanced efficiency of seeding new tumors upon xenotransplantation into mice and express cell surface markers of the normal stem cells in the tissue of origin. In a tissue reside normal stem cells and progenitor cells. A theory proposes that CSCs derive from oncogenic transformation of the normal stem cells or progenitor cells. The other possibility is that cancer cells undergo such transdifferentiation as epithelial-to-mesenchymal induced by inflammatory stroma. CSCs at distinct stages of differentiation, in addition to genome instability, also contribute to the phenotypic heterogeneity of the cancer cell population, especially in later stages of tumor progression. As stem cells are resistant to chemicals, CSCs may be the underlying cause of recurrence of the tumor, years and even decades after its debulking.

Cells in tumor stroma account for the rest of the cellular heterogeneity within a tumor. Among them are immune inflammatory cells, including macrophage subtypes, mast cells, neutrophils, and T and B cells. These immune inflammatory cells release such effectors as growth factors, proangiogenic factors, proinvasive matrix-degrading enzymes and proinflammatory cytokines to promote tumor development and progression. The adaptive arm of the immune system, supported by innate immunity, is responsible for detection and targeting of infectious agents. The innate arm is involved in debris cleaning and wound healing, which calls for angiogenesis, matrix remodeling and epithelial/stromal growth. Therefore, while some immune inflammatory cells are tumor-antagonizing, the subclasses of the innate immune inflammatory cells involved in wound healing and tissue house-cleaning are tumor-promoting.

Tumor-associated stromal cells fuel growing tumors. Evidence shows that stem and progenitor cells originating from neighboring normal tissues and from bone marrow join tumor stroma to supply tumor growth. Other tumor stromal cells include epithelial cells, pericytes and fibroblasts.

6.3 Frontiers of Conventional Treatment: Drug Cocktail Cotargeting Multiple Hallmarks; Personalized Targeted Therapy

Drugs developed by modern pharmaceutical companies have been very specific, meaning that a drug interferes with one or two targets in particular pathways. The fewer off-targets a drug has, the less nonspecific toxicity it will incur. Mechanism-based targeted therapies that deliberately direct drugs toward the molecular targets involved in a cancer hallmark have been developed for more than two decades. However, signal transduction pathways are typically densely overlapping. Partially redundant signaling pathways therefore underlie a hallmark capability. The effectiveness of targeted therapies that block single pathways has thus been found transitory as cancer cells surviving the drugs with residual function would adapt to regain the hallmark capability and renew tumor growth. Means of tumor adaptation include genetic mutation, epigenetic reprogramming and stroma remodeling. Furthermore, cancer cells can trade off a hallmark capability for the others. For example, glioblastomas treated with antiangiogenic drugs were found to show increased invasion and local metastases [Norden *et al.*, 2009]. Adaptive resistance of cancer cells via pathway redundancy or hallmark tradeoffs manifests as clinical relapse. A cocktail of mechanism-based drugs that cotarget a selection of hallmarks rationally offers more effective and durable cancer care.

So far, a few dozen drugs targeting cancer-causing mutations have been developed. If the cancer genome matches the targets of the available cancer drugs, targeted therapies will be the first line of treatment. If none in the repertoire of the available drugs targets the patient's mutations, chemotherapy or radiotherapy will be the treatment of choice. Chemotherapeutic agents crosslink to DNA, causing cell cycle arrest. Chemotherapy is therefore cytotoxic to fast dividing cells, including not only tumors but also cells in bone marrow, digestive tract and hair follicles. Immunosuppression, peptic ulceration and hair loss are among the common adverse side effects of chemotherapy. Radiation therapy directs beams of ionizing particles such as gamma rays, X-rays and beta particles at tumors, breaking DNA and causing cell death. Radiotherapy is commonly combined with surgery and chemotherapy for cancer care.

Specific genetic mutations and thus drug targets of a cancer have traditionally been identified through comparisons between cancer cells from patients and those from matched controls. The mutations identified this way are common mutations shared by the patients. Individual mutational differences from patient to patient are ignored. As whole genome sequencing is becoming clinically practical, a trend of targeted cancer therapy is to identify patient-specific genetic mutations by comparing the cancer genome from the tumor with the normal genome from adjacent normal tissue or the saliva of the same patient [The Cancer Genome Atlas Research Network, 2012]. Drugs are then searched for their interoperability on the cancer cells bearing the identified genetic causes. Note that the same gene is expressed to different levels in different tissues. Drugs developed for a cancer, e.g. lung cancer, therefore do not necessarily work for a different cancer, e.g. liver cancer. Available targeting drugs are currently a bottleneck for personalized targeted therapy. Another recent advance is cancer immunotherapies which use patient's immune system to fight cancer. In particular, cell-based immunotherapy works to (1) activate cancer antigen presentation of dendritic cells; (2) stimulate production of T/B cells; and (3) overcome the immunosuppression of cancer cells.

6.4 TCM Carbuncle-Treating, TCM Mediating Formulas; TCM Cold Herbs Against Neoplasms

If a tumor lacks the hallmark capability of invasion and metastasis, it is called benign. It is malignant otherwise. In a nationwide, cross-sectional study of TCM use, where a total of 100,679 TCM cancer prescriptions are available, we find that, for commonplace benign neoplasms, the TCM formulas that have been heavily (i.e. overrepresentation test $p < 0.05$) prescribed are carbuncle-treating ($p = 0.0006$), mediating ($p = 0.003$) and blood-regulating ($p = 0.04$) formulas. The TCM single herbs that have been heavily prescribed for those benign neoplasms are mild–cold ($p = 0.005$) in TCM herb nature. For commonplace malignant neoplasms, the TCM formulas that have been heavily prescribed are carbuncle-treating ($p = 0.0004$), mediating ($p = 0.003$), tonifying ($p = 0.009$) and dryness-treating ($p = 0.04$) formulas. And the TCM single herbs that have been heavily prescribed for those malignant neoplasms are cold ($p = 7 \times 10^{-13}$) and mild–warm ($p = 0.005$) in TCM nature. *P* values here are from tests of overrepresentation against the distribution of the set of all registered TCM formulas or herbs in the single-payer national health insurance program which covers 99.6% of Taiwan's residents.

In TCM, carbuncle-treating formulas have been developed to treat various endogenous wounds (e.g. visceral swelling) and exogenous injuries (e.g. a cutaneous abscess). Causes of endogenous wounds are the seven emotional extremes: joy, anger, sorrow, fear, love, hate and desire. TCM carbuncle-treating formulas are said to help detoxify, drain and heal the lesion. TCM mediating formulas are meant for the *shao yang zheng,* which is characterized by: (1) neither interior nor exterior; (2) neither cold nor warm; (3) neither excess nor deficiency. That is to say, *shao yang* syndromes manifest the dynamic interactions between immune defense and pathological progression. A TCM mediating formula may contain both warm and cold herbs; the former are said to activate immune function and the latter to suppress remission. TCM blood-regulating formulas treat thrombosis and hemorrhage. They are said to promote blood flow and reduce pain. TCM tonifying formulas treat conditions of *qi*/blood depletion, visceral impairment and *yin–yang* bias by enhancing *qi* and blood, nourishing viscera and restoring the *yin–yang* balance. TCM dryness-treating formulas moisten dried mucosa of the respiratory and digestive systems caused by low humidity or visceral impairment. Note that dryness, including dry mouth, dry eyes, dry skin, dry cough and constipation, is among the side effects of chemo/radiotherapy. TCM cold herbs are considered to suppress inflammation, reduce oxidative stress and lower catabolism. TCM may mix cold and mild–warm herbs to fine-tune the coldness of the prescription. In sum, the proproliferative hallmarks of cancer seem to be targeted by carbuncle-treating formulas and cold herbs, the angiogenic hallmark by blood-regulating formulas, the invasive–metastatic and tumor-promoting inflammation hallmarks by mediating formulas, the deregulated bioenergetics hallmark by cold herbs, and the genome instability hallmark by tonifying formulas. Furthermore, the tumor-supportive microenvironment is thought to be targeted by carbuncle-treating formulas.

The average number of GMP-certified formulas (herbs) in a cancer prescription is found to be two (four), independent of cancer types. Weights of the ingredients (i.e. formulas and herbs) are also essential, as two cancers can be prescribed the

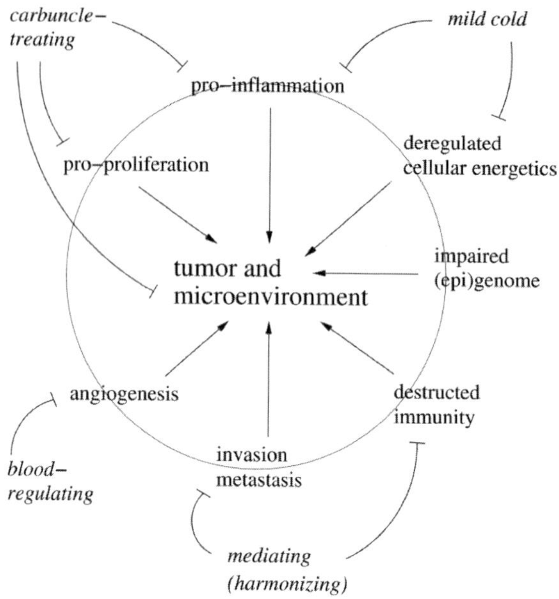

FIGURE 6.1a
Cancer hallmarks and the prescribed TCM formulas and herbs for benign neoplasms. Multiple ingredients in a TCM prescription are a feature of Chinese herbal medicine. As the hallmarks are interdependent, a TCM ingredient can cotarget one or two hallmarks. Abnormalities in gene functions and activities can arise from genetic and epigenetic impairments. Multiple compounds in a TCM ingredient may target a hallmark through concurrent receptor inhibitions and chromatin modifications. Pointed arrows indicate promotion; blunt arrows indicate suppression.

same combination of ingredients but with different weights in the ingredients. We find that the weight distribution goes like 100:66:52:44:38:34 from the heaviest to the lightest ingredient in a six-ingredient prescription for benign neoplasms and that it is 100:71:58:50:45:41 for malignant neoplasms [Chiu *et al.*, 2012]. The weight distribution of the ingredients in prescriptions for benign neoplasms decreases drastically quickly, indicating that a benign tumor prescription relies on few dominant ingredients while the ingredients in the prescriptions for malignant tumors

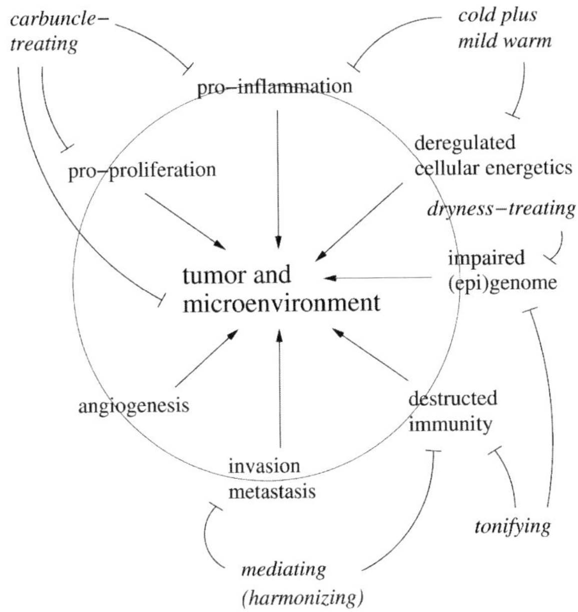

FIGURE 6.1b
Cancer hallmarks and the prescribed TCM formulas and herbs for malignant neoplasms. Multiple ingredients in a TCM prescription are a feature of Chinese herbal medicine. As the hallmarks are interdependent, a TCM ingredient can cotarget one or two hallmarks. Abnormalities in gene functions and activities can arise from genetic and epigenetic impairments. Multiple compounds in a TCM ingredient may target a hallmark through concurrent receptor inhibitions and chromatin modifications. Pointed arrows indicate promotion; blunt arrows indicate suppression.

are of relatively uniform importance. Specific formula–formula, formula–herb and herb–herb combinations for individual cancers depend on the cancer tissues of origin, as different cell types express different levels of receptors and organize different conformations of chromatin. Signs, symptoms and prognoses of tumors arising from different anatomic sites also differ even though they share many of the cancer hallmarks. TCM herbalism appears to have empirically identified organ/tissue-specific herbs, in that TCM prescriptions for the neoplasms originating from a

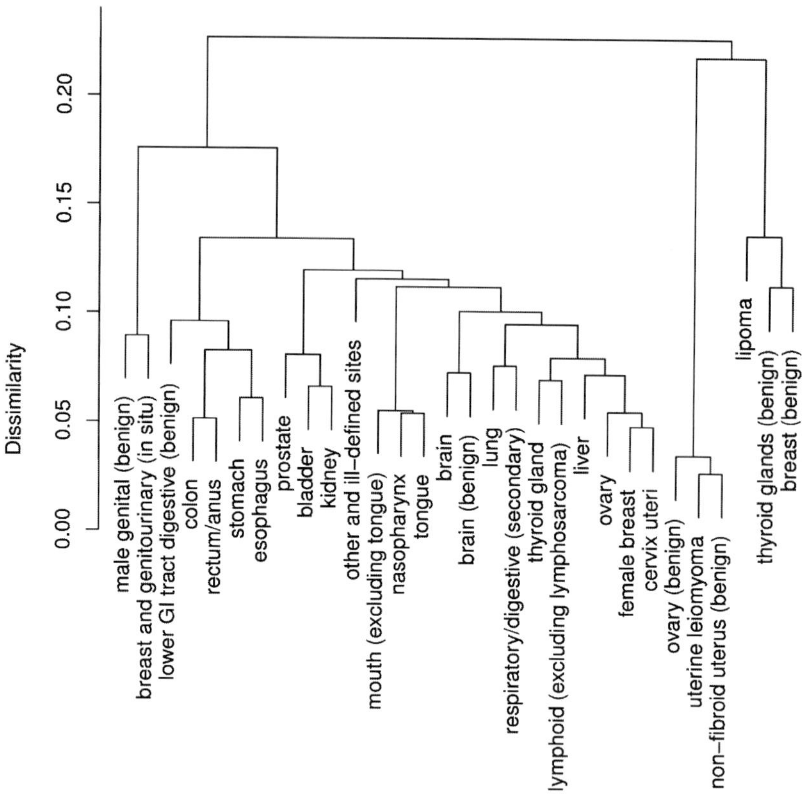

FIGURE 6.2
Clustering of TCM cancer prescriptions. Prescriptions which are similar in terms of ingredients and their relative weights in the prescription fall within branches of the tree. Prescriptions for benign neoplasms separate from those for malignant ones. Furthermore, prescriptions for neoplasms of closely related physiology/anatomy cluster together. The vertical axis measures pairwise distance or dissimilarity between prescriptions.

physiological system are similar. For example, TCM prescriptions for the digestive system (or female reproductive system) share many of the primary ingredients. Prescriptions for the neoplasms that are not in this chapter can therefore be extrapolated from existing ones.

6.5 Uterine Leiomyoma: *Gui Zhi Fu Ling Wan* and *Yi Mu Cao*

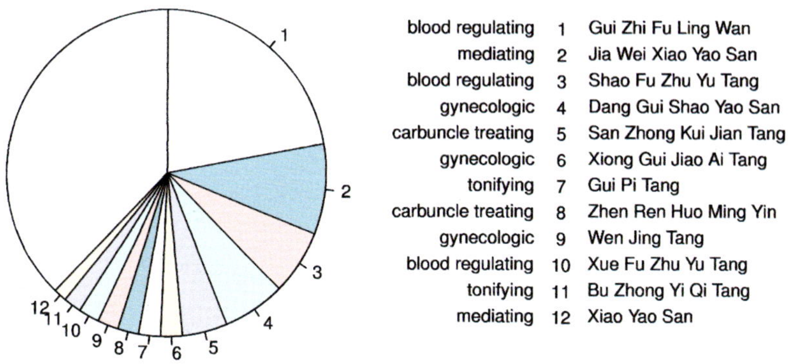

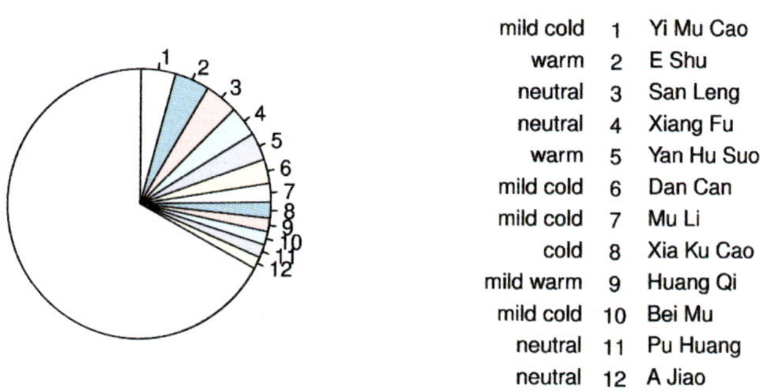

FIGURE 6.3a
A uterine leiomyoma or fibroid (ICD-9 = 218) is a benign tumor originating from the smooth muscle layer of the uterus. Uterine fibroids are treated by TCM gynecologic (p = 0.008) and blood-regulating (p = 0.04) formulas. The top 12 ingredients are shown. The areas of the pies indicate the relative weights of the formulas and herbs in the prescription for the condition. *P* values are from over-representation tests.

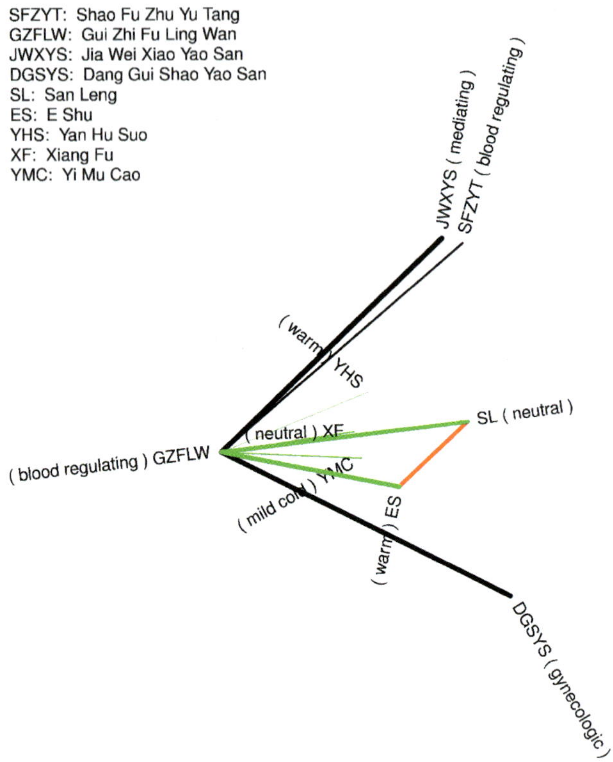

FIGURE 6.3b
The commonest TCM formula pair is GZFLW–JWXYS, the commonest formula–herb pair is GZFLW–ES and the commonest herb pair is ES–SL for the treatment of uterine leiomyoma. The thickness of the line indicates the prevalence of the pair. Formula pairs are in black, formula–herb pairs in green and herb pairs in red. The TCM pharmacotherapeutic categories of the formulas and the TCM natures of the herbs are shown in parentheses.

6.6 Benign Nonfibroid Neoplasm of the Uterus: *Gui Zhi Fu Ling Wan* and *E Shu*

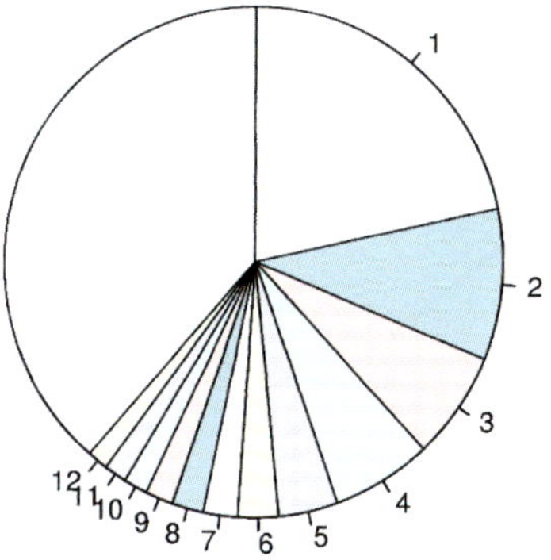

blood regulating	1	Gui Zhi Fu Ling Wan
mediating	2	Jia Wei Xiao Yao San
gynecologic	3	Dang Gui Shao Yao San
blood regulating	4	Shao Fu Zhu Yu Tang
carbuncle treating	5	San Zhong Kui Jian Tang
carbuncle treating	6	Zhen Ren Huo Ming Yin
blood regulating	7	Xue Fu Zhu Yu Tang
fire purging	8	Qing Wei San
gynecologic	9	Xiong Gui Jiao Ai Tang
tonifying	10	Liu Wei Di Huang Wan
tonifying	11	Gui Pi Tang
mediating	12	Xiao Yao San

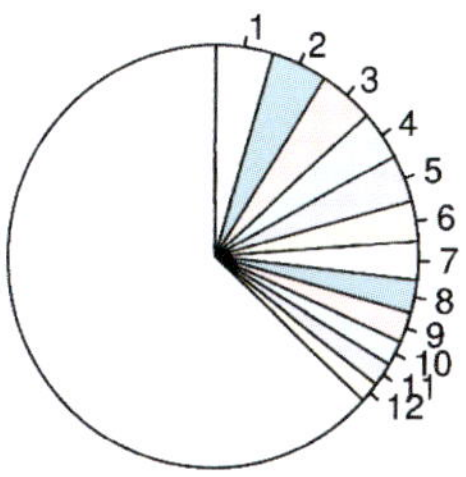

warm	1	E Shu
mild cold	2	Yi Mu Cao
neutral	3	San Leng
neutral	4	Xiang Fu
warm	5	Yan Hu Suo
cold	6	Xia Ku Cao
mild cold	7	Dan Can
warm	8	Chuan Qi
mild cold	9	Mu Li
cold	10	Yu Jin
cold	11	Pu Gong Ying
neutral	12	Tao Ren

FIGURE 6.4a
Benign neoplasms other than fibroids of the uterus (ICD-9 = 219) are treated by TCM blood-regulating formulas ($p = 0.04$). The Top 12 ingredients are shown. The areas of the pies indicate the relative weights of the formulas and herbs in the prescription for the condition. *P* values are from overrepresentation tests.

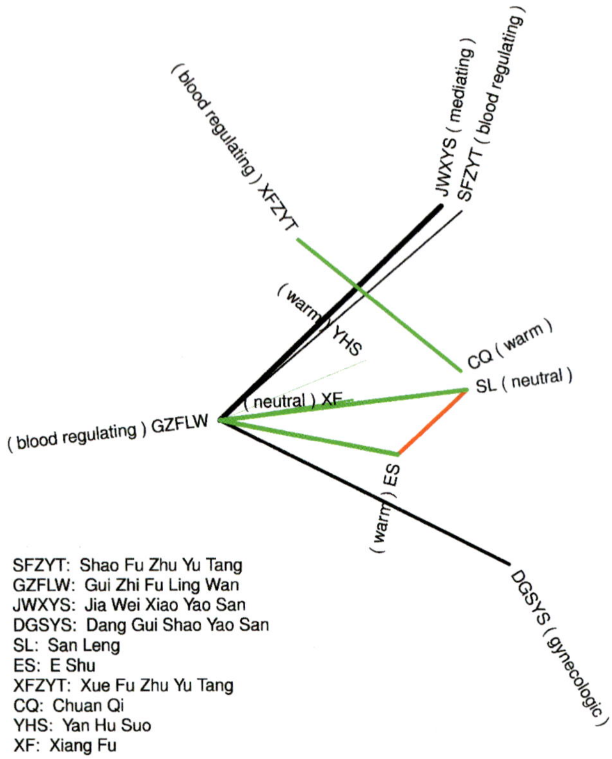

FIGURE 6.4b

The commonest TCM formula pair is GZFLW–JWXYS; the commonest formula–herb pair is GZFLW–ES, followed by XFZYT–CQ; and the commonest herb pair is ES–SL for the treatment of benign nonfibroid neoplasms of the uterus. The thickness of the line indicates the prevalence of the pair. Formula pairs are in black, formula–herb pairs in green and herb pairs in red. The TCM pharmacotherapeutic categories of the formulas and the TCM natures of the herbs are shown in parentheses.

6.7 Benign Neoplasm of the Ovary: *Gui Zhi Fu Ling Wan* and *Yi Mu Cao*

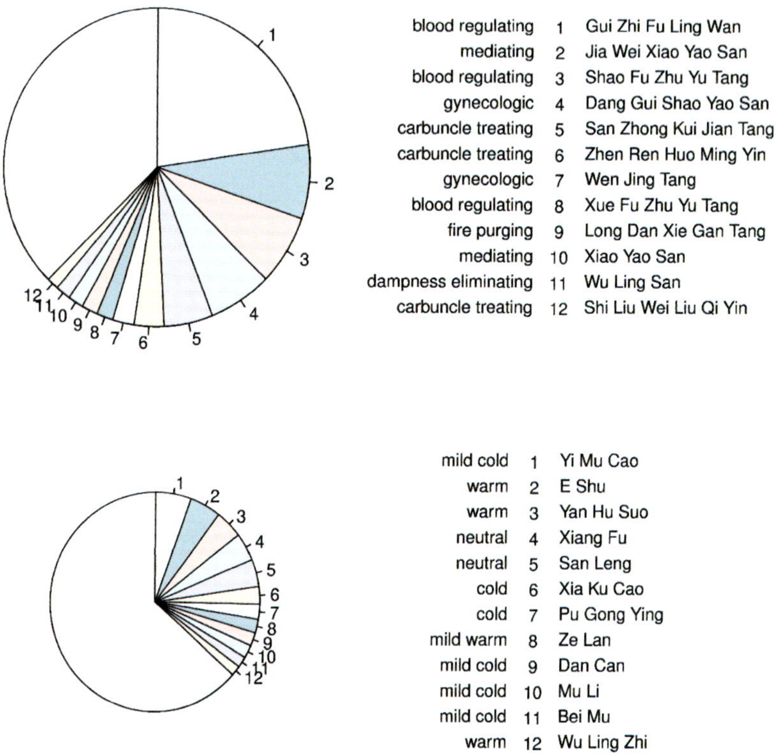

FIGURE 6.5a
Benign neoplasms of the ovary (ICD-9 = 220) are treated by TCM carbuncle-treating ($p = 0.01$) and blood-regulating ($p = 0.04$) formulas. The top 12 ingredients are shown. The areas of the pies indicate the relative weights of the formulas and herbs in the prescription for the condition. *P* values are from overrepresentation tests.

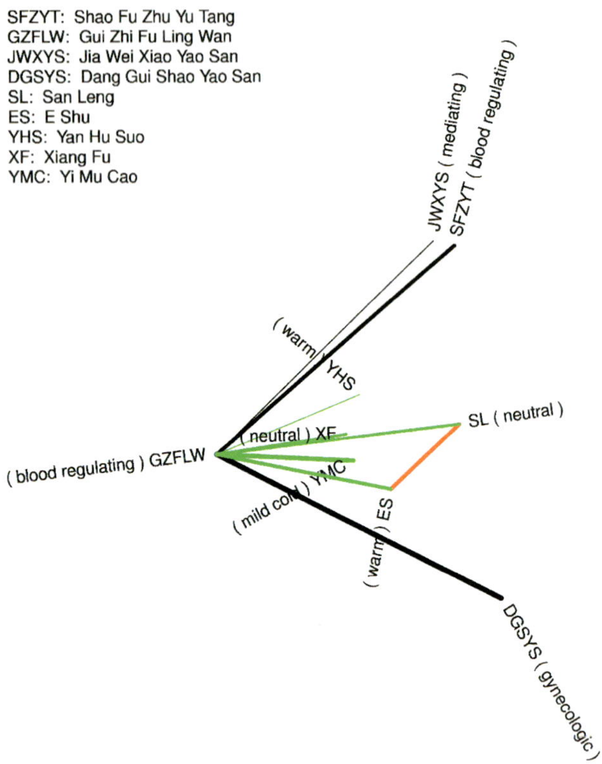

FIGURE 6.5b
The commonest TCM formula pair is GZFLW–DGSYS, the commonest formula–herb pair is GZFLW–YMC, followed by GZFLW–ES, and the commonest herb pair is ES–SL for the treatment of benign neoplasms of the ovary. The thickness of the line indicates the prevalence of the pair. Formula pairs are in black, formula–herb pairs in green and herb pairs in red. The TCM pharmacotherapeutic categories of the formulas and the TCM natures of the herbs are shown in parentheses.

6.8 Benign Neoplasm of the Thyroid Gland: *San Zhong Kui Jian Tang* and *Xia Ku Cao*

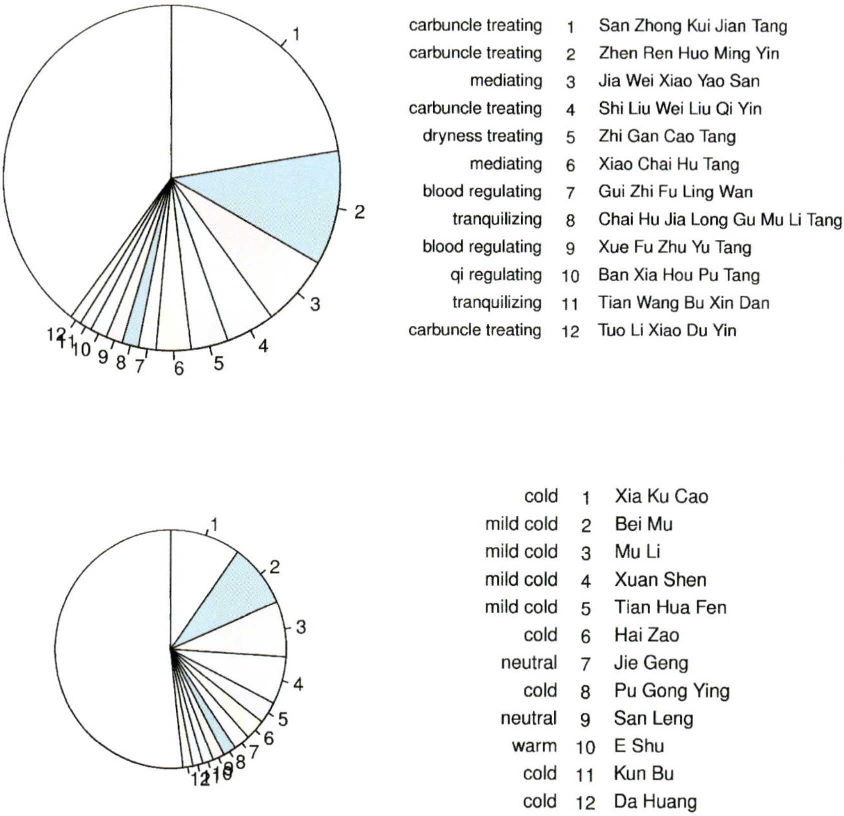

FIGURE 6.6a
Benign neoplasms of the thyroid gland (ICD-9 = 226) are treated by TCM carbuncle-treating ($p = 0.0008$) and tranquilizing ($p = 0.04$) formulas. The top 12 ingredients are shown. The areas of the pies indicate the relative weights of the formulas and herbs in the prescription for the condition. P values are from overrepresentation tests.

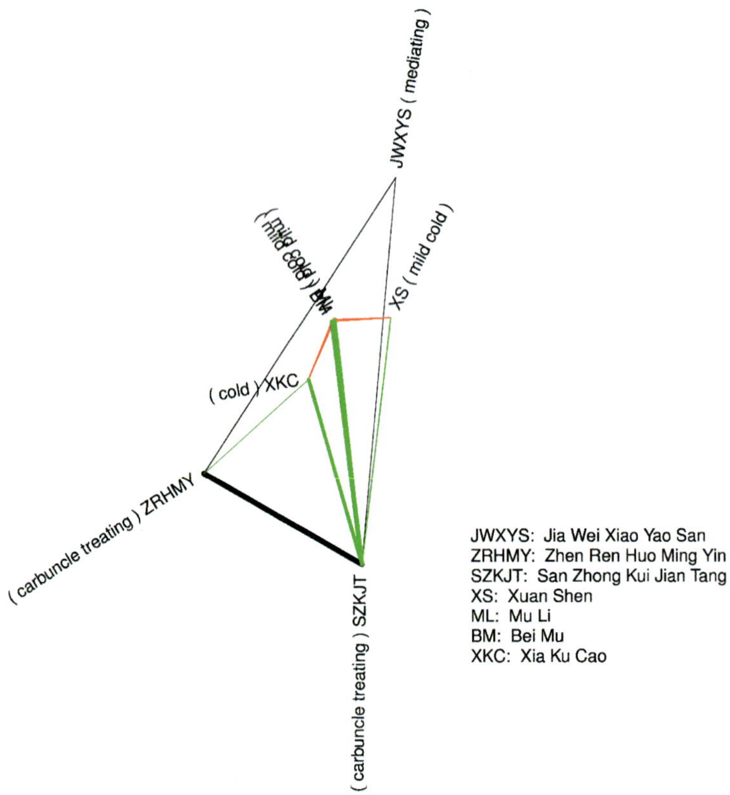

FIGURE 6.6b

The commonest TCM formula pair is SZKJT–ZRHMY, the commonest formula–herb pair is SZKJT–BM, followed by SZKJT–XKC, and the commonest herb pair is BM–ML, followed by BM–XKC, for the treatment of benign neoplasms of the thyroid glands. The thickness of the line indicates the prevalence of the pair. Formula pairs are in black, formula–herb pairs in green and herb pairs in red. The TCM pharmacotherapeutic categories of the formulas and the TCM natures of the herbs are shown in parentheses.

6.9 Benign Neoplasm of the Breast: *Jia Wei Xiao Yao San* and *Pu Gong Ying*

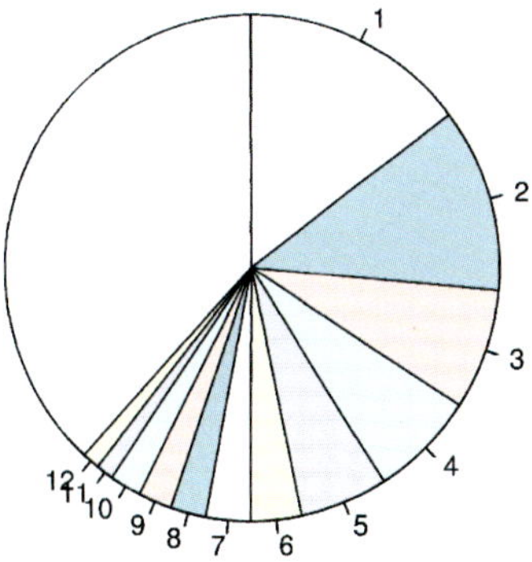

mediating	1	Jia Wei Xiao Yao San
carbuncle treating	2	San Zhong Kui Jian Tang
carbuncle treating	3	Zhen Ren Huo Ming Yin
carbuncle treating	4	Shi Liu Wei Liu Qi Yin
mediating	5	Xiao Chai Hu Tang
mediating	6	Chai Hu Shu Gan Tang
mediating	7	Xiao Yao San
blood regulating	8	Gui Zhi Fu Ling Wan
blood regulating	9	Xue Fu Zhu Yu Tang
exterior relieving	10	Jing Fang Bai Du San
exterior relieving	11	Gui Zhi Tang
carbuncle treating	12	Qian Jin Nei Tuo San

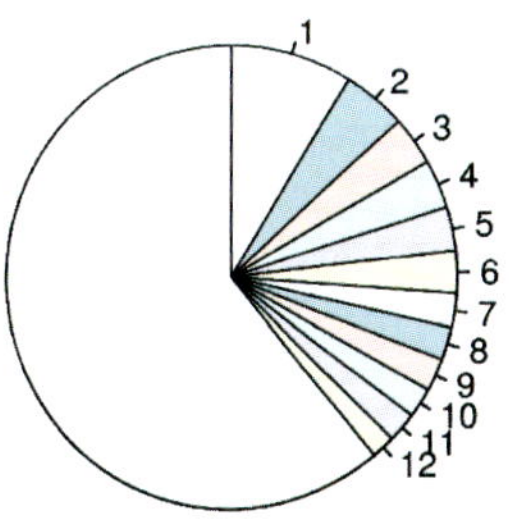

cold	1	Pu Gong Ying
mild cold	2	Bei Mu
cold	3	Xia Ku Cao
mild cold	4	Mu Li
neutral	5	Xiang Fu
mild cold	6	Tian Hua Fen
neutral	7	Mai Ya
cold	8	Yu Jin
warm	9	Yan Hu Suo
mild cold	10	Xuan Shen
neutral	11	Wang Bu Liu Xing
warm	12	E Shu

FIGURE 6.7a

Benign neoplasms of the breast (ICD-9 = 217) are treated by TCM carbuncle-treating ($p = 0.0008$) and mediating ($p = 0.03$) formulas. The top 12 ingredients are shown. The areas of the pies indicate the relative weights of the formulas and herbs in the prescription for the condition. *P* values are from overrepresentation tests.

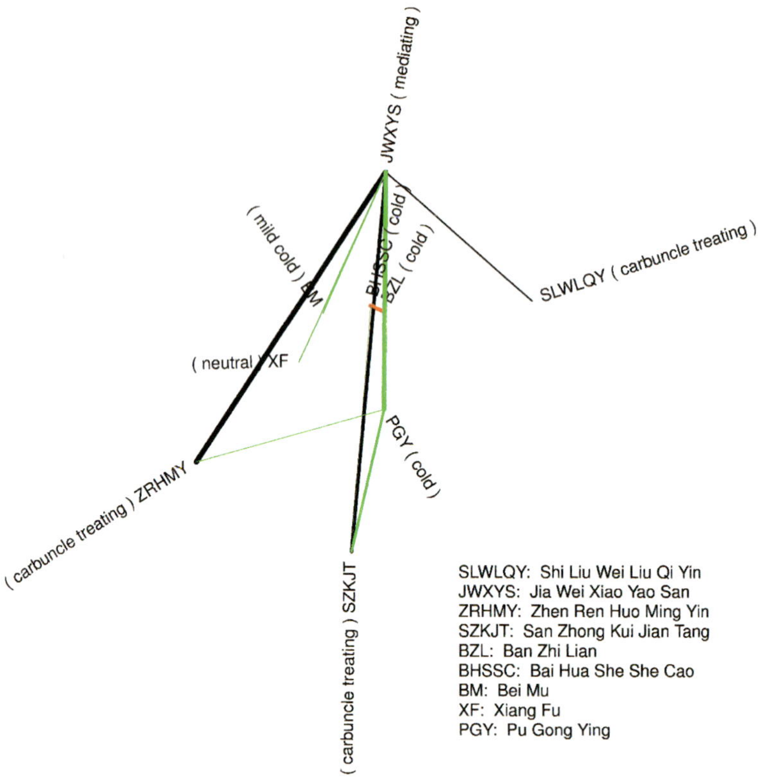

FIGURE 6.7b

The commonest TCM formula pair is JWXYS–ZRHMY, the commonest formula–herb pair is JWXYS–PGY, followed by SZKJT–PGY, and the commonest herb pair is BZL–BHSSC for the treatment of benign neoplasms of the breast. The thickness of the line indicates the prevalence of the pair. Formula pairs are in black, formula–herb pairs in green and herb pairs in red. The TCM pharmacotherapeutic categories of the formulas and the TCM natures of the herbs are shown in parentheses.

6.10 Lipoma: *San Zhong Kui Jian Tang* and *Bai Jie Zi*

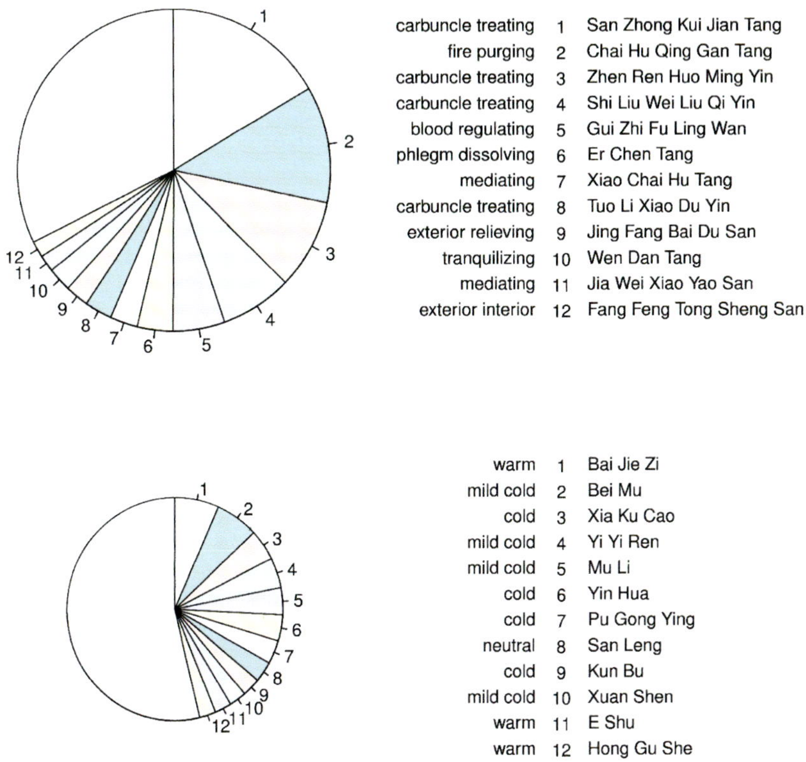

FIGURE 6.8a
Lipomas (ICD-9 = 214) are benign adipose tumors (fatty lumps) between skin and the underlying muscle layer. They are treated by TCM carbuncle-treating formulas ($p = 0.0008$). The top 12 ingredients are shown. The areas of the pies show the relative weights of the formulas and herbs in the prescription for the condition. *P* values are from overrepresentation tests.

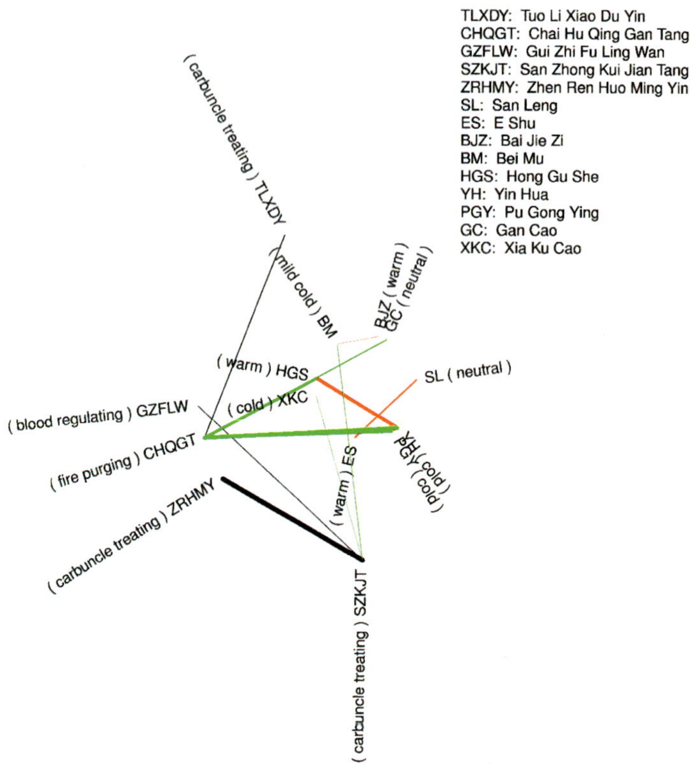

FIGURE 6.8b
The commonest TCM formula pair is SZKJT–ZRHMY, the commonest formula–herb pair is CHQGT–YH, followed by CHQGT–HGS, and the commonest herb pair is HGS–YH for the treatment of lipomas. The thickness of the line indicates the prevalence of the pair. Formula pairs are in black, formula–herb pairs in green and herb pairs in red. The TCM pharmacotherapeutic categories of the formulas and the TCM natures of the herbs are shown in parentheses.

6.11 Benign Neoplasm of Male Genital Organs: *Ji Sheng Shen Qi Wan* and *Che Qian Zi*

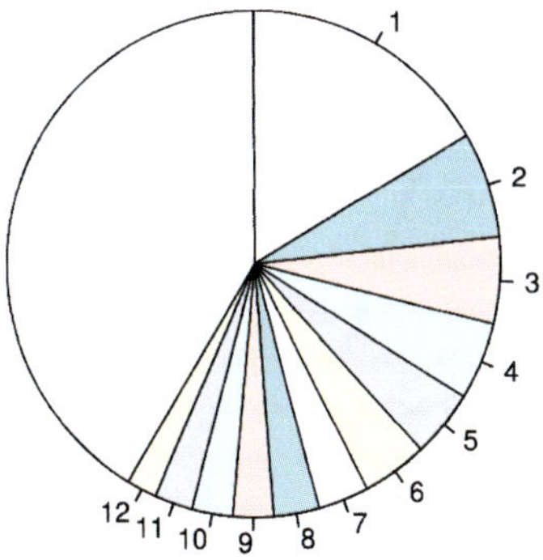

tonifying	1	Ji Sheng Shen Qi Wan
dampness eliminating	2	Zhu Ling Tang
dampness eliminating	3	Wu Ling San
astringing	4	Sang Piao Shao San
tonifying	5	Zhi Bai Di Huang Wan
fire purging	6	Qing Xin Lian Zi Yin
tonifying	7	Liu Wei Di Huang Wan
tonifying	8	Ba Wei Di Huang Wan
carbuncle treating	9	San Zhong Kui Jian Tang
astringing	10	Jin Suo Gu Jing Wan
tonifying	11	Bu Zhong Yi Qi Tang
dampness eliminating	12	Ba Zheng San

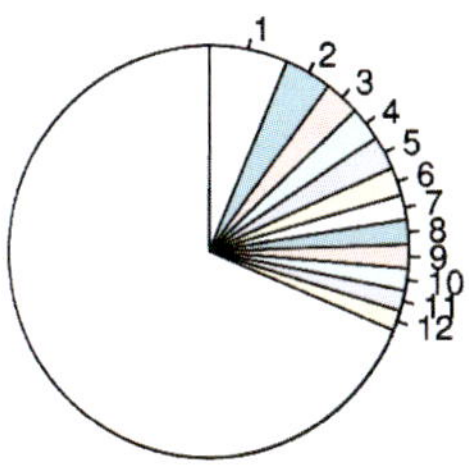

mild cold	1	Che Qian Zi
mild warm	2	Fu Pen Zi
warm	3	Wu Yao
cold	4	Dong Kui Zi
cold	5	Bai Mao Gen
warm	6	Yi Zhi Ren
mild cold	7	Dan Can
cold	8	Huang Bai
neutral	9	Fu Ling
cold	10	Zhi Mu
warm	11	Yin Yang Huo
hot	12	Fu Zi

FIGURE 6.9a
Benign neoplasms of male genital organs (ICD-9 = 222) are treated by TCM tonifying ($p = 0.01$), astringing ($p = 0.04$) or dampness-eliminating ($p = 0.05$) formulas. The top 12 ingredients are shown. The areas of the pies show the relative weights of the formulas and herbs in the prescription for the condition. *P* values are from overrepresentation tests.

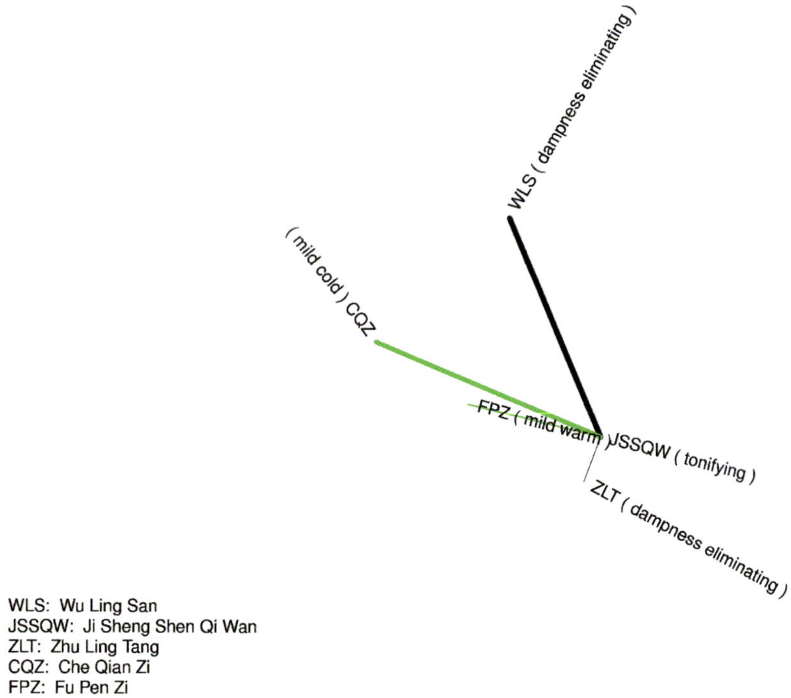

FIGURE 6.9b
The commonest TCM formula pair is JSSQW–WLS and the commonest formula–herb pair is JSSQW–CQZ for the treatment of benign neoplasms of male genital organs. The thickness of the line indicates the prevalence of the pair. Formula pairs are in black and formula–herb pairs in green. The TCM pharmacotherapeutic categories of the formulas and the TCM natures of the herbs are shown in parentheses.

6.12 Benign Neoplasm of the Lower GI Tract Digestive System: *Ban Xia Xie Xin Tang* and *Yan Hu Suo*

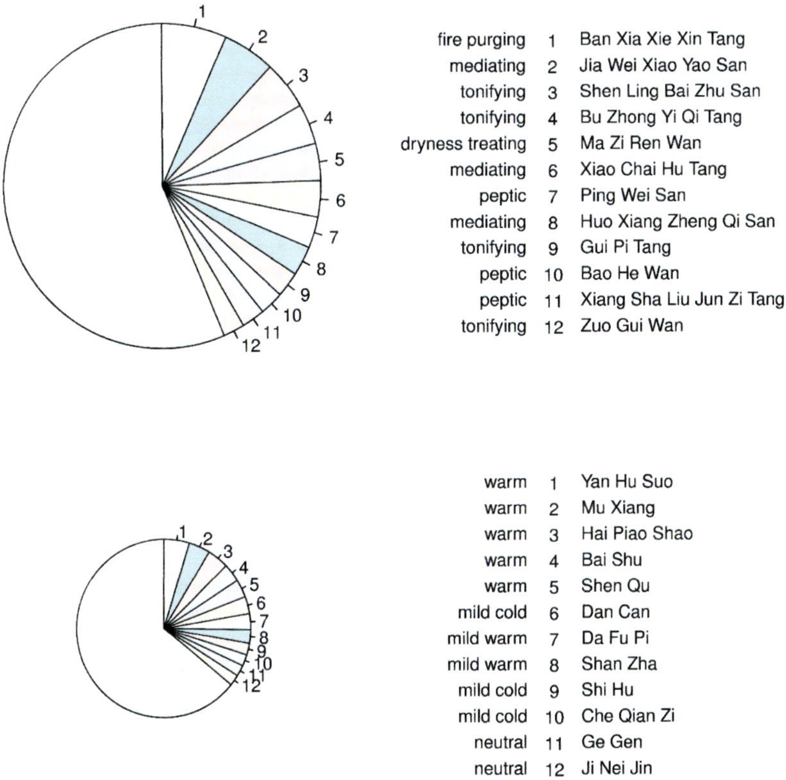

FIGURE 6.10a

Benign neoplasms of the digestive system excluding the lips, oral cavity and pharynx (ICD-9 = 211) are treated by TCM peptic ($p = 0.008$) and mediating ($p = 0.03$) formulas. The top 12 ingredients are shown. The areas of the pies indicate the relative weights of the formulas and herbs in the prescription for the condition. *P* values are from overrepresentation tests.

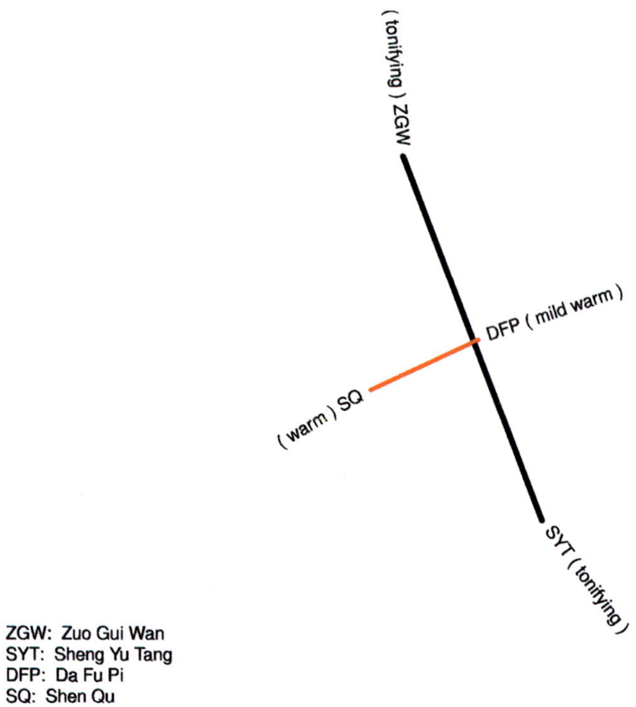

FIGURE 6.10b

The commonest TCM formula pair is ZGW–SYT and the commonest herb pair is DFP–SQ for the treatment of benign neoplasms of the lower GI tract digestive system. The thickness of the line indicates the prevalence of the pair. Formula pairs are in black and herb pairs in red. The TCM pharmacotherapeutic categories of the formulas and the TCM natures of the herbs are shown in parentheses.

6.13 Carcinoma *in Situ* of the Breast and Genitourinary System: *Ji Sheng Shen Qi Wan* and *Pu Gong Ying*

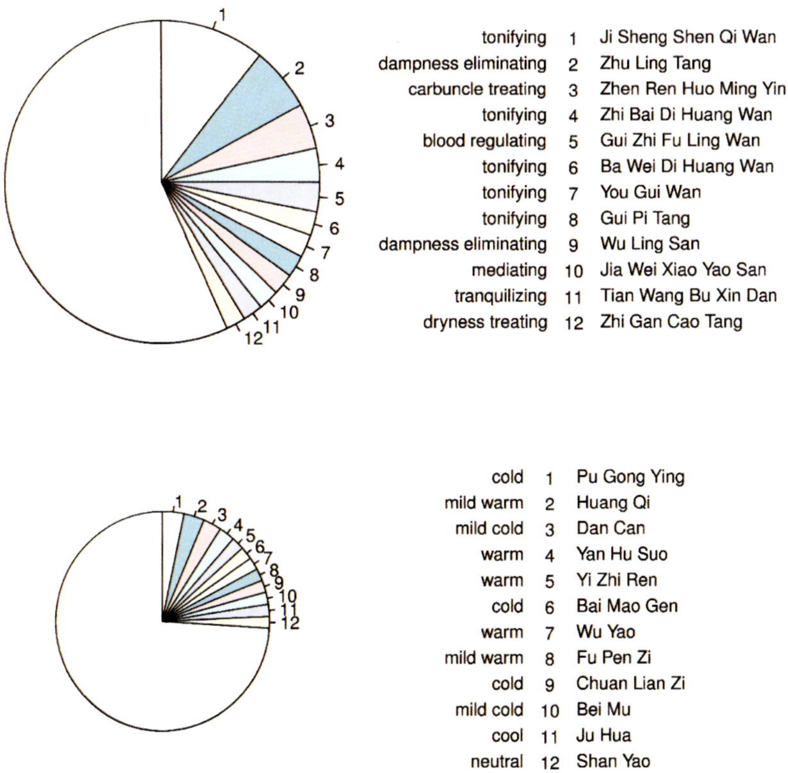

FIGURE 6.11a
Carcinoma *in situ* is considered an early form of cancer which, if left untreated, may become malignant. Carcinomas *in situ* of the breast and genitourinary system (ICD-9 = 233) are treated by TCM tonifying formulas ($p = 0.01$). The top 12 ingredients are shown. The areas of the pies indicate the relative weights of the formulas and herbs in the prescription for the condition. *P* values are from over-representation tests.

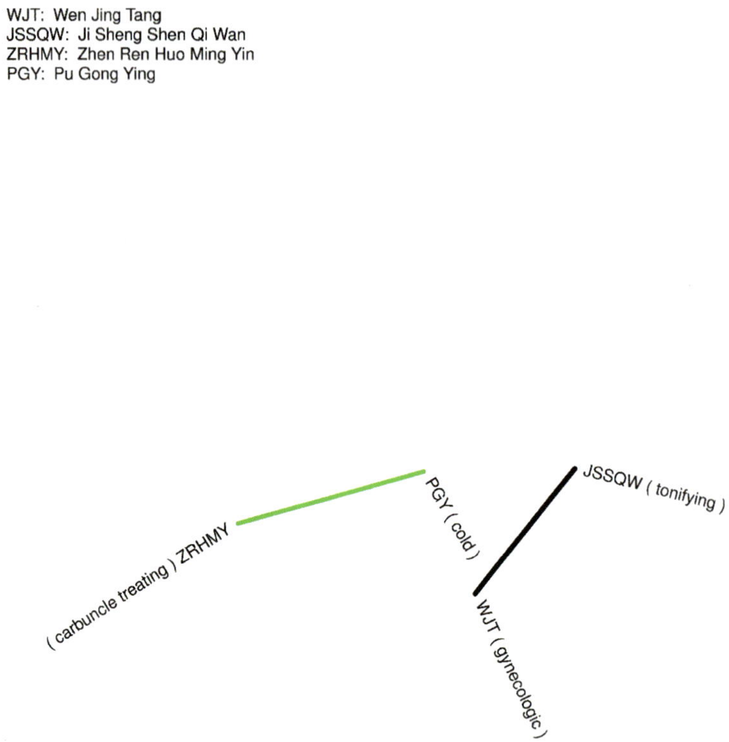

FIGURE 6.11b

The commonest TCM formula pair is JSSQW–WJT and the commonest formula–herb pair is ZRHMY–PGY for the treatment of carcinomas *in situ* of the breast and genitourinary system. The thickness of the line indicates the prevalence of the pair. Formula pairs are in black and formula–herb pairs in green. The TCM pharmacotherapeutic categories of the formulas and the TCM natures of the herbs are shown in parentheses.

6.14 Benign Neoplasm of the Brain and Other Parts of the Nervous System: *Zhen Ren Huo Ming Yin* and *Bei Mu*

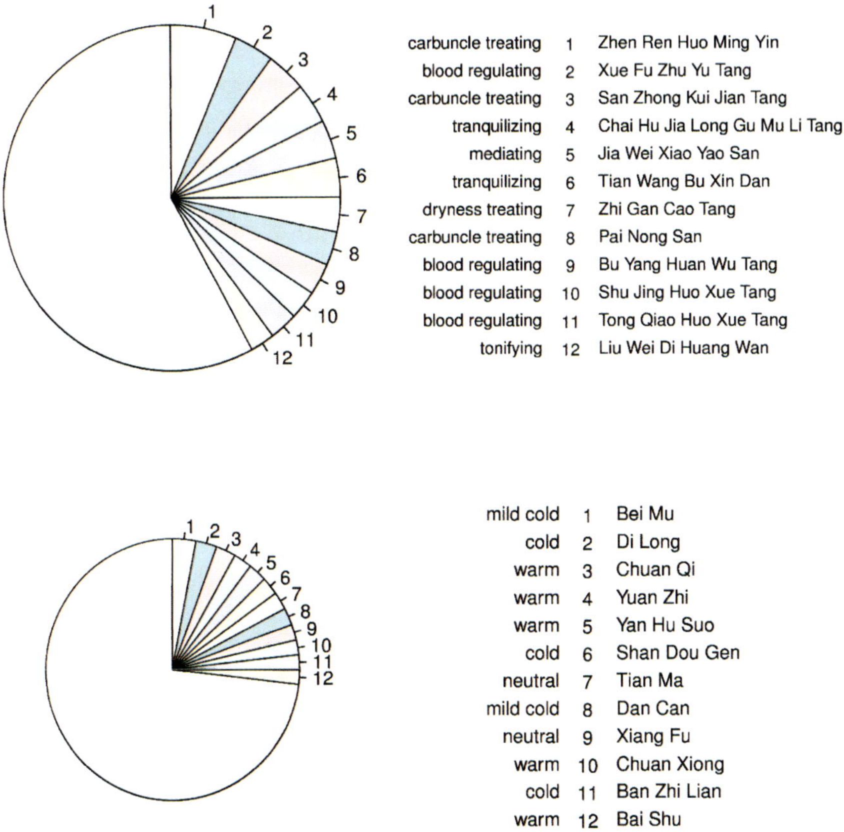

FIGURE 6.12a
Benign neoplasms of the brain and other parts of the nervous system (ICD-9 = 225) are treated by TCM blood-regulating ($p = 0.006$), carbuncle-treating ($p = 0.01$) or tranquilizing ($p = 0.05$) formulas. The top 12 ingredients are shown. The areas of the pies indicate the relative weights of the formulas and herbs in the prescription for the condition. P values are from overrepresentation tests.

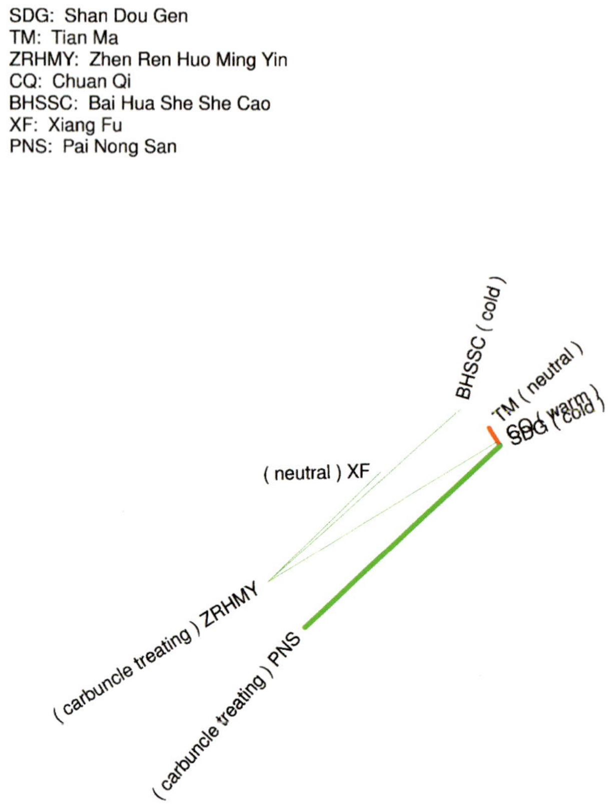

FIGURE 6.12b
The commonest TCM formula–herb pair is PNS–SDG, followed by ZRHMY–XF, and the commonest herb pair is SDG–TM for the treatment of benign neoplasms of the brain and other parts of the nervous system. The thickness of the line indicates the prevalence of the pair. Formula–herb pairs are in green and herb pairs in red. The TCM pharmacotherapeutic categories of the formulas and the TCM natures of the herbs are shown in parentheses.

6.15 Malignant Neoplasm of the Female Breast: *Jia Wei Xiao Yao San* and *Pu Gong Ying*

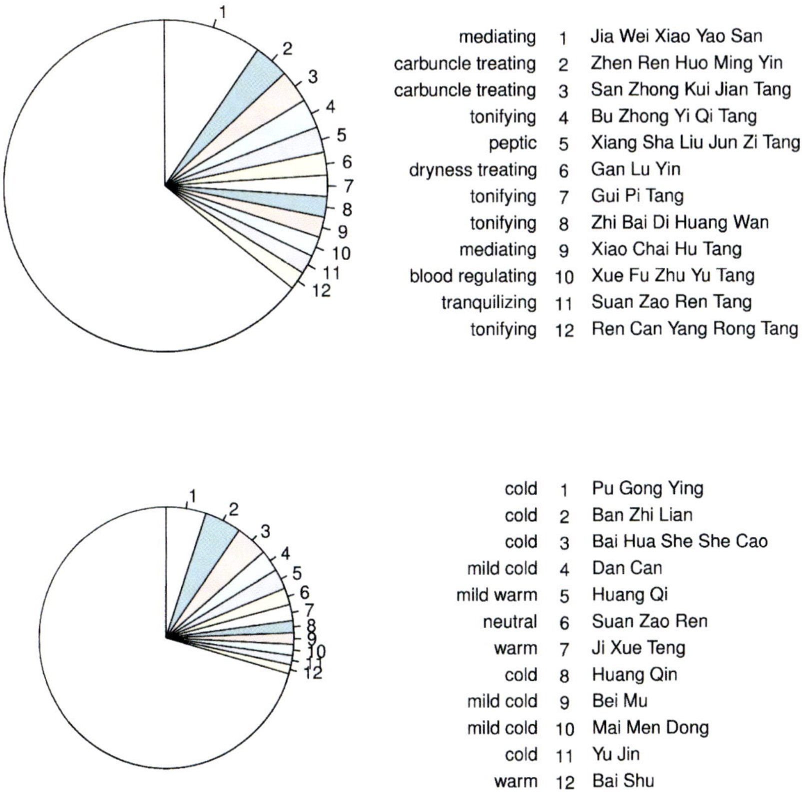

FIGURE 6.13a
Malignant neoplasms of the female breast (ICD-9 = 174) might be treated by TCM tonifying formulas ($p = 0.06$). The top 12 ingredients are shown. The areas of the pies indicate the relative weights of the formulas and herbs in the prescription for the condition. *P* values are from overrepresentation tests.

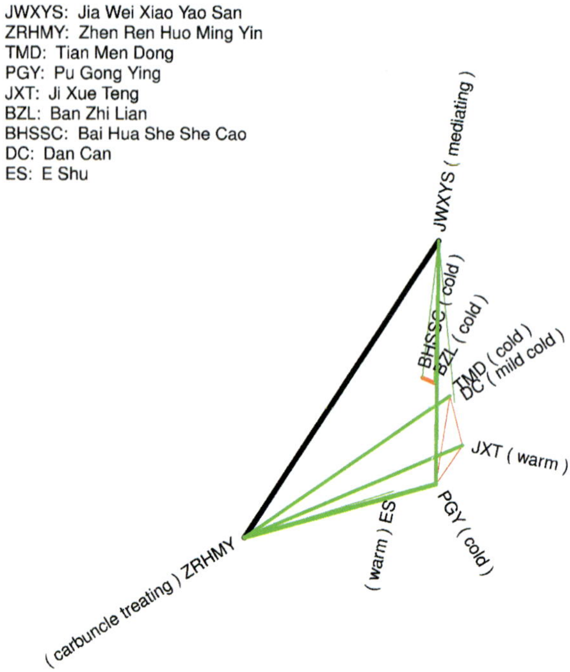

FIGURE 6.13b

The commonest TCM formula pair is ZRHMY–JWXYS, the commonest formula–herb pair is ZRHMY–PGY, followed by JWXYS–PGY and ZRHMY–JXT, and the commonest herb pair is BZL–BHSSC, followed by PGY–JXT and PGY–TMD, for the treatment of malignant neoplasms of the female breast. The thickness of the line indicates the prevalence of the pair. Formula pairs are in black, formula–herb pairs in green and herb pairs in red. The TCM pharmacotherapeutic categories of the formulas and the TCM natures of the herbs are shown in parentheses.

6.16 Malignant Neoplasm of the Liver and Intrahepatic Bile Ducts: *Jia Wei Xiao Yao San* and *Bai Hua She She Cao*

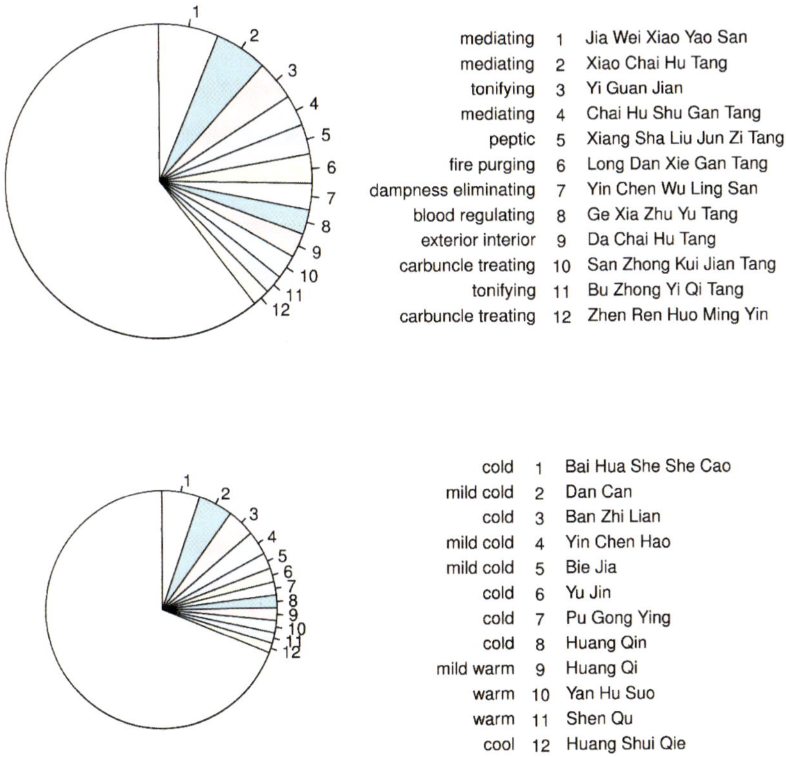

FIGURE 6.14a
Malignant neoplasms of the liver and intrahepatic bile ducts (ICD-9 = 155) are treated by TCM mediating formulas ($p = 0.03$) and TCM cold herbs ($p = 0.04$). The top 12 ingredients are shown. The areas of the pies indicate the relative weights of the formulas and herbs in the prescription for the condition. *P* values are from overrepresentation tests.

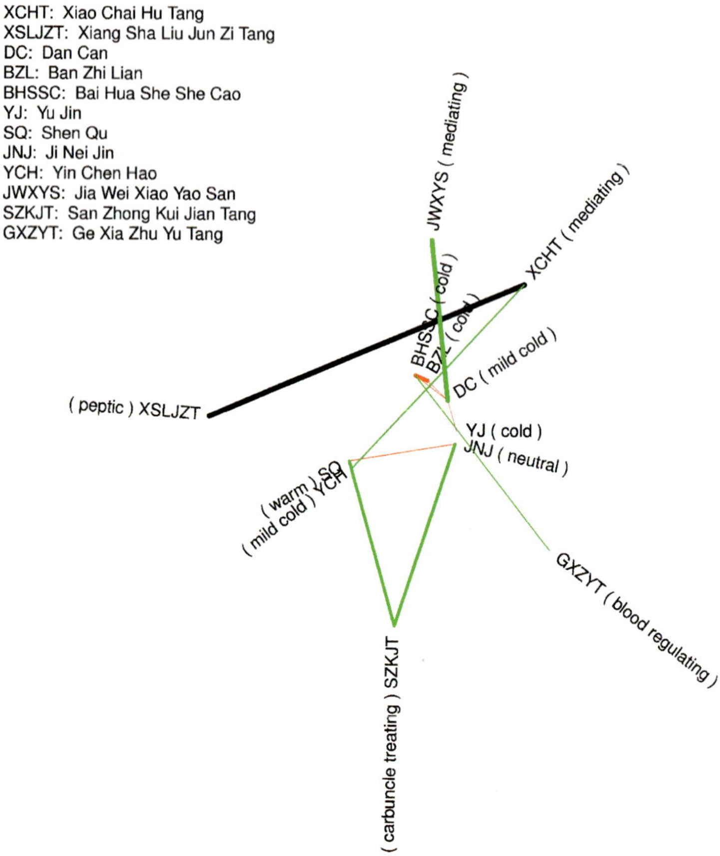

FIGURE 6.14b

The commonest TCM formula pair is XSLJZT–XCHT, the commonest formula–herb pair is XWXYS–DC, followed by SZKJT–JNJ, and the commonest herb pair is BZL–BHSSC, followed by JNJ–SQ, for the treatment of malignant neoplasms of the liver and intrahepatic bile ducts. The thickness of the line indicates the prevalence of the pair. Formula pairs are in black, formula–herb pairs in green and herb pairs in red. The TCM pharmacotherapeutic categories of the formulas and the TCM natures of the herbs are shown in parentheses.

6.17 Malignant Neoplasm of the Nasopharynx: *Gan Lu Yin* and *Xuan Shen*

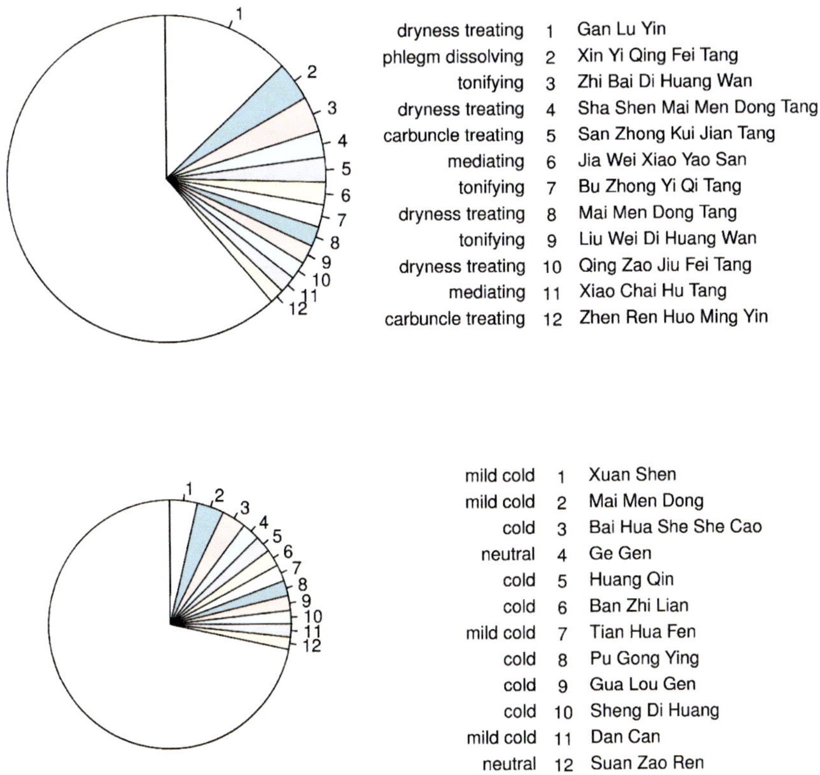

FIGURE 6.15a
Malignant neoplasms of the nasopharynx (ICD-9 = 147) are treated by TCM dryness-treating formulas ($p = 0.006$) and TCM cold herbs ($p = 0.04$). The top 12 ingredients are shown. The areas of the pies indicate the relative weights of the formulas and herbs in the prescription for the condition. *P* values are from over-representation tests.

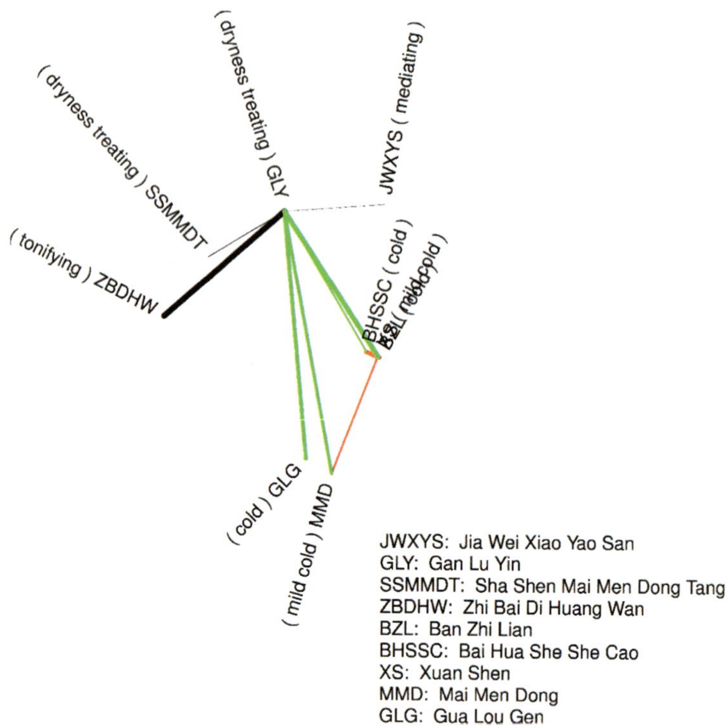

FIGURE 6.15b

The commonest TCM formula pair is GLY–ZBDHW, the commonest formula–herb pair is GLY–XS, followed by GLY–GLG, and the commonest herb pair is BZL–BHSSC for the treatment of malignant neoplasms of the nasopharynx. The thickness of the line indicates the prevalence of the pair. Formula pairs are in black, formula–herb pairs in green and herb pairs in red. The TCM pharmacotherapeutic categories of the formulas and the TCM natures of the herbs are shown in parentheses.

6.18 Malignant Neoplasm of the Colon: *Xiang Sha Liu Jun Zi Tang* and *Ban Zhi Lian*

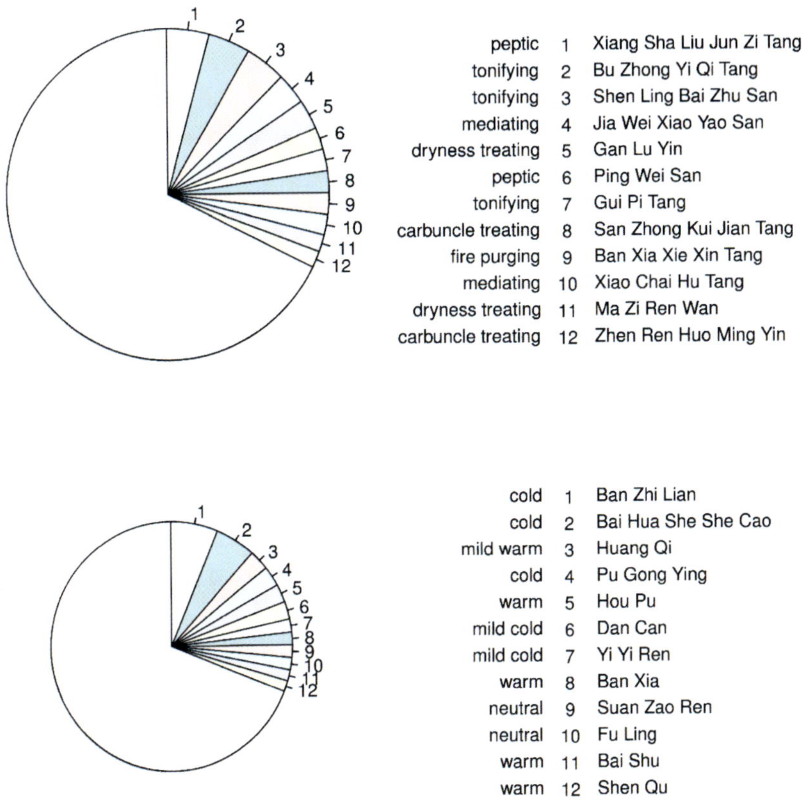

FIGURE 6.16a
Malignant neoplasms of the colon (ICD-9 = 153) might be treated by TCM dryness-treating formulas ($p = 0.06$). The top 12 ingredients are shown. The areas of the pies indicate the relative weights of the formulas and herbs in the prescription for the condition. *P* values are from overrepresentation tests.

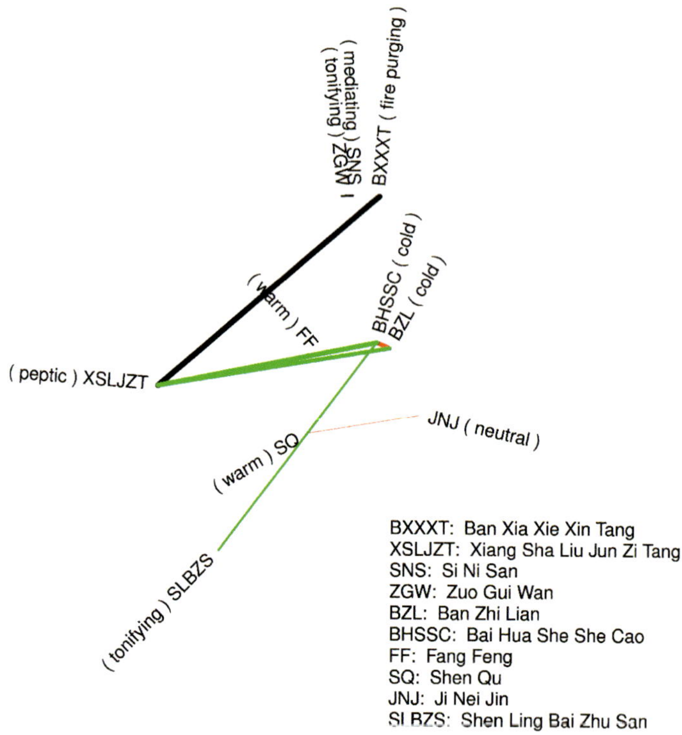

FIGURE 6.16b
The commonest TCM formula pair is XSLJZT–BXXXT, the commonest formula–herb pair is XSLJZT–BHSSC and the commonest herb pair is BZL–BHSSC for the treatment of malignant neoplasms of the colon. The thickness of the line indicates the prevalence of the pair. Formula pairs are in black, formula–herb pairs in green and herb pairs in red. The TCM pharmacotherapeutic categories of the formulas and the TCM natures of the herbs are shown in parentheses.

6.19 Malignant Neoplasm of the Rectum and Anus: *Xiang Sha Liu Jun Zi Tang* and *Bai Hua She She Cao*

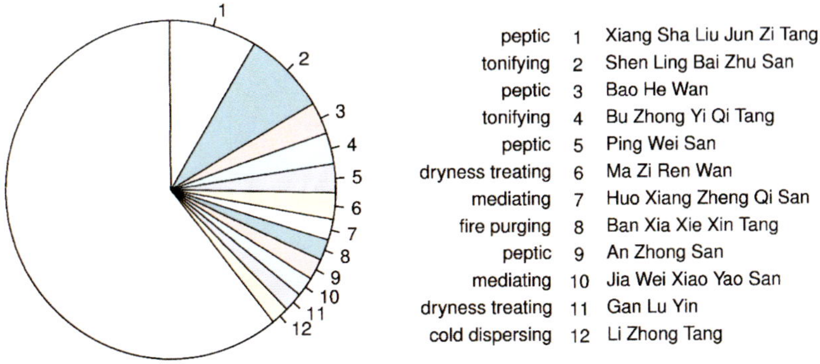

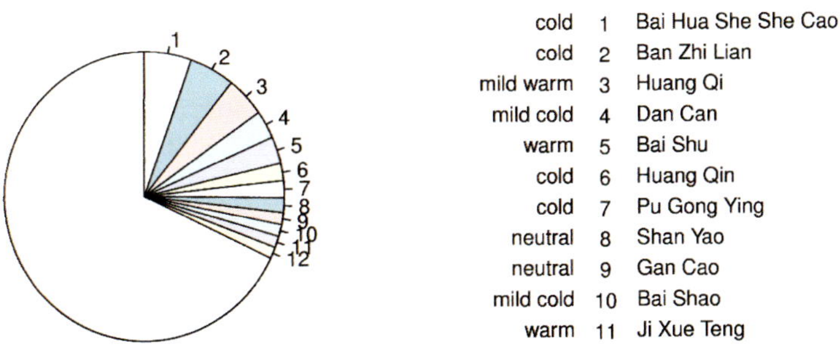

FIGURE 6.17a
Malignant neoplasms of the rectum, rectosigmoid junction and anus (ICD-9 = 154) are treated by TCM peptic formulas (p = 0.0006). The top 12 ingredients are shown. The areas of the pies indicate the relative weights of the formulas and herbs in the prescription for the condition. P values are from overrepresentation tests.

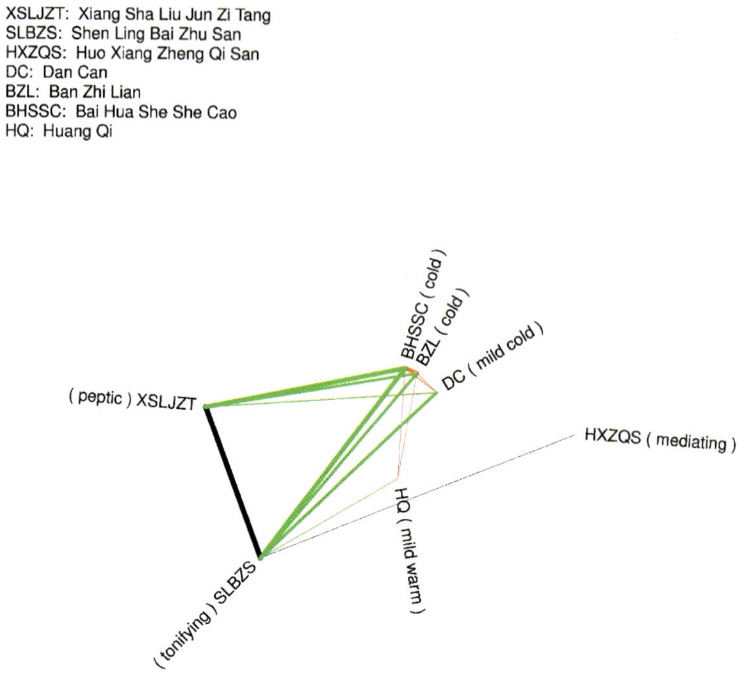

FIGURE 6.17b

The commonest TCM formula pair is XSLJZT–SLBZS, the commonest formula–herb pair is XSLJZT–BHSSC, followed by SLBZS–BHSSC, SLBZS–DC and SLBZS–BZL, and the commonest herb pair is BZL–BHSSC, followed by BHSSC–DC and BZL–DC, for the treatment of malignant neoplasms of the rectum, rectosigmoid junction and anus. The thickness of the line indicates the prevalence of the pair. Formula pairs are in black, formula–herb pairs in green and herb pairs in red. The TCM pharmacotherapeutic categories of the formulas and the TCM natures of the herbs are shown in parentheses.

6.20 Malignant Neoplasm of the Trachea, Bronchus and Lung: *Bai He Gu Jin Tang* and *Ban Zhi Lian*

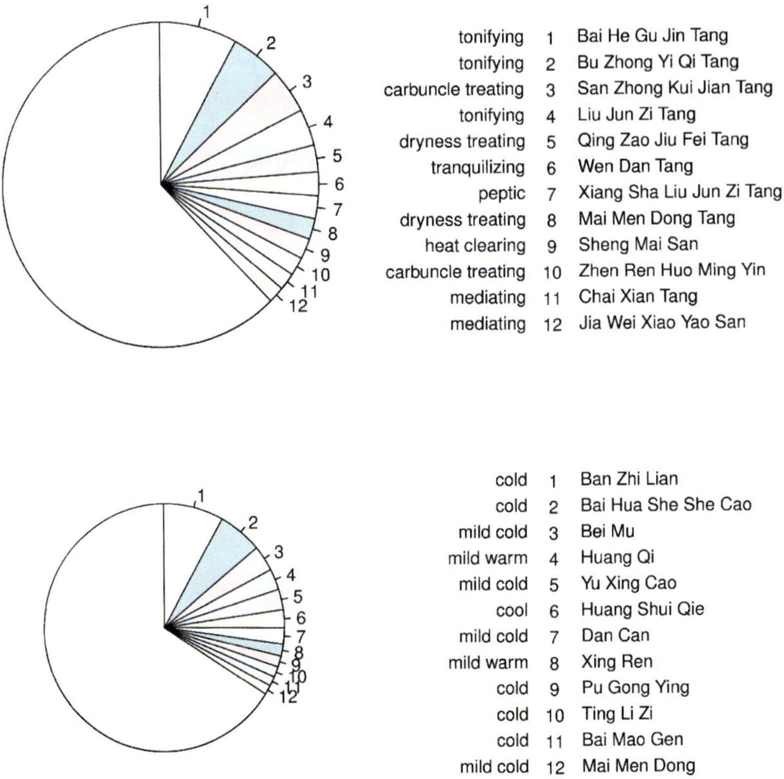

FIGURE 6.18a
Malignant neoplasms of the trachea, bronchus and lung (ICD-9 = 162) are treated by TCM cold herbs ($p = 0.04$) and might also be treated by TCM dryness-treating formulas ($p = 0.06$). The top 12 ingredients are shown. The areas of the pies indicate the relative weights of the formulas and herbs in the prescription for the condition. *P* values are from overrepresentation tests.

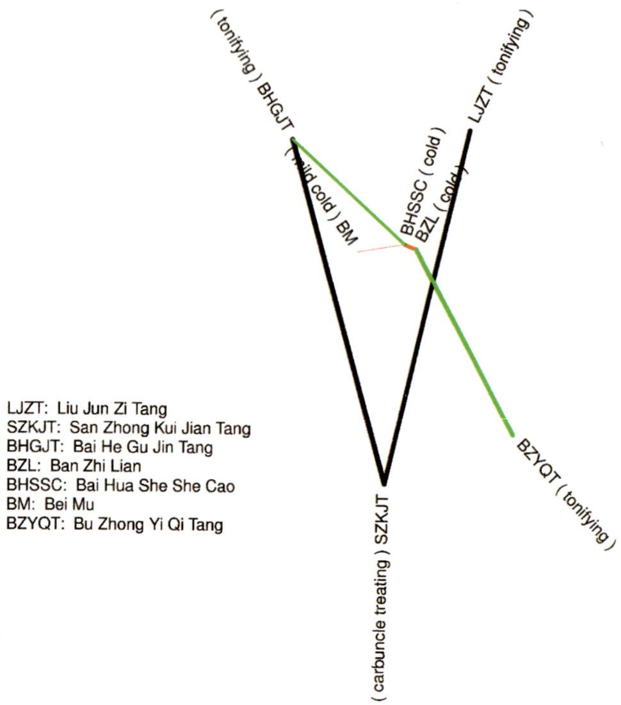

FIGURE 6.18b

The commonest TCM formula pair is SZKJT–BHGJT, the commonest formula–herb pair is BZYQT–BZL and the commonest herb pair is BZL–BHSSC for the treatment of malignant neoplasms of the trachea, bronchus and lung. The thickness of the line indicates the prevalence of the pair. Formula pairs are in black, formula–herb pairs in green and herb pairs in red. The TCM pharmacotherapeutic categories of the formulas and the TCM natures of the herbs are shown in parentheses.

6.21 Malignant Neoplasm of the Cervix Uteri: *Jia Wei Xiao Yao San* and *Bai Hua She She Cao*

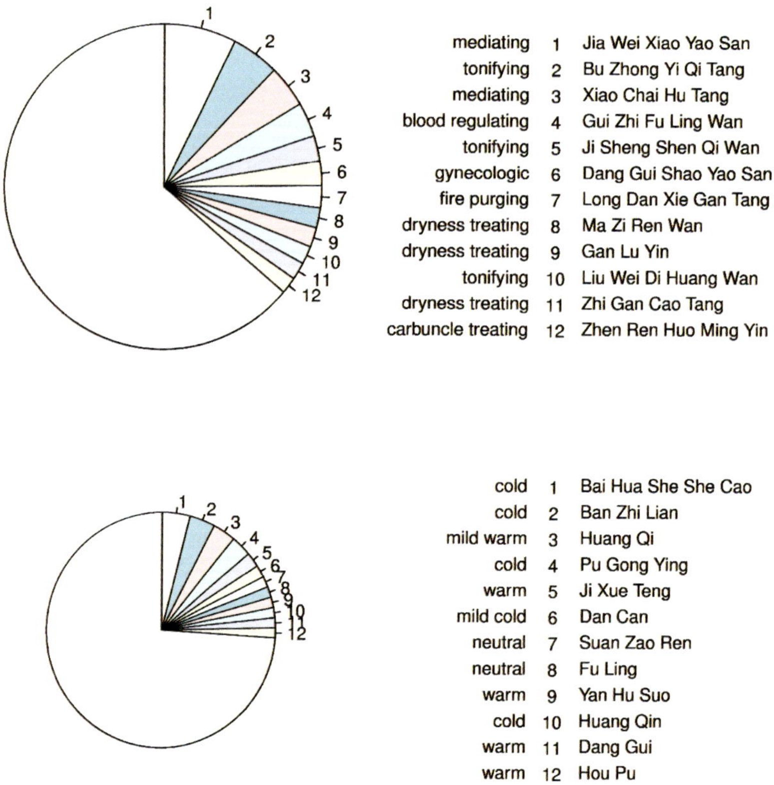

FIGURE 6.19a
Malignant neoplasms of the cervix uteri (ICD-9 = 180) are treated by TCM dryness-treating formulas ($p = 0.006$). The top 12 ingredients are shown. The areas of the pies indicate the relative weights of the formulas and herbs in the prescription for the condition. *P* values are from overrepresentation tests.

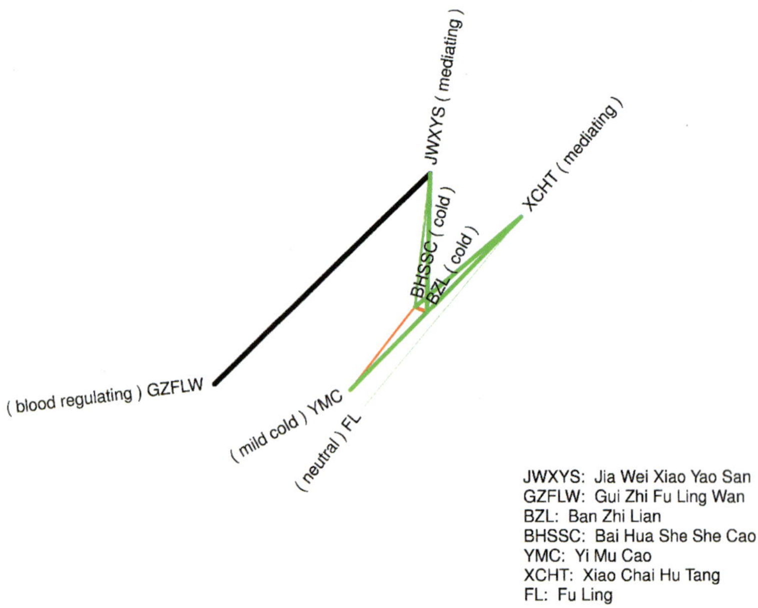

FIGURE 6.19b

The commonest TCM formula pair is JWXYS–GZFLW, the commonest formula–herb pair is JWXYS–BZL, followed by XCHT–BHSSC and XCHT–YMC, and the commonest herb pair is BZL–BHSSC for the treatment of malignant neoplasms of the cervix uteri. The thickness of the line indicates the prevalence of the pair. Formula pairs are in black, formula–herb pairs in green and herb pairs in red. The TCM pharmacotherapeutic categories of the formulas and the TCM natures of the herbs are shown in parentheses.

6.22 Malignant Neoplasm of the Stomach: *Ban Xia Xie Xin Tang* and *Ban Zhi Lian*

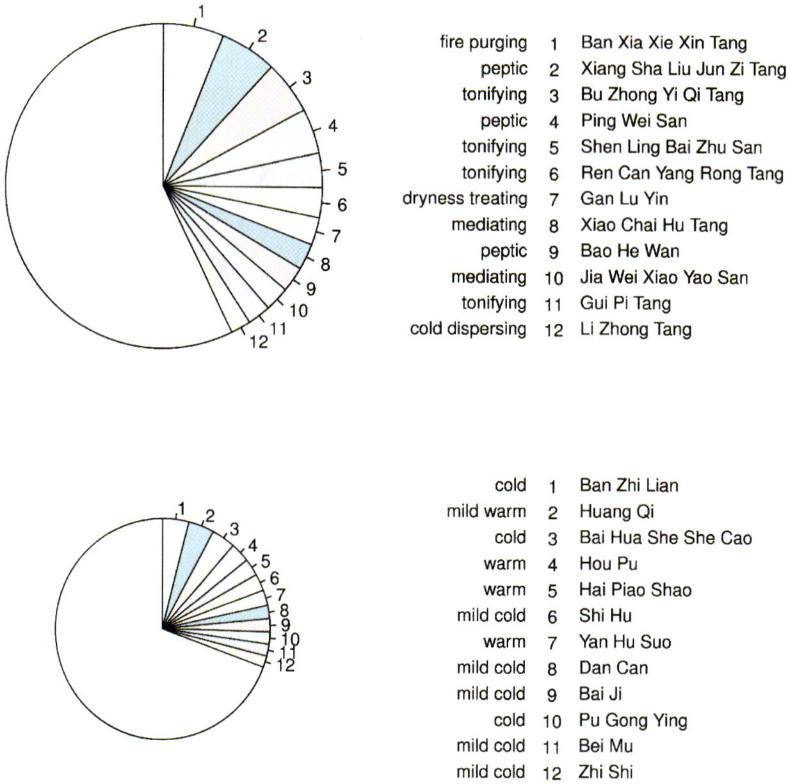

FIGURE 6.20a
Malignant neoplasms of the stomach (ICD-9 = 151) are treated by TCM peptic formulas ($p = 0.008$) and TCM mild–cold herbs ($p = 0.02$). The top 12 ingredients are shown. The areas of the pies indicate the relative weights of the formulas and herbs in the prescription for the condition. P values are from overrepresentation tests.

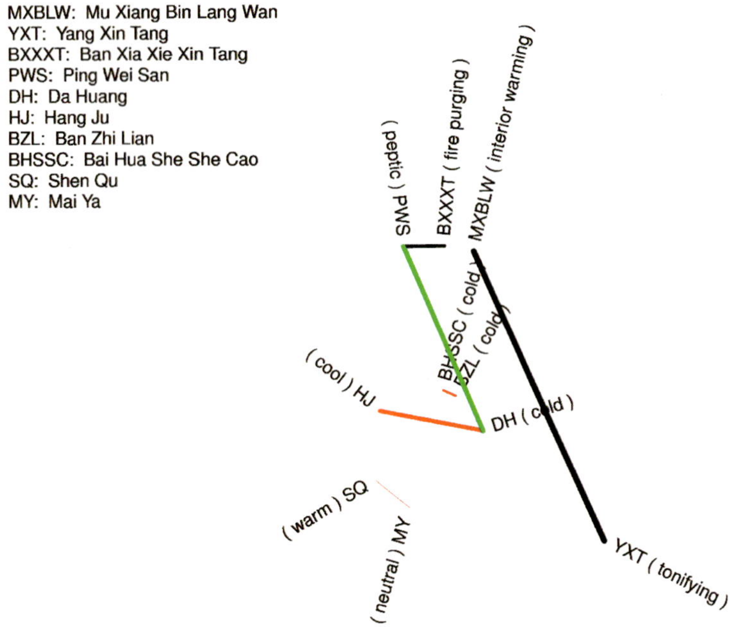

FIGURE 6.20b
The commonest TCM formula pair is MXBLW–YXT, the commonest formula–herb pair is PWS–DH and the commonest herb pair is DH–HJ for the treatment of malignant neoplasms of the stomach. The thickness of the line indicates the prevalence of the pair. Formula pairs are in black, formula–herb pairs in green and herb pairs in red. The TCM pharmacotherapeutic categories of the formulas and the TCM natures of the herbs are shown in parentheses.

6.23 Malignant Neoplasm of the Prostate: *Ji Sheng Shen Qi Wan* and *Huang Bai*

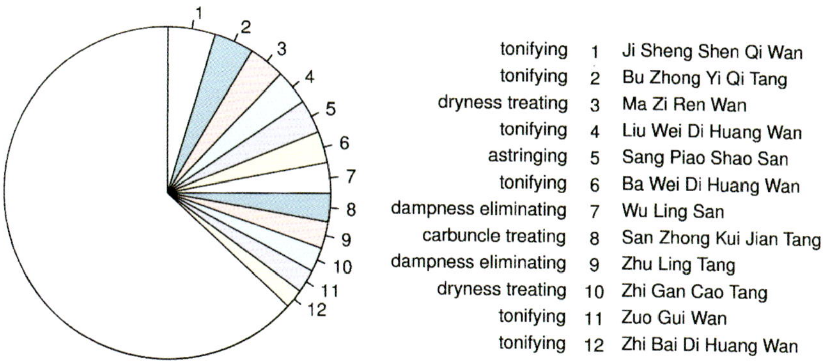

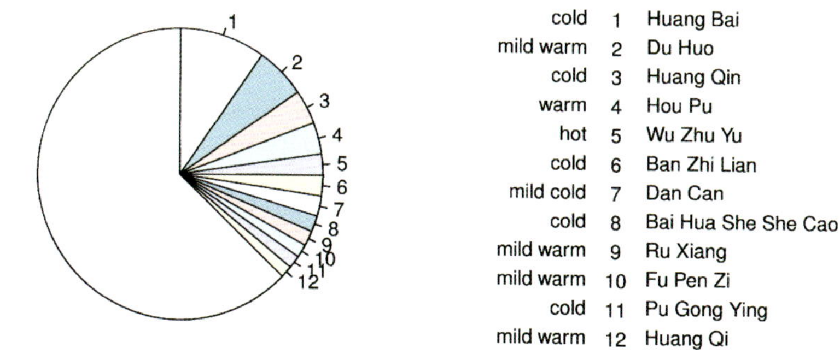

FIGURE 6.21a
Malignant neoplasms of the prostate (ICD-9 = 185) are treated by TCM tonifying formulas ($p = 0.002$) and TCM mild–warm herbs ($p = 0.004$). The top 12 ingredients are shown. The areas of the pies indicate the relative weights of the formulas and herbs in the prescription for the condition. *P* values are from overrepresentation tests.

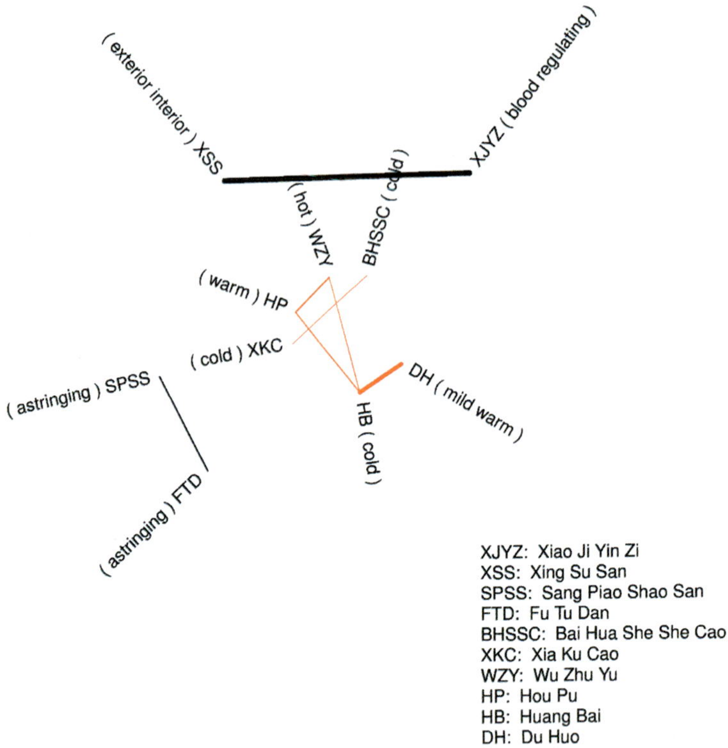

FIGURE 6.21b
The commonest TCM formula pair is XJYZ–XSS and the commonest herb pair is HB–DH, followed by HP–WZY and HP–HB, for the treatment of malignant neoplasms of the prostate. The thickness of the line indicates the prevalence of the pair. Formula pairs are in black and herb pairs in red. The TCM pharmacotherapeutic categories of the formulas and the TCM natures of the herbs are shown in parentheses.

6.24 Malignant Neoplasm of the Ovary and Other Uterine Adnexa: *Gui Zhi Fu Ling Wan* and *Ban Zhi Lian*

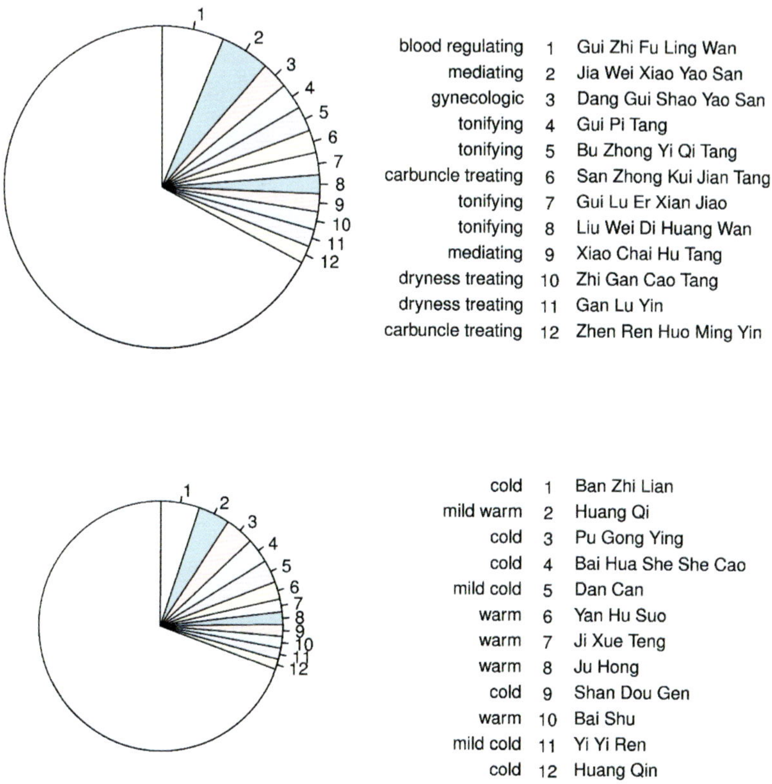

FIGURE 6.22a
Malignant neoplasms of the ovary and other uterine adnexa (ICD-9 = 183) might be treated by TCM tonifying formulas ($p = 0.06$). The top 12 ingredients are shown. The areas of the pies indicate the relative weights of the formulas and herbs in the prescription for the condition. P values are from overrepresentation tests.

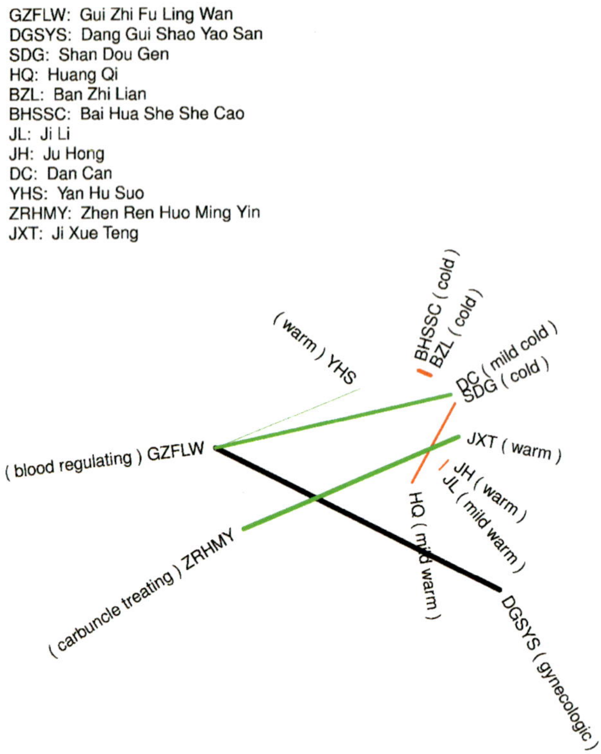

FIGURE 6.22b

The commonest TCM formula pair is GZFLW–DGSYS, the commonest formula–herb pair is ZRHMY–JXT and the commonest herb pair is BZL–BHSSC, followed by HQ–SDG, for the treatment of malignant neoplasms of the ovary and other uterine adnexa. The thickness of the line indicates the prevalence of the pair. Formula pairs are in black, formula–herb pairs in green and herb pairs in red. The TCM pharmacotherapeutic categories of the formulas and the TCM natures of the herbs are shown in parentheses.

6.25 Malignant Neoplasm of the Bladder: *Ji Sheng Shen Qi Wan* and *Ban Zhi Lian*

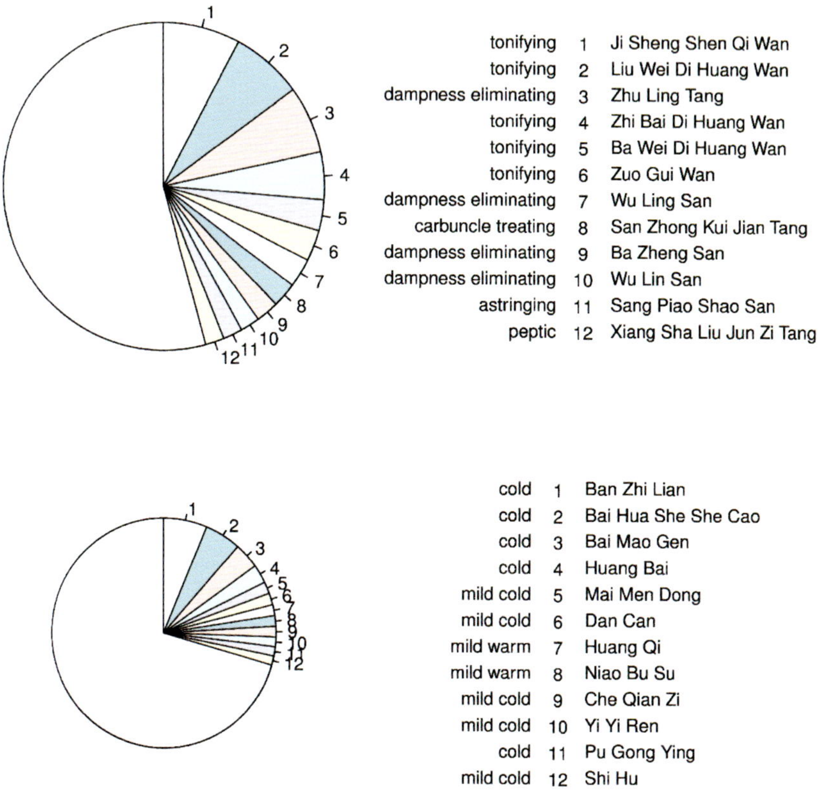

FIGURE 6.23a

Malignant neoplasms of the bladder (ICD-9 = 188) are treated by TCM dampness-eliminating ($p = 0.007$), tonifying ($p = 0.01$) formulas and TCM mild–cold ($p = 0.02$) herbs. The top 12 ingredients are shown. The areas of the pies indicate the relative weights of the formulas and herbs in the prescription for the condition. *P* values are from overrepresentation tests.

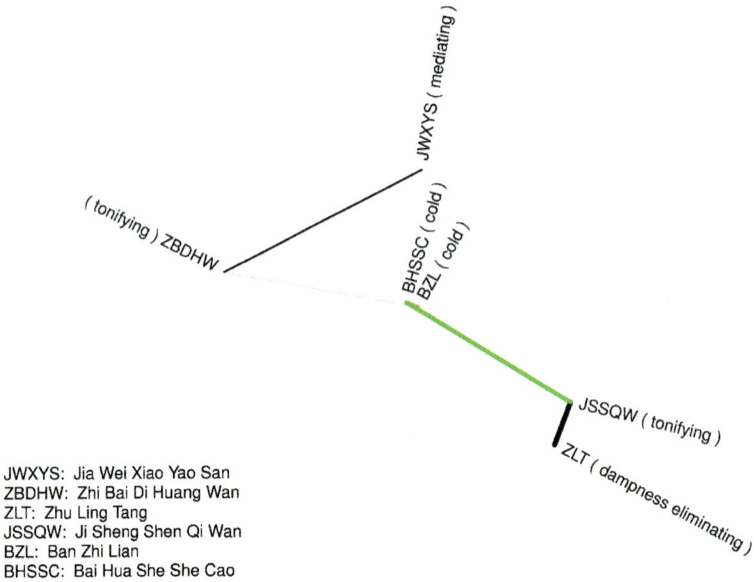

FIGURE 6.23b

The commonest TCM formula pair is JSSQW–ZLT, the commonest formula–herb pair is JSSQW–BHSSC and the commonest herb pair is BZL–BHSSC for the treatment of malignant neoplasms of the bladder. The thickness of the line indicates the prevalence of the pair. Formula pairs are in black, formula–herb pairs in green and herb pairs in red. The TCM pharmacotherapeutic categories of the formulas and the TCM natures of the herbs are shown in parentheses.

6.26 Malignant Neoplasm of the Thyroid Gland: *Jia Wei Xiao Yao San* and *Xuan Shen*

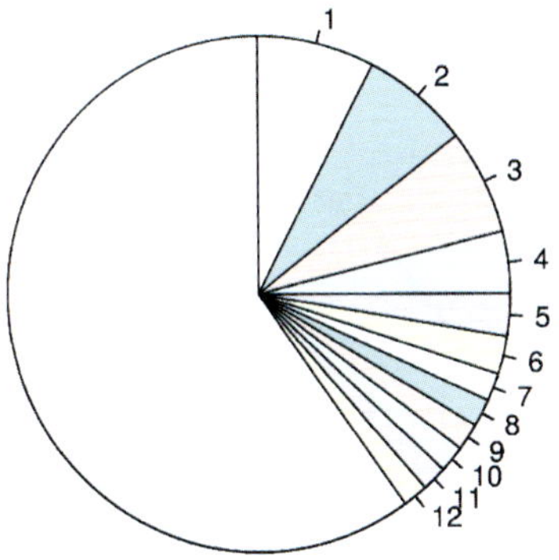

mediating	1	Jia Wei Xiao Yao San
carbuncle treating	2	San Zhong Kui Jian Tang
dryness treating	3	Zhi Gan Cao Tang
carbuncle treating	4	Zhen Ren Huo Ming Yin
mediating	5	Xiao Chai Hu Tang
carbuncle treating	6	Shi Liu Wei Liu Qi Yin
mediating	7	Xiao Yao San
tonifying	8	Gui Pi Tang
tonifying	9	Yi Guan Jian
peptic	10	Xiang Sha Liu Jun Zi Tang
blood regulating	11	Gui Zhi Fu Ling Wan
blood regulating	12	Xue Fu Zhu Yu Tang

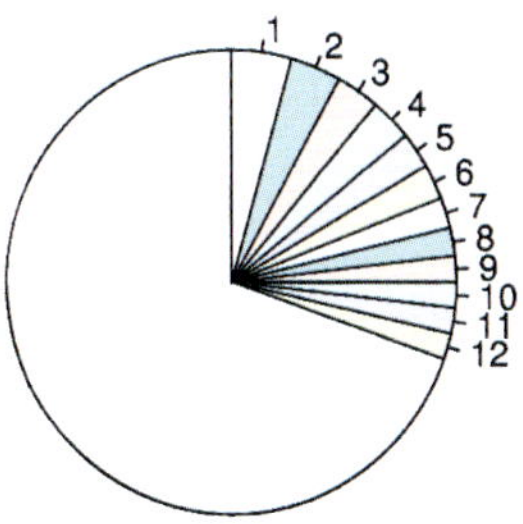

mild cold	1	Xuan Shen
cold	2	Xia Ku Cao
cold	3	Bai Hua She She Cao
cold	4	Ban Zhi Lian
neutral	5	Suan Zao Ren
mild cold	6	Bei Mu
mild cold	7	Tian Hua Fen
cold	8	Pu Gong Ying
neutral	9	Dang Shen
cold	10	Bai He
mild warm	11	Huang Qi
neutral	12	Gan Cao

FIGURE 6.24a
Malignant neoplasms of the thyroid gland (ICD-9 = 193) are treated by TCM carbuncle-treating ($p = 0.01$) and mediating ($p = 0.02$) formulas. The top 12 ingredients are shown. The areas of the pies indicate the relative weights of the formulas and herbs in the prescription for the condition. P values are from overrepresentation tests.

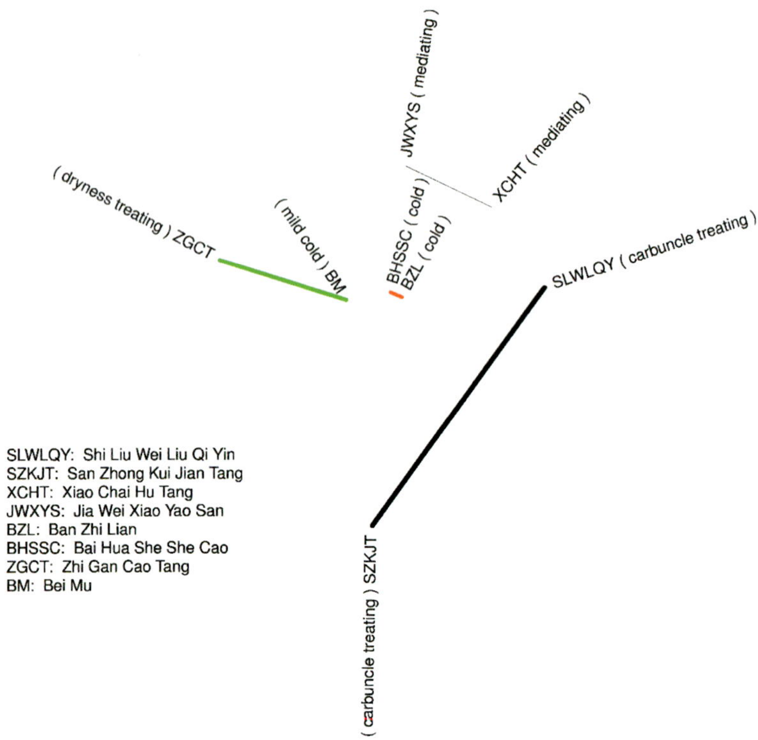

FIGURE 6.24b
The commonest TCM formula pair is SZKJT–SLWLQY, the commonest formula–herb pair is ZGCT–BM and the commonest herb pair is BZL–BHSSC for the treatment of malignant neoplasms of the thyroid gland. The thickness of the line indicates the prevalence of the pair. Formula pairs are in black, formula–herb pairs in green and herb pairs in red. The TCM pharmacotherapeutic categories of the formulas and the TCM natures of the herbs are shown in parentheses.

6.27 Secondary Malignant Neoplasm of the Respiratory and Digestive Systems: *Chai Xian Tang* and *Mai Men Dong*

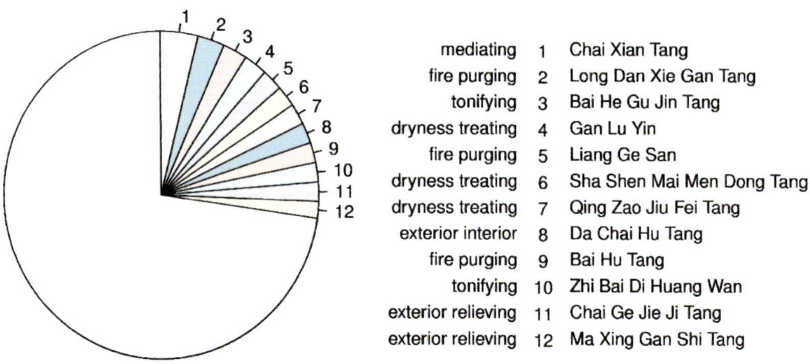

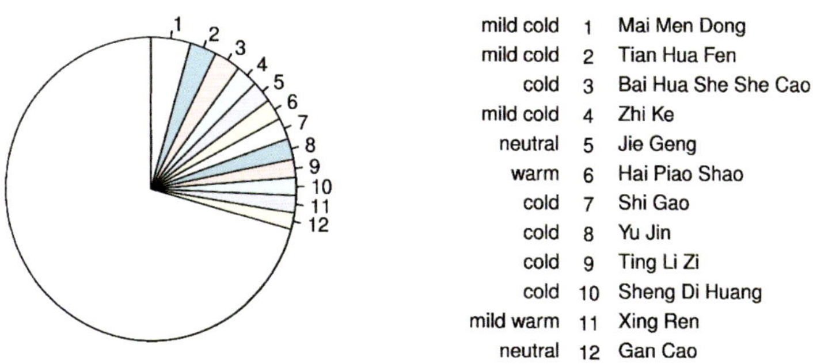

FIGURE 6.25a
Secondary malignant neoplasms of the respiratory and digestive systems (ICD-9 = 197) are treated by TCM dryness-treating formulas ($p = 0.006$). The top 12 ingredients are shown. The areas of the pies indicate the relative weights of the formulas and herbs in the prescription for the condition. *P* values are from overrepresentation tests.

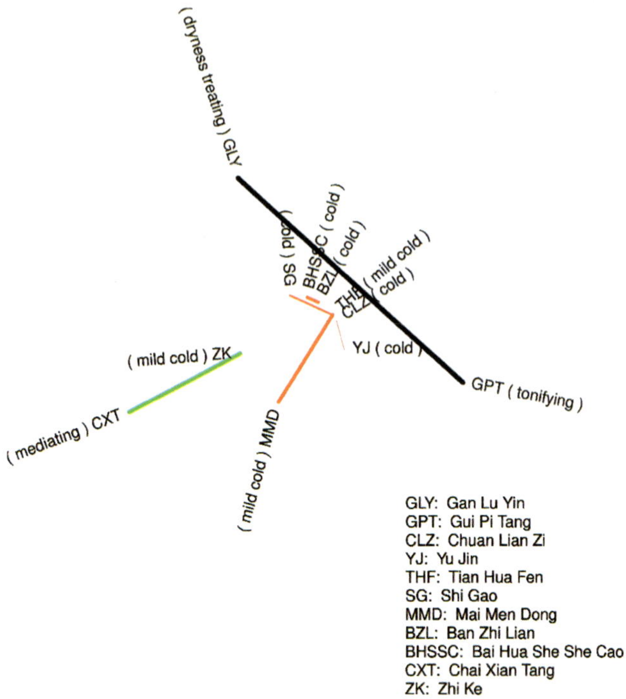

FIGURE 6.25b

The commonest TCM formula pair is GLY–GPT, the commonest formula–herb pair is CXT–ZK and the commonest herb pair is MMD–THF, followed by BZL–BHSSC, for the treatment of secondary malignant neoplasms of the respiratory and digestive systems. The thickness of the line indicates the prevalence of the pair. Formula pairs are in black, formula–herb pairs in green and herb pairs in red. The TCM pharmacotherapeutic categories of the formulas and the TCM natures of the herbs are shown in parentheses.

6.28 Malignant Neoplasm of the Mouth: *Gan Lu Yin* and *Ban Zhi Lian*

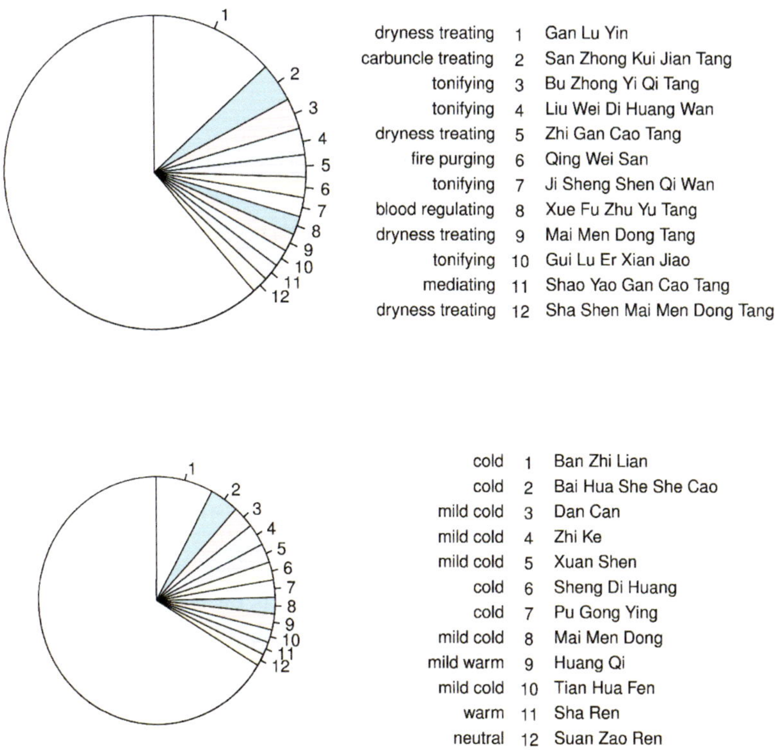

FIGURE 6.26a
Malignant neoplasms of the mouth excluding the lips, tongue, salivary glands, gums and mouth floor (ICD-9 = 145) are treated by TCM dryness-treating formulas ($p = 0.006$). The top 12 ingredients are shown. The areas of the pies indicate the relative weights of the formulas and herbs in the prescription for the condition. *P* values are from overrepresentation tests.

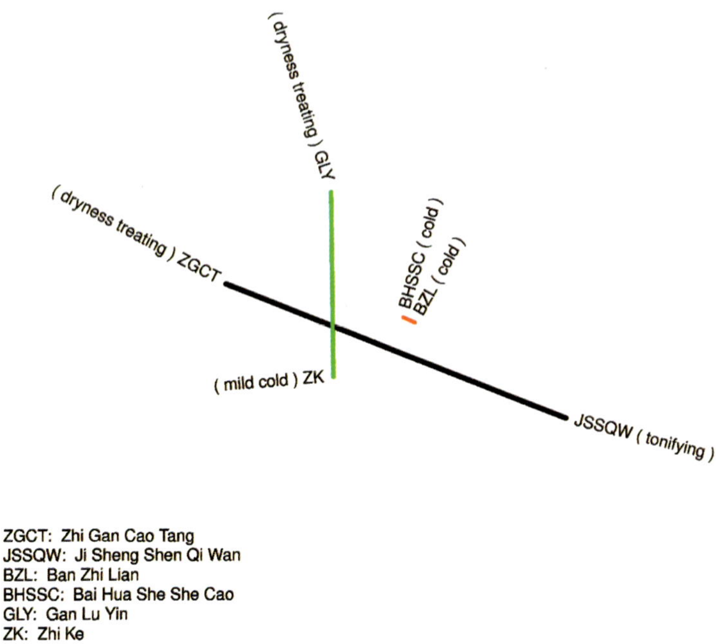

FIGURE 6.26b

The commonest TCM formula pair is JSSQW–ZGCT, the commonest formula–herb pair is GLY–ZK and the commonest herb pair is BZL–BHSSC for the treatment of malignant neoplasms of the mouth excluding the lips, tongue, salivary glands, gums and mouth floor. The thickness of the line indicates the prevalence of the pair. Formula pairs are in black, formula–herb pairs in green and herb pairs in red. The TCM pharmacotherapeutic categories of the formulas and the TCM natures of the herbs are shown in parentheses.

6.29 Malignant Neoplasm of the Tongue: *Gan Lu Yin* and *Dan Can*

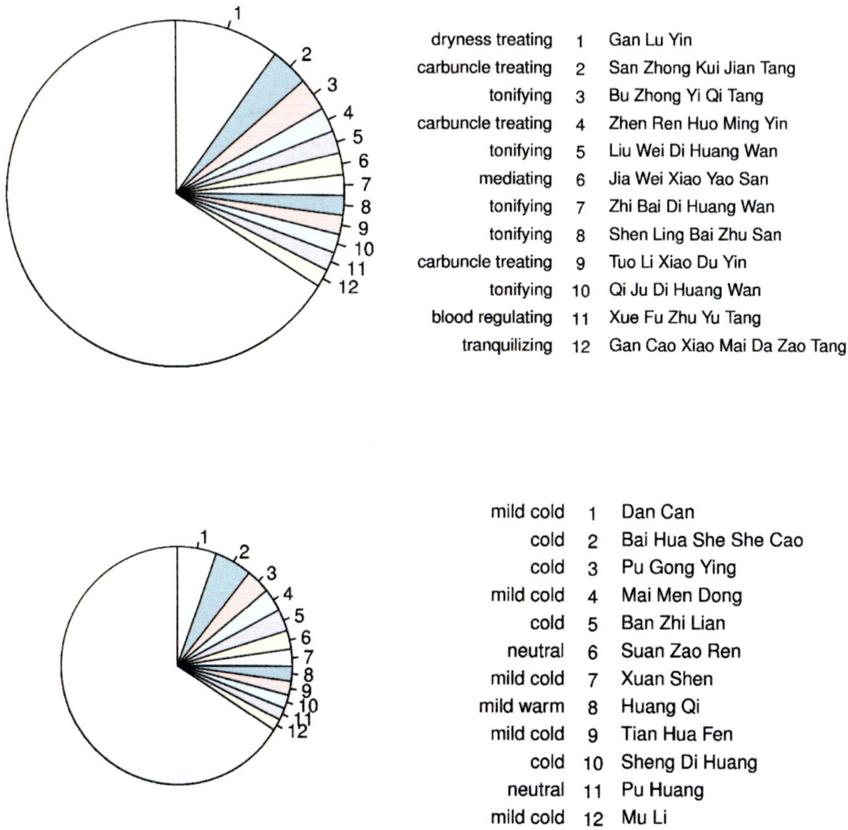

FIGURE 6.27a

Malignant neoplasms of the tongue (ICD-9 = 141) are treated by TCM carbuncle-treating (p = 0.01), tonifying (p = 0.01) formulas and TCM mild–cold (p = 0.02) herbs. The top 12 ingredients are shown. The areas of the pies indicate the relative weights of the formulas and herbs in the prescription for the condition. *P* values are from overrepresentation tests.

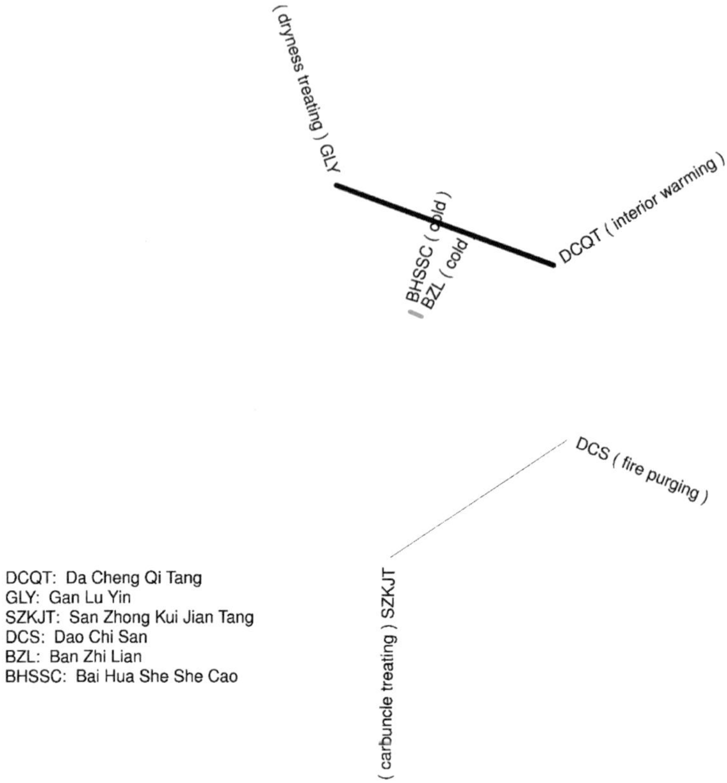

FIGURE 6.27b
The commonest TCM formula pair is GLY–DCQT and the commonest herb pair is BZL–BHSSC for the treatment of malignant neoplasms of the tongue. The thickness of the line indicates the prevalence of the pair. Formula pairs are in black and herb pairs in red. The TCM pharmacotherapeutic categories of the formulas and the TCM natures of the herbs are shown in parentheses.

6.30 Malignant Neoplasm of the Brain: *Bu Yang Huan Wu Tang* and *Tian Ma*

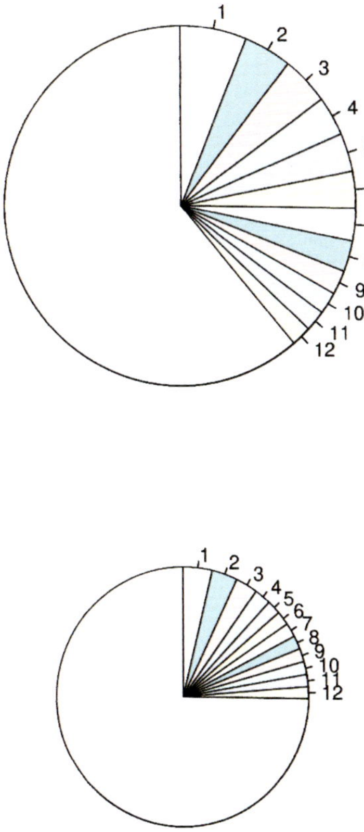

blood regulating	1	Bu Yang Huan Wu Tang
carbuncle treating	2	San Zhong Kui Jian Tang
blood regulating	3	Xue Fu Zhu Yu Tang
tonifying	4	Liu Wei Di Huang Wan
exterior relieving	5	Chuan Xiong Cha Diao San
tranquilizing	6	Chai Hu Jia Long Gu Mu Li Tang
tranquilizing	7	Tian Wang Bu Xin Dan
mediating	8	Xiao Chai Hu Tang
cold dispersing	9	Zhen Wu Tang
mediating	10	Jia Wei Xiao Yao San
wind expelling	11	Tian Ma Gou Teng Yin
tonifying	12	Zhi Bai Di Huang Wan

neutral	1	Tian Ma
mild cold	2	Dan Can
cold	3	Bai Hua She She Cao
cool	4	Shuang Gou Teng
hot	5	Fu Zi
mild warm	6	Huang Qi
warm	7	Yuan Zhi
warm	8	Wei Ling Xian
neutral	9	He Ye
warm	10	E Shu
cold	11	Di Long
neutral	12	Suan Zao Ren

FIGURE 6.28a
Malignant neoplasms of the brain (ICD-9 = 191) are treated by TCM tranquilizing formulas ($p = 0.05$). The top 12 ingredients are shown. The areas of the pies indicate the relative weights of the formulas and herbs in the prescription for the condition. *P* values are from overrepresentation tests.

WYSQS: Wu Yao Shun Qi San
BYHWT: Bu Yang Huan Wu Tang
DH: Da Huang
DC: Dan Can
SZR: Suan Zao Ren
BHSSC: Bai Hua She She Cao
ES: E Shu
ML: Mu Li
XKC: Xia Ku Cao

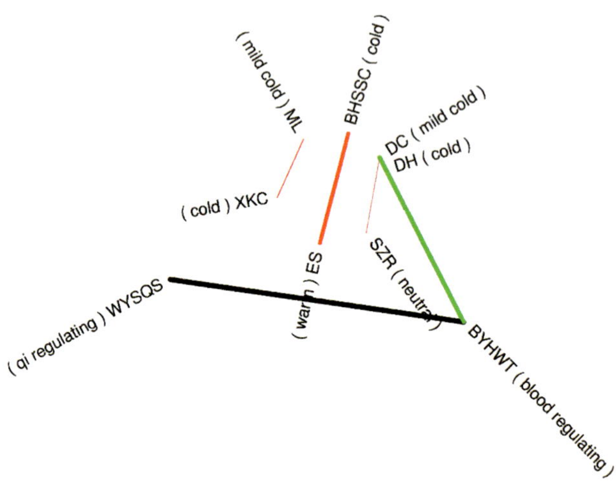

FIGURE 6.28b
The commonest TCM formula pair is BYHWT–WYSQS, the commonest formula–herb pair is BYHWT–DC and the commonest herb pair is BHSSC–ES, followed by ML–XKC, DC–SZR and DC–DH, for the treatment of malignant neoplasms of the brain. The thickness of the line indicates the prevalence of the pair. Formula pairs are in black, formula–herb pairs in green and herb pairs in red. The TCM pharmacotherapeutic categories of the formulas and the TCM natures of the herbs are shown in parentheses.

6.31 Malignant Neoplasm of Lymphoid and Histiocytic Tissue: *San Zhong Kui Jian Tang* and *Pu Gong Ying*

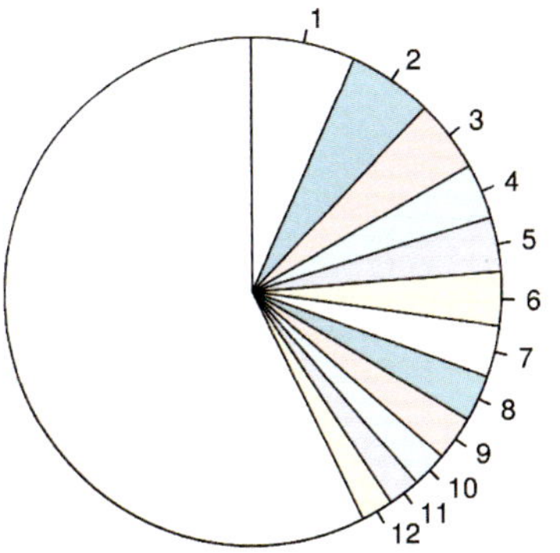

carbuncle treating	1	San Zhong Kui Jian Tang
carbuncle treating	2	Zhen Ren Huo Ming Yin
mediating	3	Xiao Chai Hu Tang
tonifying	4	Shen Ling Bai Zhu San
peptic	5	Xiang Sha Liu Jun Zi Tang
tonifying	6	Qi Ju Di Huang Wan
tonifying	7	Bu Zhong Yi Qi Tang
dryness treating	8	Zhi Gan Cao Tang
tranquilizing	9	Wen Dan Tang
tonifying	10	Liu Wei Di Huang Wan
mediating	11	Jia Wei Xiao Yao San
exterior interior	12	Chai Hu Gui Zhi Tang

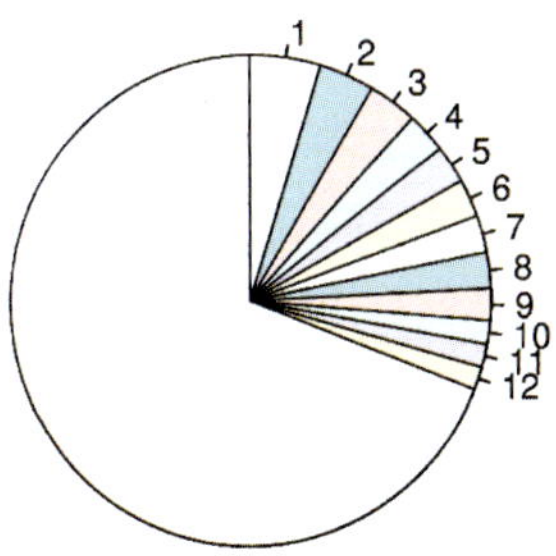

cold	1	Pu Gong Ying
cold	2	Bai Hua She She Cao
cold	3	Xia Ku Cao
mild cold	4	Bei Mu
cold	5	Ban Zhi Lian
mild cold	6	Dan Can
mild cold	7	Xuan Shen
warm	8	Ji Xue Teng
mild warm	9	Huang Qi
warm	10	Bai Shu
cold	11	Ban Lan Gen
mild cold	12	Tian Hua Fen

FIGURE 6.29a
Malignant neoplasms of the lymphoid and histiocytic tissue excluding lymphosarcoma and Hodgkin's disease (ICD-9 = 202) might be treated by TCM tonifying formulas ($p = 0.06$). The top 12 ingredients are shown. The areas of the pies indicate the relative weights of the formulas and herbs in the prescription for the condition. *P* values are from overrepresentation tests.

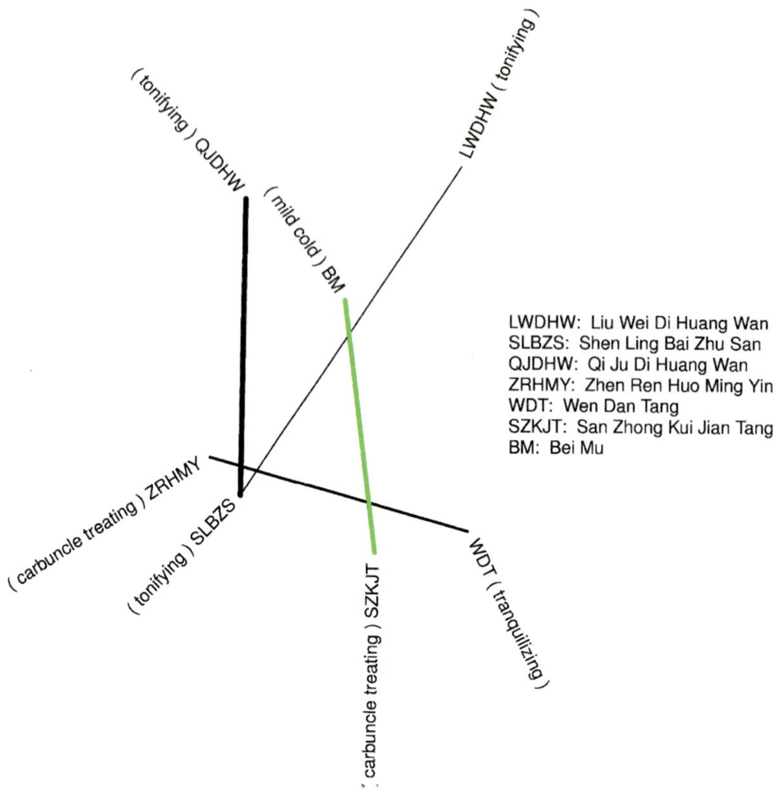

FIGURE 6.29b
The commonest TCM formula pair is SLBZS–QJDHW, followed by ZRHMY–WDT, and the commonest formula–herb pair is SZKJT–BM for the treatment of malignant neoplasms of the lymphoid and histiocystic tissue excluding lymphosarcoma and Hodgkin's disease. The thickness of the line indicates the prevalence of the pair. Formula pairs are in black and formula–herb pairs in green. The TCM pharmacotherapeutic categories of the formulas and the TCM natures of the herbs are shown in parentheses.

6.32 Malignant Neoplasm of the Kidney: *Zhu Ling Tang* and *Ban Zhi Lian*

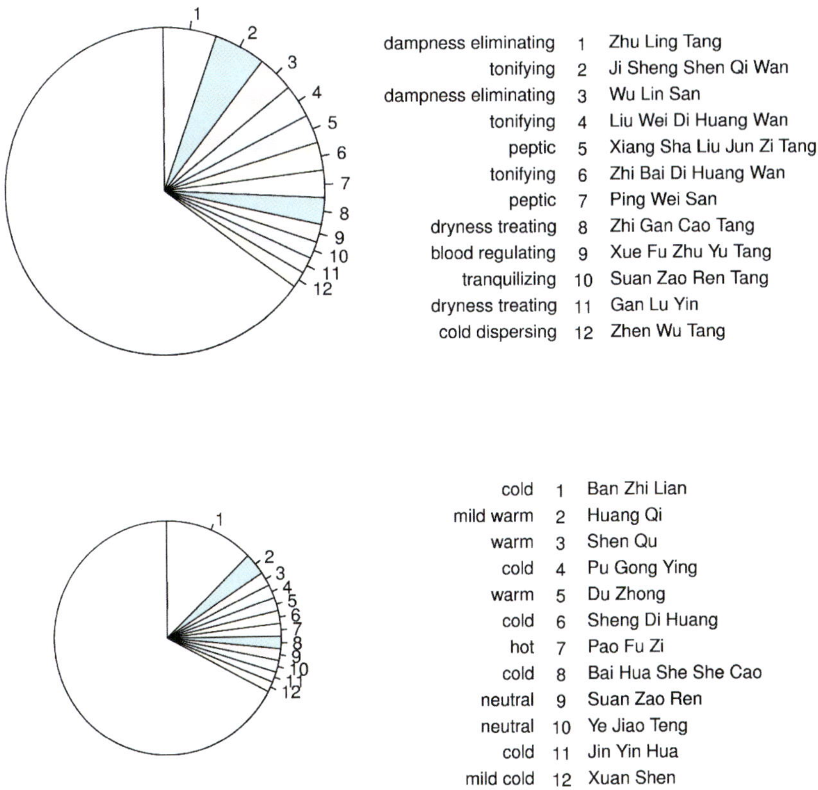

FIGURE 6.30a
Malignant neoplasms of the kidney and other, unspecified urinary organs (ICD-9 = 189) might be treated by TCM peptic formulas ($p = 0.07$). The top 12 ingredients are shown. The areas of the pies indicate the relative weights of the formulas and herbs in the prescription for the condition. *P* values are from over-representation tests.

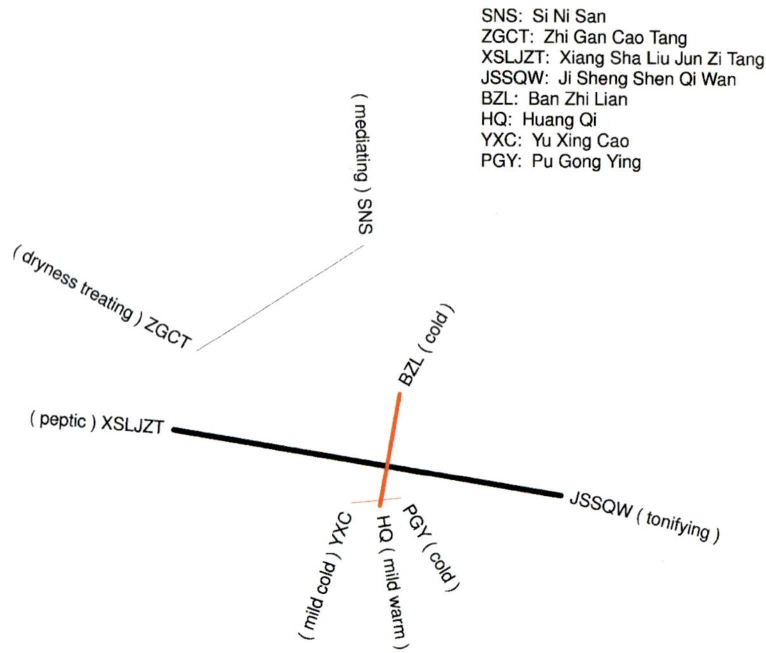

FIGURE 6.30b
The commonest TCM formula pair is JSSQW–XSLJZT and the commonest herb pair is BZL–HQ for the treatment of malignant neoplasms of the kidney and other, unspecified urinary organs. The thickness of the line indicates the prevalence of the pair. Formula pairs are in black and herb pairs in red. The TCM pharmacotherapeutic categories of the formulas and the TCM natures of the herbs are shown in parentheses.

6.33 Malignant Neoplasm of the Esophagus: *Bu Zhong Yi Qi Tang* and *Ban Zhi Lian*

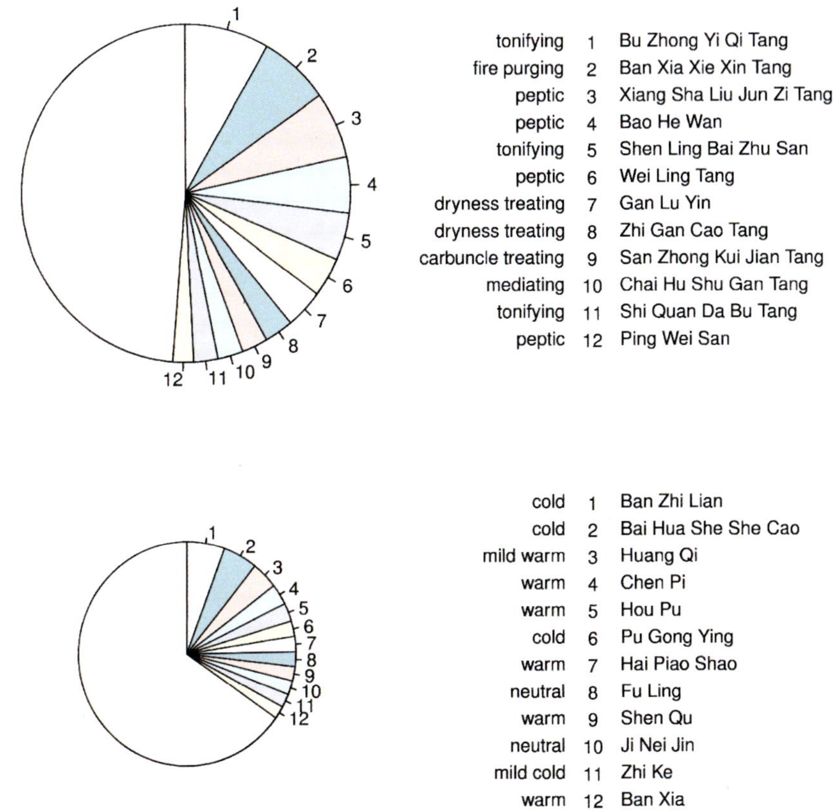

FIGURE 6.31a
Malignant neoplasms of the esophagus (ICD-9 = 150) are treated by TCM peptic formulas (p = 0.0006). The top 12 ingredients are shown. The areas of the pies indicate the relative weights of the formulas and herbs in the prescription for the condition. P values are from overrepresentation tests.

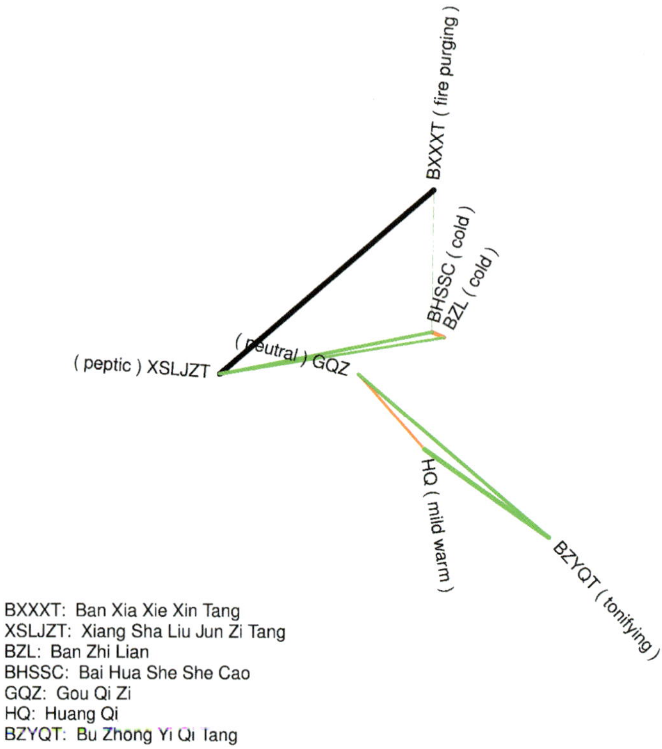

FIGURE 6.31b

The commonest TCM formula pair is XSLJZT–BXXXT, the commonest formula–herb pair is BZYQT–HQ, followed by BZYQT–GQZ and XSLJZT–BHSSC, and the commonest herb pair is BZL–BHSSC for the treatment of malignant neoplasms of the esophagus. The thickness of the line indicates the prevalence of the pair. Formula pairs are in black, formula–herb pairs in green and herb pairs in red. The TCM pharmacotherapeutic categories of the formulas and the TCM natures of the herbs are shown in parentheses.

6.34 Malignant Neoplasm of Other, Ill-Defined Sites: *Yang Yin Qing Fei Tang* and *Dan Can*

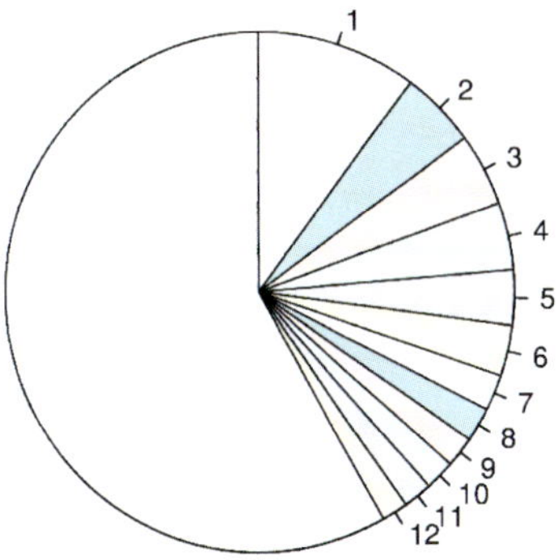

dryness treating	1	Yang Yin Qing Fei Tang
fire purging	2	Zi Yin Jiang Huo Tang
tonifying	3	Bu Zhong Yi Qi Tang
tonifying	4	Zhi Bai Di Huang Wan
carbuncle treating	5	Zhen Ren Huo Ming Yin
tonifying	6	Zuo Gui Wan
tonifying	7	Gui Lu Er Xian Jiao
dryness treating	8	Gan Lu Yin
mediating	9	Si Ni San
dryness treating	10	Zhi Gan Cao Tang
carbuncle treating	11	San Zhong Kui Jian Tang
mediating	12	Xiao Chai Hu Tang

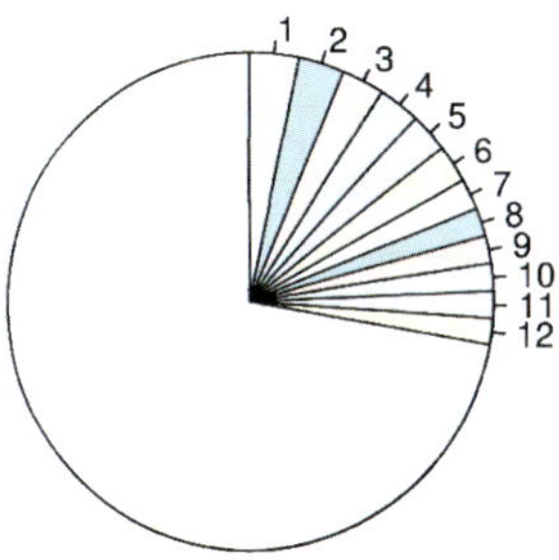

mild cold	1	Dan Can
mild warm	2	Huang Qi
cold	3	Ban Zhi Lian
mild cold	4	Xuan Shen
mild cold	5	Bei Mu
cold	6	Bai Hua She She Cao
warm	7	She Chuang Zi
neutral	8	Ge Gen
mild cold	9	Yin Chen Hao
cold	10	Jin Yin Hua
warm	11	Dang Gui
mild cold	12	Mai Men Dong

FIGURE 6.32a
Malignant neoplasms of other, ill-defined sites (ICD-9 = 195) are treated by TCM dryness-treating formulas ($p = 0.006$) and TCM mild–cold herbs ($p = 0.02$). The top 12 ingredients are shown. The areas of the pies indicate the relative weights of the formulas and herbs in the prescription for the condition. P values are from over-representation tests.

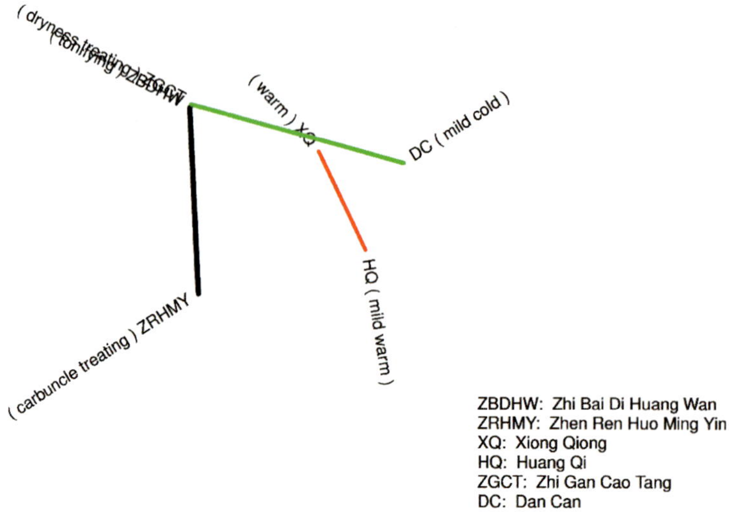

FIGURE 6.32b
The commonest TCM formula pair is ZRHMY–ZBDHW, the commonest formula–herb pair is ZGCT–DC and the commonest herb pair is HQ–XQ for the treatment of malignant neoplasms of other, ill-defined sites. The thickness of the line indicates the prevalence of the pair. Formula pairs are in black, formula–herb pairs in green and herb pairs in red. The TCM pharmacotherapeutic categories of the formulas and the TCM natures of the herbs are shown in parentheses.

7

Common Fatal Diseases

According to the June 2011 fact sheets of the World Health Organization, the top ten causes of death worldwide are: (1) ischemic heart disease; (2) stroke and other cerebrovascular diseases; (3) lower respiratory, infections; (4) chronic obstructive pulmonary disease (COPD); (5) diarrheal diseases; (6) HIV/AIDS; (7) trachea, bronchus and lung cancers; (8) tuberculosis; (9) diabetes mellitus; and (10) road traffic accidents. Major causes of death vary with the income of the country. In high-income countries, the ten leading causes of death are: (1) ischemic heart disease; (2) stroke and other cerebrovascular diseases; (3) trachea, bronchus and lung cancers; (4) Alzheimer's and other dementias; (5) lower respiratory infections; (6) COPD; (7) colon and rectum cancers; (8) diabetes mellitus; (9) hypertensive heart disease; and (10) breast cancer. The differences can reflect the distinct healthcare infrastructures, public health, regional diets and personal hygiene across regions. While modern western medicine is standard in developed countries, it may not be accessible or affordable in the rest of the world. Cost-effective traditional herbal medicines can serve as being alternative in low-income countries and complementary in developed countries. With a total of 1.1 million TCM prescriptions for the deadliest diseases, made in a whole year by about 5000 licensed TCM doctors in Taiwan, ingredients including their doses in the prescription are identified. Systematic quantification of TCM prescriptions is one of the steps toward TCM globalization.

7.1 Atherosclerosis, Hypertension, Cerebrocardiorenal Vascular Disease

Arteries are the blood vessels that carry blood away from the heart. Artery walls have three layers: intima, media and adventitia. Intima, the inner layer, contains mostly endothelial cells; media, the middle layer, comprises vascular smooth muscle cells; and adventitia, the outer layer, contains connective tissue cells. Atherosclerosis refers to a pathological condition of arteries caused by formation of plaques or lesions in artery walls. Expansion of the plaque thickens the wall, closing the lumen. Rupture of the lesion releases blood clots into the circulation, occluding blood flow. Both scenarios can cause ischemia of the tissues fed by the artery, leading to infarction. Atherosclerosis is slowly progressive, remaining clinically silent for decades before it is symptomatic. In the intima and media of atherosclerotic lesions are vascular dendritic cells, macrophages and foam cells, the last surrounding a necrotic core. Foam cells are macrophages that have phagocytosed oxidized low-density-lipoprotein (oxLDL) cholesterol. The adventitia of the lesion area has a dense population of T and B lymphocytes. Angiogenic processes in atherosclerotic lesions lead to neovessel invasion of the intima, destabilizing the plaque and precipitating rupture events. The composition and features of the plaque indicate that atherosclerosis is a complex process involving lipid retention, immune response and vascular remodeling [Galkina and Ley, 2009]. Atherogenesis is thought to be mediated by oxLDLs, which are an autoantigen. Furthermore, atherosclerosis is accelerated by chronic inflammation, which produces reactive oxygen species (ROS) and worsens vascular inflammation.

Hypertension, i.e. elevated blood pressure in the arteries, is the other chronic medical condition. Vascular remodeling by ROS is thought to play a role in the pathogenesis of hypertension

[Montezano and Touyz, 2012]. In healthy vessels, ROS participates in redox signaling for maintaining endothelial function and vascular integrity. Excessive concentrations of ROS induce endothelial cell hypertrophy, inflammatory cell infiltration, smooth muscle cell growth/fibrosis and extracellular matrix accumulation, resulting in vasoconstriction. Peripheral resistance rises as a consequence; so does blood pressure. Although animal experimental data support a causal role for oxidative stress in hypertension, human clinical trials for the antihypertensive effects of antioxidants have been less convincing, highlighting the multifactorial nature of hypertension pathogenesis. Among other prohypertensive factors are salt intake, renin–angiotensin system upregulation and sympathetic nervous system hyperactivity.

Among the cardiovascular diseases, the coronary arteries are the major sites of atherosclerotic lesions, resulting in coronary heart diseases. Among the cerebrovascular diseases, the anterior, middle and posterior cerebral arteries are the common sites of ischemia or hemorrhage, giving rise to stroke. Among the renovascular diseases, the juxtamedullary afferent arteries are the principal sites for microalbuminuria, leading to chronic kidney disease. A shared hemodynamic feature of the aforementioned arteries is that they are exposed to great pulsatile pressure and blood flow. The strained vessels are thus the sites of vascular vulnerability [Ito, 2012]. Until recently, in the fight for survival in the natural environment, humans have suffered frequent wound injuries in their lifetime. Hypotension had thus been the primary challenge for humans. The potent vasoconstrictive mechanisms that have been evolved to cope with the challenge may account for the high prevalence of hypertension among the people in modern societies.

7.2 Low-Grade Chronic Inflammation, Insulin Resistance, Metabolic Syndrome

Glucose is the primary source of energy for the growth, development and maintenance of all tissues, including muscle, liver, fat and brain. Adipose tissues are increasingly recognized as not only energy storage depots but also endocrine organs. In particular, the enlarged adipocytes in the abdomens of obese individuals, relative to the normal adipocytes in the abdomens of lean individuals, secrete abnormal proportions of cytokines called adipokines. Many of the adipokines, including leptin, TNF-alpha and IL-6, are proinflammatory. Some hypertrophied adipocytes that are overfed can expand no more — due, for example, to hypoxia. They die through apoptosis or necrosis. As a result, macrophages infiltrate obese adipose tissues to remove the debris via phagocytosis. Visceral fat obesity, characterized by adipocyte hypertrophy, immune cell infiltration and proinflammatory cytokine production through adipose tissue remodeling, induces a state of low-grade chronic inflammation called metabolic inflammation.

Insulin is an anabolic hormone secreted by the pancreas. It functions to activate uptake of glucose from the blood by muscle, fat and liver cells. Along the signaling pathway initiated by TNF-alpha, JNK is activated. JNK, however, inhibits the insulin receptor pathway via deactivation of insulin receptor substrate IRS-1. IL-6 has also been found to be associated with insulin signaling impairment via IRS-1 inhibition. The comprehensive picture of insulin signaling impairment can be complex. The proinflammatory cytokines, released by adipocytes and inflammatory cells from visceral and ectopic fats, are believed to induce signaling pathways that converse to inhibit the insulin receptor pathway, leading to insulin resistance.

When insulin loses its glucose absorbing effect on metabolic tissues, plasma glucose builds up. Chronic hyperglycemia is one of the hallmarks of diabetes. As glucose is the main source of energy for cells, persistent high concentrations of blood glucose can drive up ROS production in noninsulin target cells. Deleterious effects of chronic oxidative stress are thought to contribute to the secondary complications of diabetes, including retinopathy, neuropathy, nephropathy, cardiovascular disease, cerebrovascular disease and peripheral vascular disease. Diabetics are also vulnerable to infection due to hyperglycemia-induced neutrophil dysfunction.

7.3 Oligemic/Hypoxic Insults, Blood–Brain Barrier Breakdown, Cerebrodegenerative Disease

Dementia, including Alzheimer's disease, shares many of the risk factors for cardiovascular, carotid artery and cerebrovascular diseases. Vascular dysfunctions have therefore been increasingly recognized as a mechanism contributing to dementia. The vascular components in a neurovascular unit of cerebral microcirculation are pericytes and endothelial cells. The neural components include astrocytes, microglia and neurons. Astrocyte processes ensheath pericytes, which in turn ensheath endothelial cells. Microglia are the resident macrophages that sense neuronal injury. The endothelial cells along brain vessels are densely stitched together to form a barrier, called the blood–brain barrier (BBB), that restricts the passage of many more solutes than elsewhere. BBB is not only a physical barrier but also a system of cellular transporters for ions, peptides and nutrients, acting to protect the brain from common bacterial infections.

Disruption of the BBB — due, for example, to previous cerebrovascular insults — can detach pericytes, leaving a BBB breach. Plasma constituents such as albumin and red blood cells (RBCs) leak into brain parenchyma, yielding vasogenic edema, which causes hypoperfusion and hypoxia of the affected brain region. The iron in RBCs is pro-oxidant and elevates ROS. Both oligemia/hypoxia and increased oxidative stress cause neuronal injury and synaptic dysfunction, leading to neuron loss [Zlokovic, 2011]. Activated microglia, in response to oligemic injury, are proinflammatory and aggravate microneurovascular degeneration. Cognitive decline such as memory loss and learning impairment due to neuron loss are among the signs and symptoms of neurodegenerative diseases.

Amyloid beta is a proteolyzed product of APP, which is expressed in many tissues, especially in neuron synapses. The primary function of APP is unknown. However, amyloid beta levels in the normal brain are kept low. In addition to the enzymatic degradation of amyloid beta in many tissues, amyloid beta is transported from the brain across the BBB into blood by the receptor-related proteins LRP1 and LRP2 on the BBB. Amyloid beta in the systemic circulation is cleared by the liver and kidneys. On the other hand, amyloid beta in blood can re-enter the brain by RAGE on the BBB. In Alzheimer's disease, impaired amyloid beta clearance causes accumulation amyloid beta in the brain's interstitial fluid, forming amyloid beta oligomers, which are neurotoxic. Aggregates of amyloid beta, together with astrocytes, microglia and degenerative neural structures, form plaques, which are a characteristic of Alzheimer's-stricken brains.

7.4 Tobacco Smoke, Chronic Obstructive Pulmonary Disease, Tuberculosis

The lung exposes a large surface area to the atmosphere for the exchange of oxygen and carbon dioxide. Pollutants in the air, including cigarette smoke, ozone, nitrogen dioxide and combustion particulates, can be hazardous to the lung under long-term exposure. Tobacco smoking is a particular threat to the lung, as a puff of smoke contains more than $10^{15–17}$ oxidant/free radical molecules.

Although the half-life of free radicals is less than 1 s, large quantities of inhaled free radicals quickly deplete the endogenous antioxidants which function to neutralize oxidative toxicities. An oxidant–antioxidant imbalance in favor of oxidants activates the cellular processes involved in the pathogenesis of chronic obstructive pulmonary disease (COPD). Damage to epithelial cells, endothelial cells, extracellular matrix (ECM) and fibroblasts can cause mucus hypersecretion, endothelial leakage, ECM fragmentation and abnormal tissue repair, respectively, concomitant with secretion of proinflammatory cytokines. Infiltration of inflammatory cells increase protease release, which exacerbates pulmonary tissue remodeling. Damage to bronchi causes airway narrowing, leading to chronic bronchitis. Damage to alveoli causes air sac destruction, resulting in emphysema. Both conditions hinder oxygenation. Smoking cessation is an effective means of halting or slowing COPD-related morbidity and mortality.

Airborne pathogens once inhaled can infect the lung. Depending on the pathogens and the infected cell types in the lung, symptoms differ and prognosis varies. For example, *Mycobacterium tuberculosis* invades and replicates within alveolar macrophages. In response, T and B lymphocytes surround the infected macrophages to wall off *M. tuberculosis*. The bacteria become dormant and the patient remains asymptomatic. When the patient becomes immunodeficient, the tuberculosis turns active. Patients who suffer from active tuberculosis without treatment are contagious. Inflammatory lung diseases due to other bacterial or viral infections are called pneumonia.

7.5 Steatosis, Alcohol, Chronic Liver Disease and Cirrhosis

Cirrhosis refers to a progressive and permanent fibrotic degeneration of the liver. The causes of cirrhosis are (1) deregulated lipid metabolism, (2) alcoholism, (3) viral infections and (4) hepatotoxic agents. Inflammatory responses of the body to the chronic insult(s) lead to excessive formation of fibrous connective tissue, which obliterates the liver parenchyma.

Overnutrition marked by hyperlipidemia and/or hyperglycemia predisposes lipid metabolism deregulation in modern societies. The liver is the major organ that metabolizes lipids. When the supply of fatty acids to hepatocytes overwhelms fatty acid utilization, abnormal retention of lipids in the form of intracytoplasmic droplets of triglycerides occurs in the hepatocytes. When more than 5%–10% of the liver weight is fat, a condition of a fatty liver called steatosis develops. Note that peripheral insulin resistance can cause delivery of fatty acids from adipose tissues to the liver, contributing to steatosis. Ballooning of hepatocytes by excess unmetabolized fat induces hepatic necrosis. Inflammatory response activates hepatic stellate cells, which play a role in liver fibrosis.

Alcoholic beverages contain ethanol. About 80% of consumed alcohol is processed by the liver. Metabolism of alcohol produces NADH and raises the NADPH/$NADP^+$ ratio in hepatocytes. Both NADH and NADPH/$NADP^+$ promote fatty acid synthesis. Furthermore, NADH, being an oxidant, poses an oxidative stress challenge to the liver. Abstinence from alcohol can prevent and even reverse alcoholic hepatitis. Chronic infection of the liver by hepatotrophic viruses, such as hepatitis B and C viruses, can also lead to cirrhosis.

7.6 Pathophysiology-Specific TCM Formulas and Herbs for the Common Fatal Diseases

Inflammatory stimuli such as oxidants, oxLDLs, glucose toxicity and pathogens cause stress and damage to the endothelial cells of the large and medium arteries, leading to vascular diseases, including ischemic heart disease, stroke, dementia, atherosclerosis, hypertensive heart and renal disease, hypertensive heart disease and hypertension. Using the set of all reimbursable formulas (or herbs) as the control, we find that TCM wind-expelling ($p = 0.00002$) and blood-regulating ($p = 0.001$) formulas are overrepresented in the TCM prescriptions for the vascular diseases. Obesity and diabetes are metabolic syndromes. Kidney diseases, in particular nephrotic syndrome, are strongly linked to diabetes. We find the dominant TCM formulas for the metabolic syndrome to be TCM tonifying formulas ($p = 0.03$). COPD, acute bronchitis/bronchiolitis, tuberculosis and pneumonia are diseases of the lung that has been damaged by airborne free radicals, pollutants or pathogens. TCM exterior-relieving ($p = 0.008$) and dryness-treating ($p = 0.03$) formulas and TCM mild–cold ($p = 0.003$) herbs are the commonest ingredients. Chronic liver disease and cirrhosis are treated by TCM mediating formulas ($p = 0.02$) and mild–cold herbs ($p = 0.003$).

Sudden alteration of a condition typifies a wind syndrome in TCM. Examples of TCM wind syndrome are stroke and heart attack. According to a school of TCM practices, i.e. Hejian Liu (c.1110–1200 CE), an inappropriate and irregular life style can set the TCM heart on fire; raging TCM heart flares ravage TCM kidney *yin*. The agitating wind, when unvented, causes seizure. TCM fire corresponds to ROS, immune response and inflammation in modern western medicine. Blood stasis in TCM is a slow-down or stoppage of blood flow. TCM blood-regulating formulas are said to help remove microclots in the circulation. TCM tonifying formulas are believed to help tissue repair and strengthen immune defense. The exterior in TCM encompasses the body parts that are exposed to the environment. Exopathic diseases such as infection afflict the exterior first. If unsuccessfully treated, pathogens progress through TCM meridians to the interior. Once the pathogens entrench the viscera (i.e. the five *zang* organs), the patient is said to be half-dead. TCM exterior-relieving formulas aim to terminate pathogens on the exterior. Lack of bodily fluids characterizes a TCM dry syndrome. The causes of dryness are heat and fire. TCM dry syndromes are treated by sweet, cold and moisturizing TCM herbs. TCM mediating formulas address diseases affecting the *shao yang* meridian, which borders the exterior and interior. *Shao yang* syndrome is also characterized by alternating cold and warm syndromes, manifesting an ongoing battle between the pathogen and immunity. TCM cold and mild–cold herbs are thought to be anti-inflammatory.

TCM prescriptions for the common fatal diseases, through weighted combination of the ingredients, are sensitive to the mechanisms and sites of pathogenesis. For example, prescriptions for the hypertension-related diseases cluster together in the hierarchical tree. Lung diseases form a cluster, while tuberculosis clusters with lung cancer, which clusters with other cancers. A typical TCM prescription for a common fatal disease

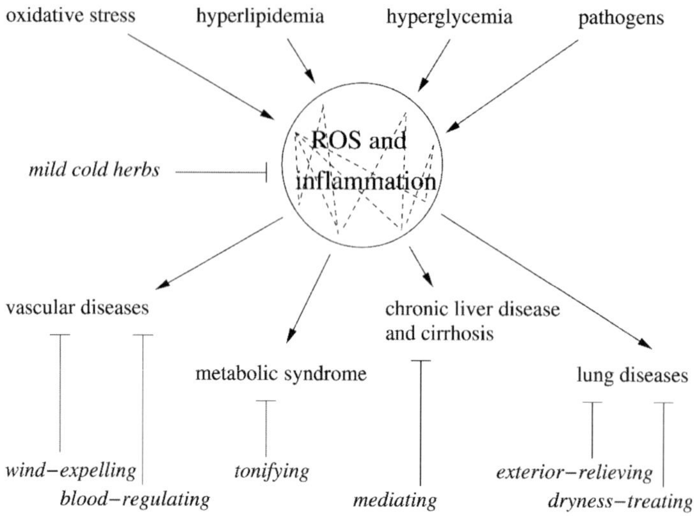

FIGURE 7.1

Common fatal diseases and the prescribed TCM formulas and herbs. Vascular diseases include ischemic heart disease, stroke, dementia, atherosclerosis, hypertensive heart and renal disease, hypertensive heart disease and essential hypertension. Metabolic syndrome includes obesity, diabetes and kidney diseases. Lung diseases include COPD, acute bronchitis and bronchiolitis, tuberculosis and pneumonia. Pointed arrows indicate promotion; blunt arrows indicate suppression. Note the dashed lines connecting the arrows.

consists of two formulas and three herbs. The weights of the ingredients in a typical prescription for a common fatal disease are 100:71:58:50:45, following a power law. The weights from the heaviest to the next-heaviest ingredient in the prescriptions for pediatric patients decreases drastically: 100:65:50:42:36. Consultation with the doctor or pharmacist is required to prevent potential adverse interactions between herbal and conventional medicines.

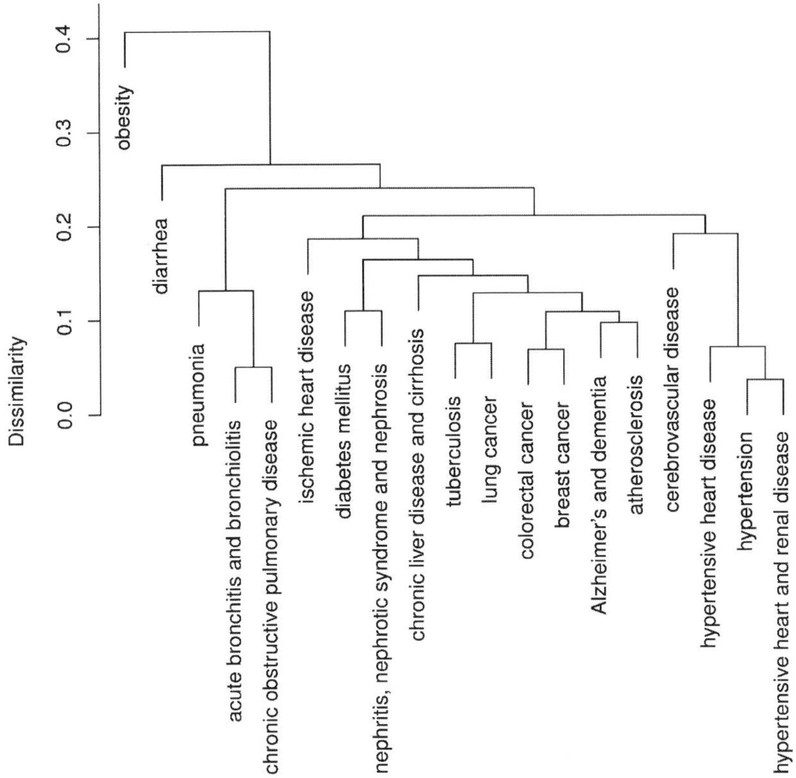

FIGURE 7.2

Clustering of TCM prescriptions for common fatal diseases and related conditions. Prescriptions which are similar, in terms of ingredients and relative weights of the ingredients in the prescription, fall within a branch of the tree in the hierarchical clustering analysis. Prescriptions for vascular diseases/conditions, cancers, metabolic syndrome and lung diseases tend to cluster within separate branches. The vertical axis measures pairwise distance or dissimilarity between prescriptions.

7.7 Ischemic Heart Disease: *Xue Fu Zhu Yu Tang* and *Dan Can*

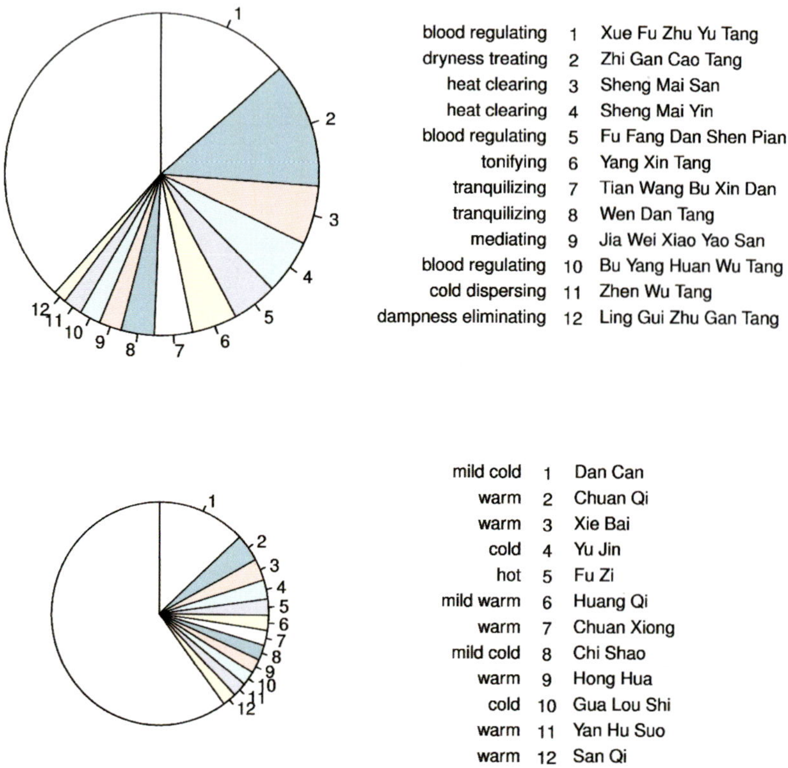

FIGURE 7.3a

Ischemic heart disease (ICD-9 = 410–414) is treated by TCM heat-clearing ($p = 0.04$), blood-regulating ($p = 0.04$) or tranquilizing ($p = 0.05$) formulas. The top 12 ingredients are shown. The areas of the pies indicate the relative weights of the formulas and herbs in the prescription for the condition. *P* values are from over-representation tests.

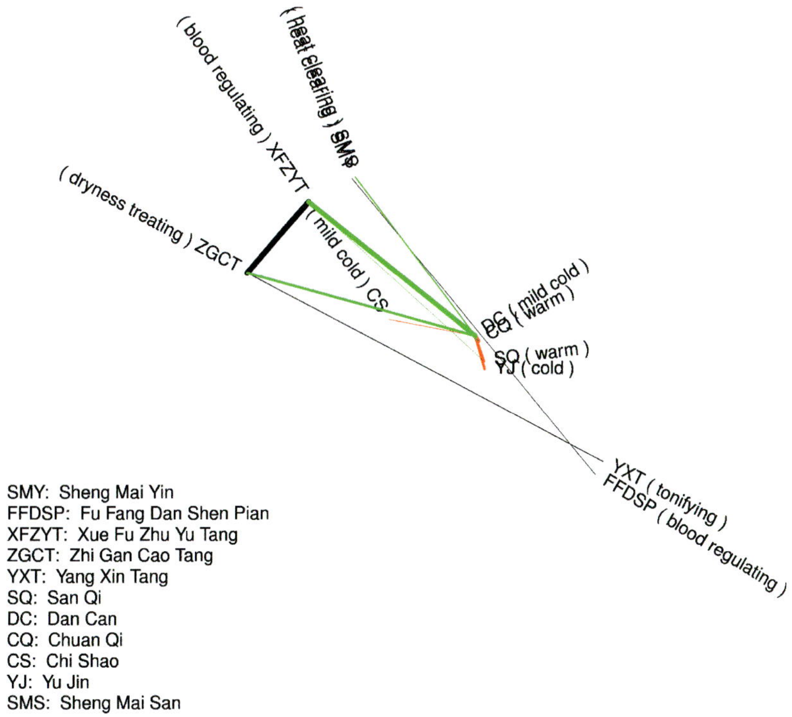

FIGURE 7.3b

The commonest TCM formula pair is XFZYT–ZGCT, the commonest formula–herb pair is XFZYT–DC and the commonest herb pair is DC–CQ, followed by DC–YJ, for the treatment of ischemic heart disease. The thickness of the line indicates the prevalence of the pair. Formula pairs are in black, formula–herb pairs in green and herb pairs in red. The TCM pharmacotherapeutic categories of the formulas and the TCM natures of the herbs are shown in parentheses.

7.8 Cerebrovascular Disease: *Bu Yang Huan Wu Tang* and *Dan Can*

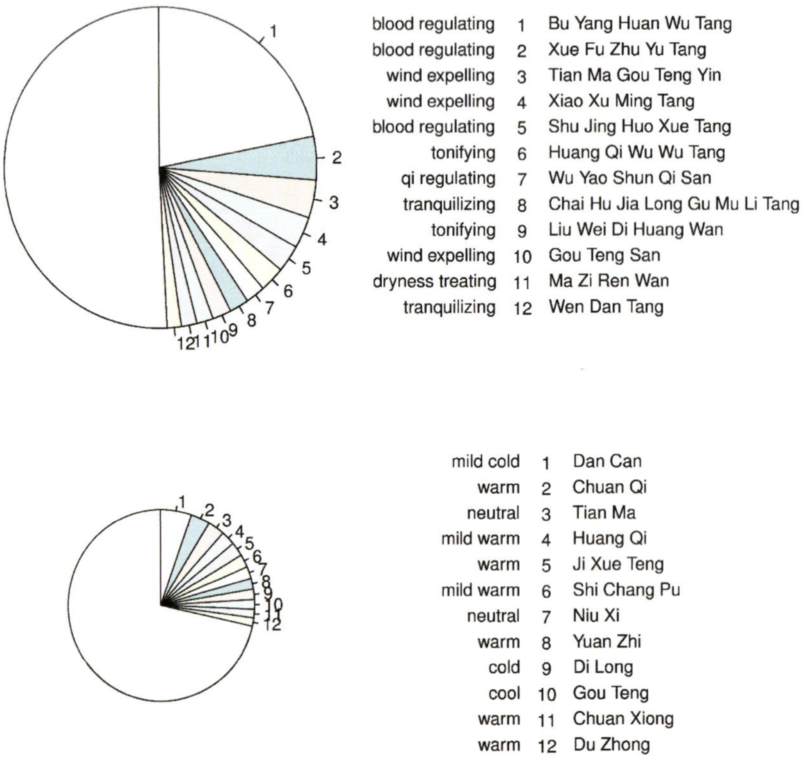

FIGURE 7.4a

Cerebrovascular disease (ICD-9 = 430–438) is treated by TCM wind-expelling ($p = 0.02$), blood-regulating ($p = 0.04$) or tranquilizing ($p = 0.05$) formulas. The top 12 ingredients are shown. The areas of the pies indicate the relative weights of the formulas and herbs in the prescription for the condition. P values are from over-representation tests.

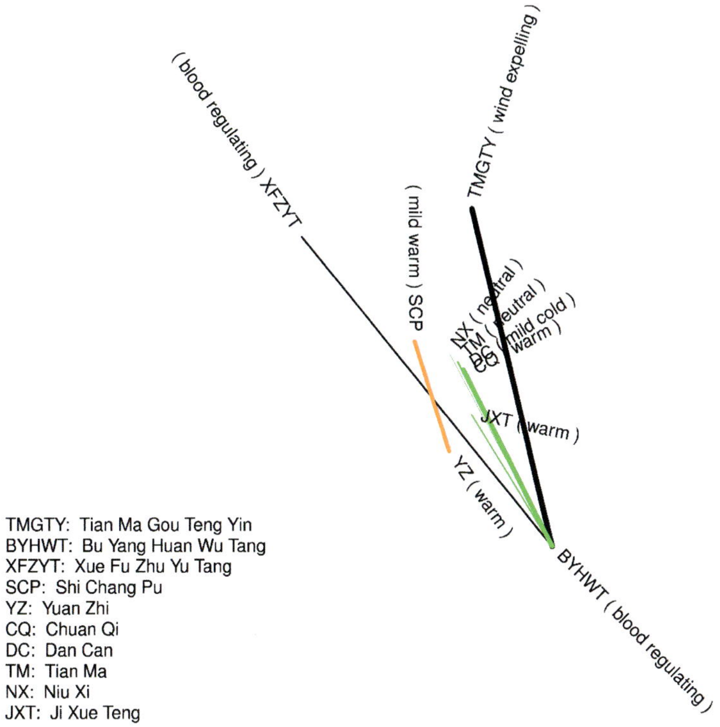

FIGURE 7.4b

The commonest TCM formula pair is BYHWT–TMGTY, the commonest formula–herb pair is BYHWT–DC, followed by BYHWT–CQ, BYHWT–TM and BYHWT–JXT, and the commonest herb pair is SCP–YZ for the treatment of stroke. The thickness of the line indicates the prevalence of the pair. Formula pairs are in black, formula–herb pairs in green and herb pairs in red. The TCM pharmacotherapeutic categories of the formulas and the TCM natures of the herbs are shown in parentheses.

7.9 Alzheimer's and Other Dementias: *Tian Wang Bu Xin Dan* and *Yuan Zhi*

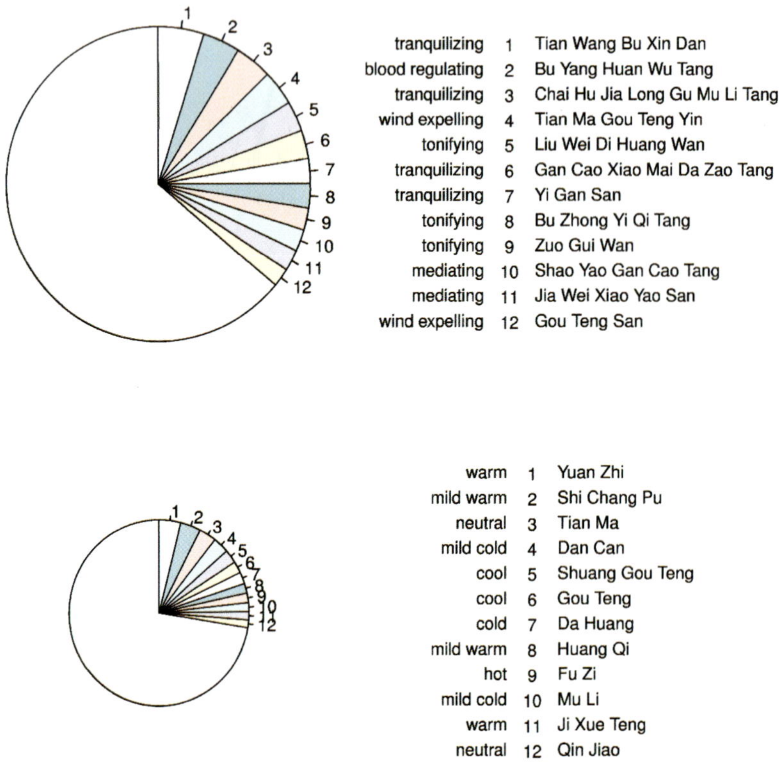

FIGURE 7.5a

Dementias, including Alzheimer's and Parkinson's disease (ICD-9 = 290, 294, 331, 332), are treated by TCM tranquilizing formulas ($p = 0.0002$). The top 12 ingredients are shown. The areas of the pies indicate the relative weights of the formulas and herbs in the prescription for the conditions. *P* values are from overrepresentation tests.

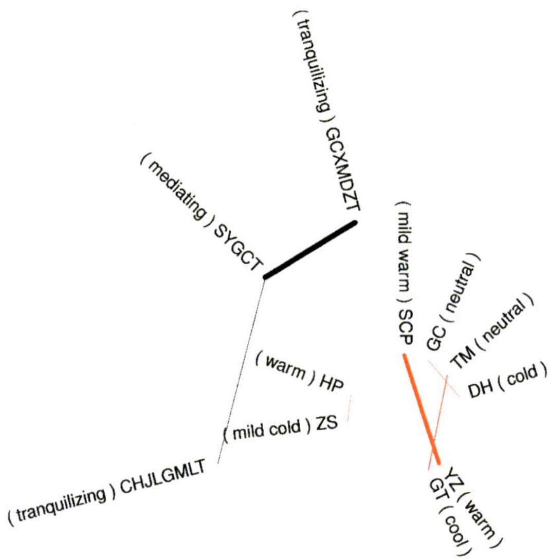

GCXMDZT: Gan Cao Xiao Mai Da Zao Tang
SYGCT: Shao Yao Gan Cao Tang
CHJLGMLT: Chai Hu Jia Long Gu Mu Li Tang
DH: Da Huang
GC: Gan Cao
TM: Tian Ma
GT: Gou Teng
SCP: Shi Chang Pu
YZ: Yuan Zhi
HP: Hou Pu
ZS: Zhi Shi

FIGURE 7.5b

The commonest TCM formula pair is GCXMDZT–SYGCT and the commonest herb pair is SCP–YZ for the treatment of Alzheimer's and other dementias. The thickness of the line indicates the prevalence of the pair. Formula pairs are in black and herb pairs in red. The TCM pharmacotherapeutic categories of the formulas and the TCM natures of the herbs are shown in parentheses.

7.10 Hypertensive Heart and Renal Disease: *Tian Ma Gou Teng Yin* and *Dan Can*

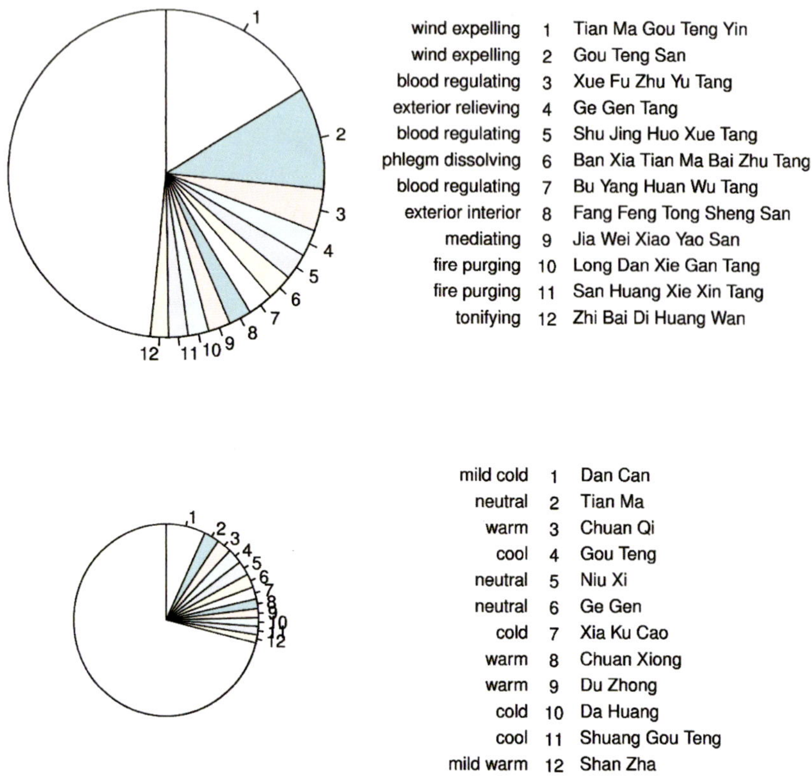

FIGURE 7.6a

Hypertensive heart and renal disease (ICD-9 = 404) is treated by TCM blood-regulating formulas ($p = 0.04$). The top 12 ingredients are shown. The areas of the pies indicate the relative weights of the formulas and herbs in the prescription for the condition. *P* values are from overrepresentation tests.

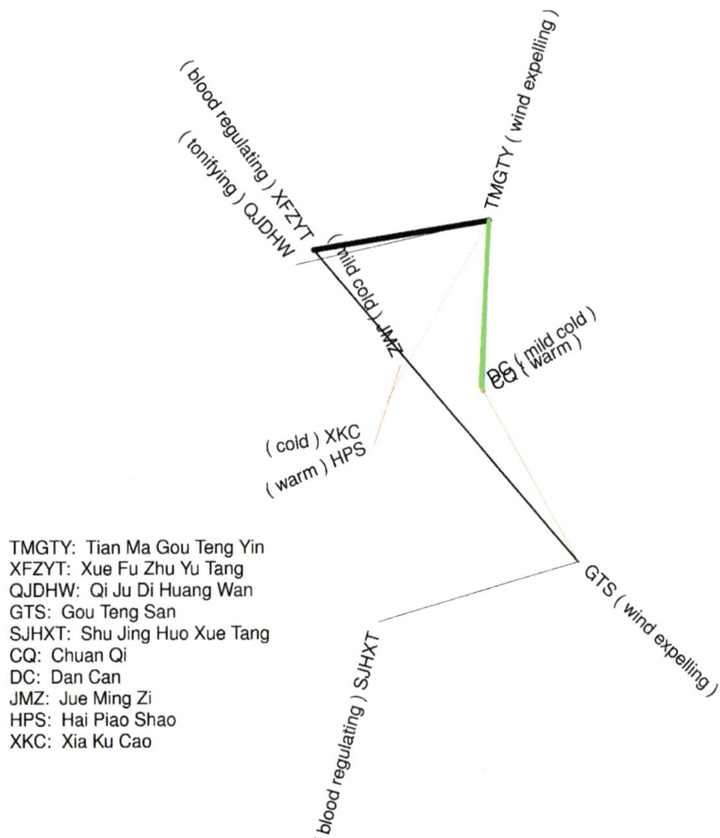

FIGURE 7.6b

The commonest TCM formula pair is TMGTY–XFZYT, the commonest formula–herb pair is TMGTY–DC, followed by TMGTY–CQ, and the commonest herb pair is CQ–DC for the treatment of hypertensive heart and renal disease. The thickness of the line indicates the prevalence of the pair. Formula pairs are in black, formula–herb pairs in green and herb pairs in red. The TCM pharmacotherapeutic categories of the formulas and the TCM natures of the herbs are shown in parentheses.

7.11 Hypertensive Heart Disease: *Tian Ma Gou Teng Yin* and *Dan Can*

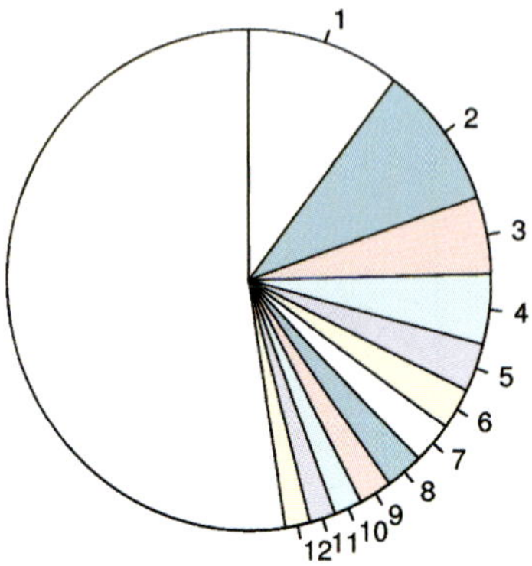

wind expelling	1	Tian Ma Gou Teng Yin
wind expelling	2	Gou Teng San
blood regulating	3	Xue Fu Zhu Yu Tang
dryness treating	4	Zhi Gan Cao Tang
blood regulating	5	Bu Yang Huan Wu Tang
tonifying	6	Qi Ju Di Huang Wan
heat clearing	7	Sheng Mai Yin
tranquilizing	8	Tian Wang Bu Xin Dan
mediating	9	Jia Wei Xiao Yao San
tranquilizing	10	Chai Hu Jia Long Gu Mu Li Tang
fire purging	11	Long Dan Xie Gan Tang
tonifying	12	Zhi Bai Di Huang Wan

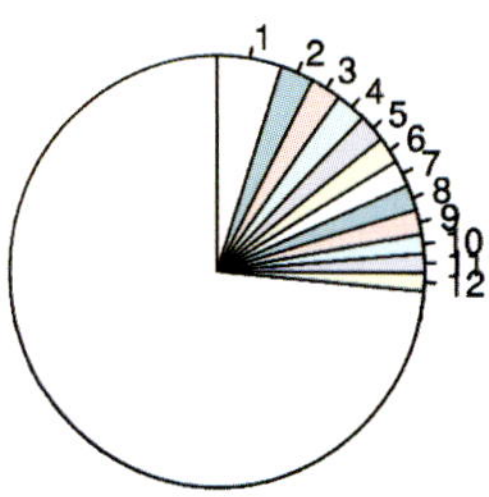

mild cold	1	Dan Can
neutral	2	Tian Ma
cool	3	Ju Hua
mild warm	4	Huang Qi
cold	5	Huang Qin
cool	6	Gou Teng
cold	7	Xia Ku Cao
neutral	8	Ge Gen
mild cold	9	Bai Ji
mild warm	10	Shan Zha
warm	11	Du Zhong
neutral	12	Niu Xi

FIGURE 7.7a

Hypertensive heart disease (ICD-9 = 402) is treated by TCM tranquilizing formulas ($p = 0.05$). The top 12 ingredients are shown. The areas of the pies indicate the relative weights of the formulas and herbs in the prescription for the condition. *P* values are from overrepresentation tests.

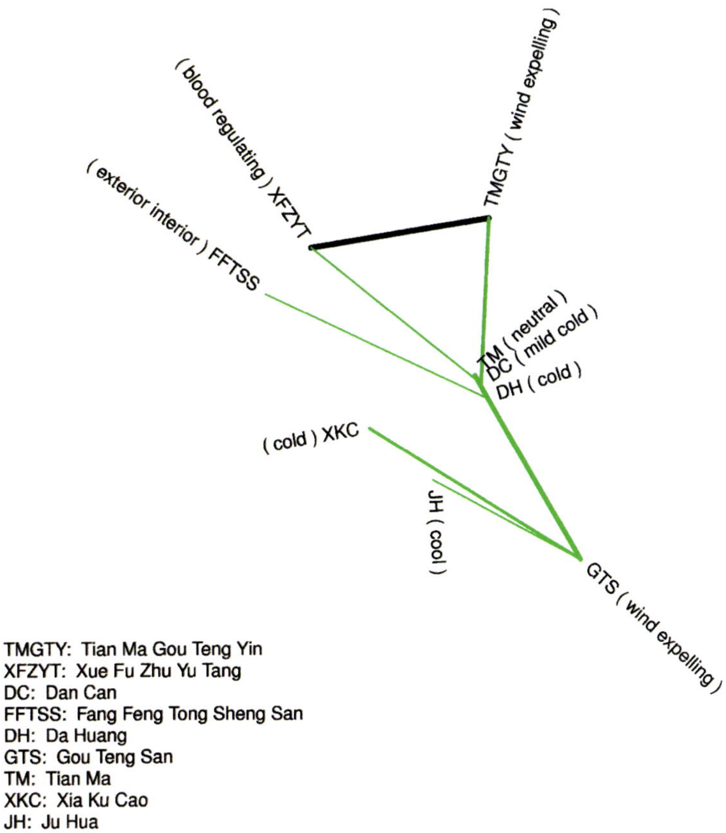

FIGURE 7.7b

The commonest TCM formula pair is TMGTY–XFZYT and the commonest formula–herb pair is GTS–TM, followed by TMGTY–DC, GTS–XKC and XFZYT–DC, for the treatment of hypertensive heart disease. The thickness of the line indicates the prevalence of the pair. Formula pairs are in black and formula–herb pairs in green. The TCM pharmacotherapeutic categories of the formulas and the TCM natures of the herbs are shown in parentheses.

7.12 Essential Hypertension: *Tian Ma Gou Teng Yin* and *Dan Can*

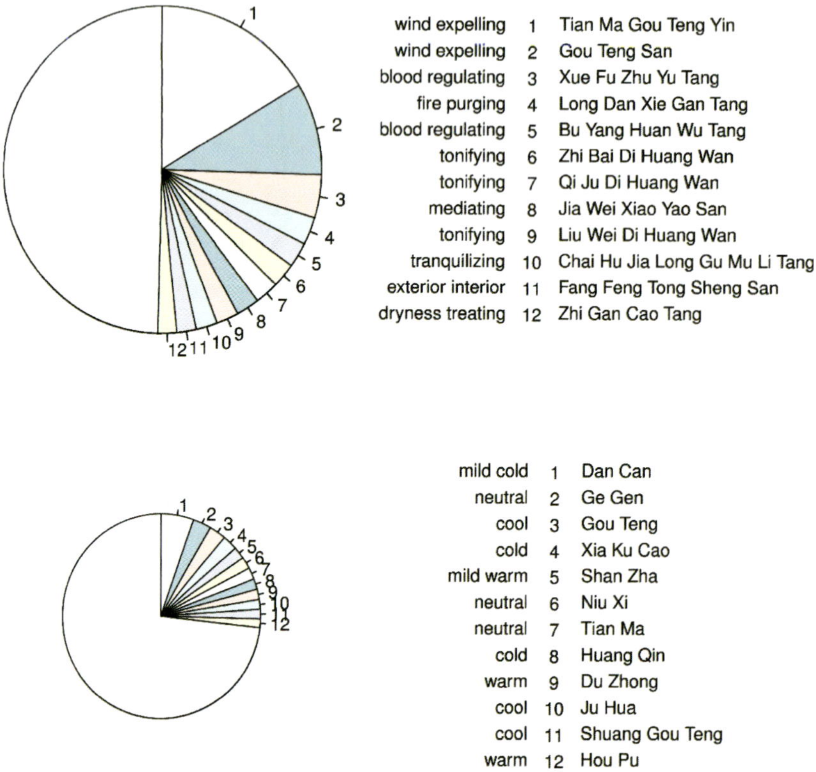

FIGURE 7.8a

Essential hypertension (ICD-9 = 401) might be treated by TCM wind-expelling formulas ($p = 0.12$). The top 12 ingredients are shown. The areas of the pies indicate the relative weights of the formulas and herbs in the prescription for the condition. *P* values are from overrepresentation tests.

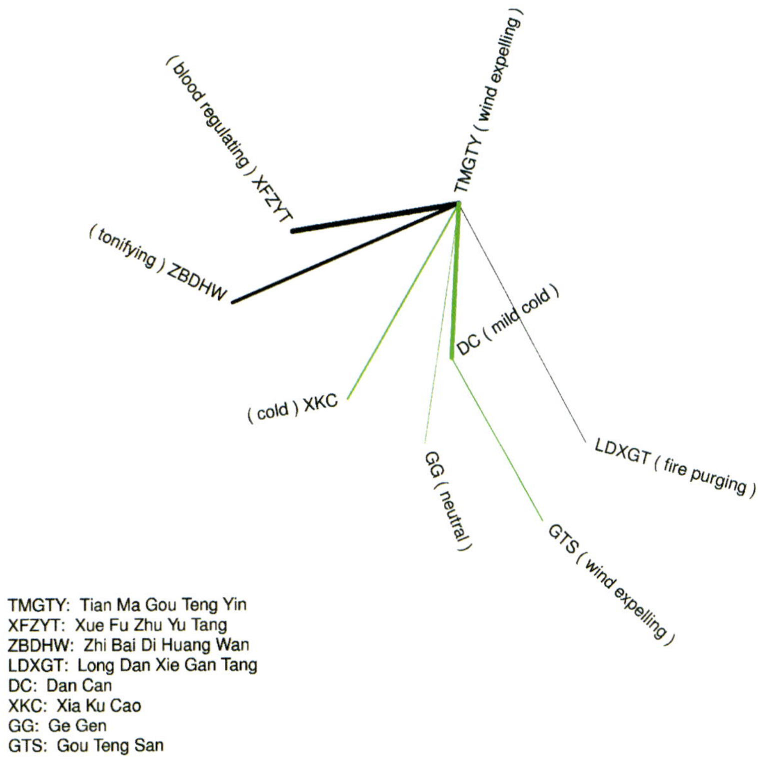

FIGURE 7.8b

The commonest TCM formula pair is TMGTY–XFZYT and the commonest formula–herb pair is TMGTY–DC for the treatment of essential hypertension. The thickness of the line indicates the prevalence of the pair. Formula pairs are in black and formula–herb pairs in green. The TCM pharmacotherapeutic categories of the formulas and the TCM natures of the herbs are shown in parentheses.

7.13 Atherosclerosis: *Jia Wei Xiao Yao San* and *Dan Can*

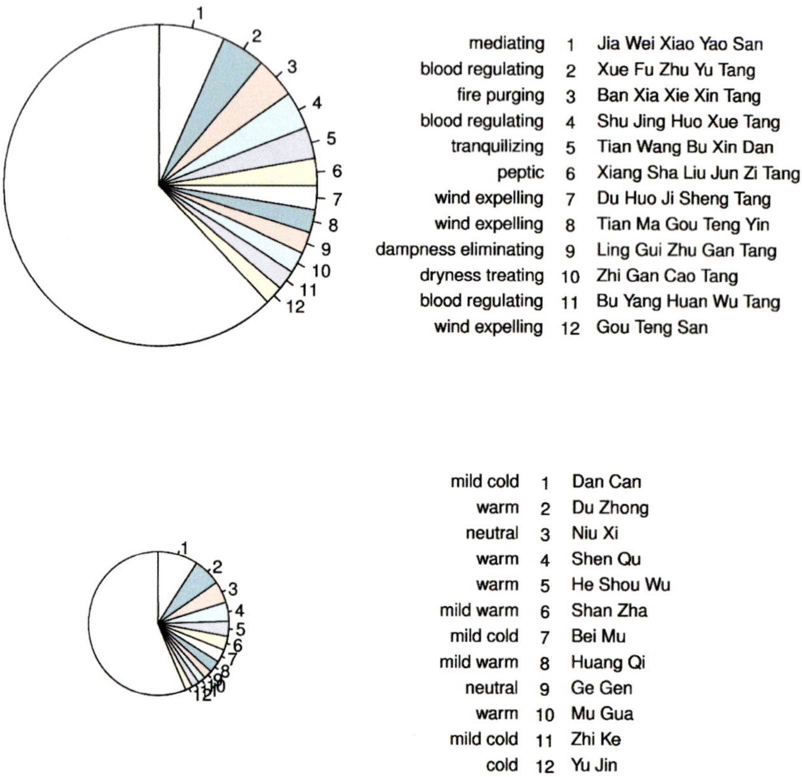

FIGURE 7.9a

Atherosclerosis (ICD-9 = 440) is treated by TCM wind-expelling ($p = 0.02$) and blood-regulating ($p = 0.04$) formulas. The top 12 ingredients are shown. The areas of the pies indicate the relative weights of the formulas and herbs in the prescription for the condition. *P* values are from overrepresentation tests.

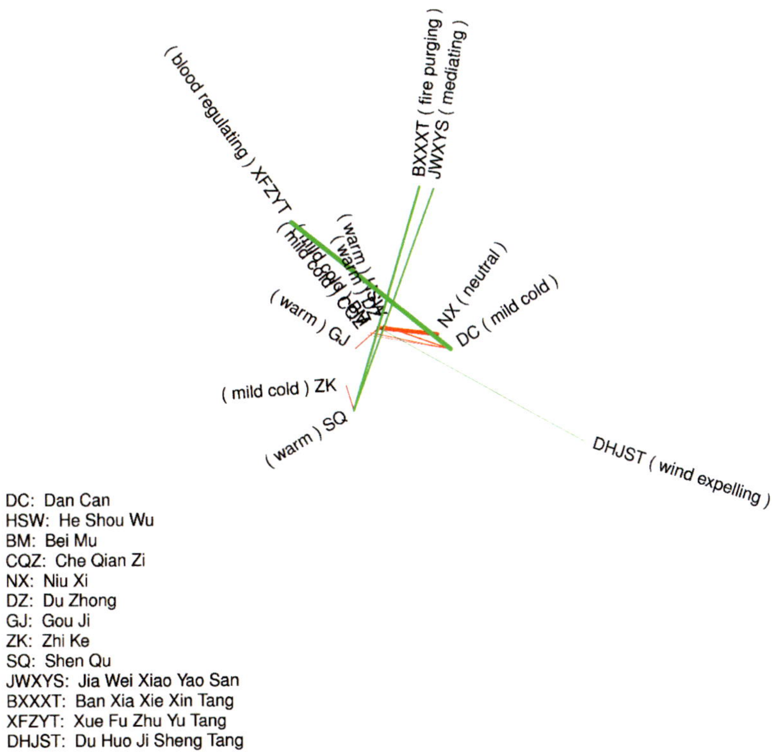

FIGURE 7.9b

The commonest TCM formula–herb pair is XFZYT–DC, followed by BXXXT–SQ, and the commonest herb pair is DZ–NX, followed by HSW–DC, DZ–GJ and ZK–SQ, for the treatment of atherosclerosis. The thickness of the line indicates the prevalence of the pair. Formula–herb pairs are in green and herb pairs in red. The TCM pharmacotherapeutic categories of the formulas and the TCM natures of the herbs are shown in parentheses.

7.14 Diabetes Mellitus: *Liu Wei Di Huang Wan* and *Tian Hua Fen*

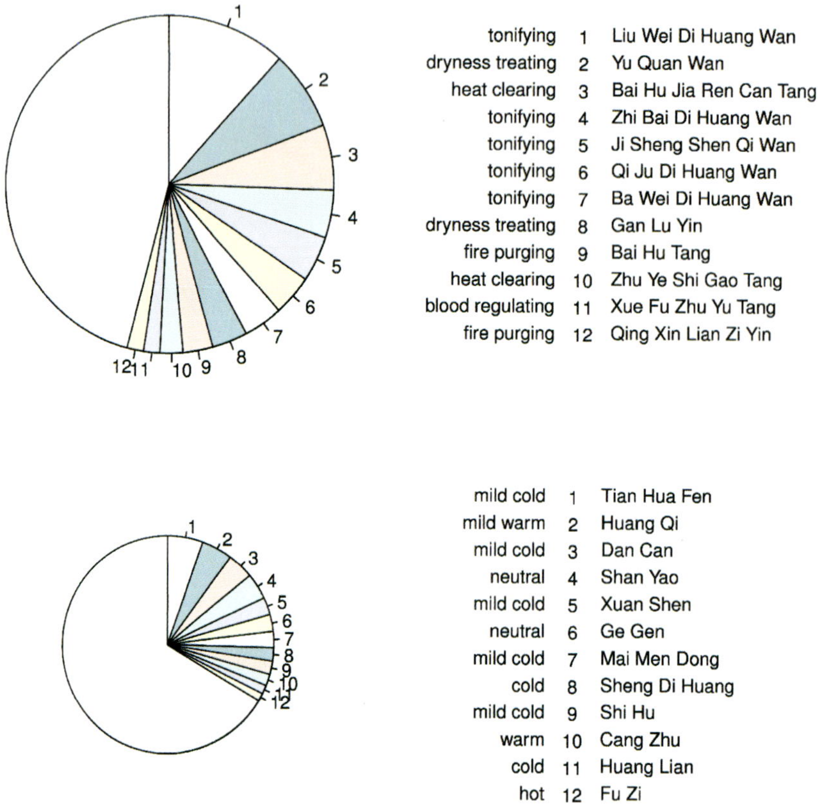

FIGURE 7.10a

Diabetes (ICD-9 = 250) is treated by TCM tonifying ($p = 0.01$) and heat-clearing ($p = 0.04$) formulas and TCM mild–cold ($p = 0.02$) herbs. The top 12 ingredients are shown. The areas of the pies indicate the relative weights of the formulas and herbs in the prescription for the condition. *P* values are from overrepresentation tests.

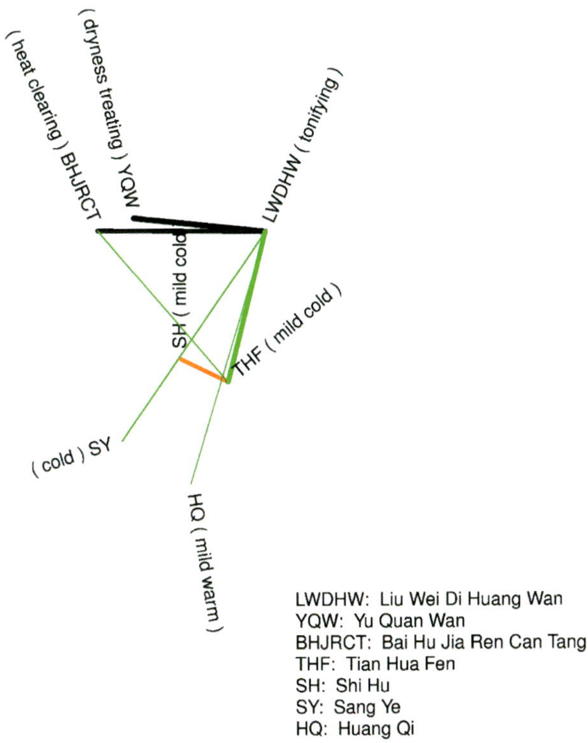

FIGURE 7.10b

The commonest TCM formula pair is LWDHW–YQW, the commonest formula–herb pair is LWDHW–THF, followed by LWDHW–SY and BHJRCT–THF, and the commonest herb pair is THF–SH for the treatment of diabetes. The thickness of the line indicates the prevalence of the pair. Formula pairs are in black, formula–herb pairs in green and herb pairs in red. The TCM pharmacotherapeutic categories of the formulas and the TCM natures of the herbs are shown in parentheses.

7.15 Nephritis, Nephrotic Syndrome and Nephrosis: *Ji Sheng Shen Qi Wan* and *Che Qian Zi*

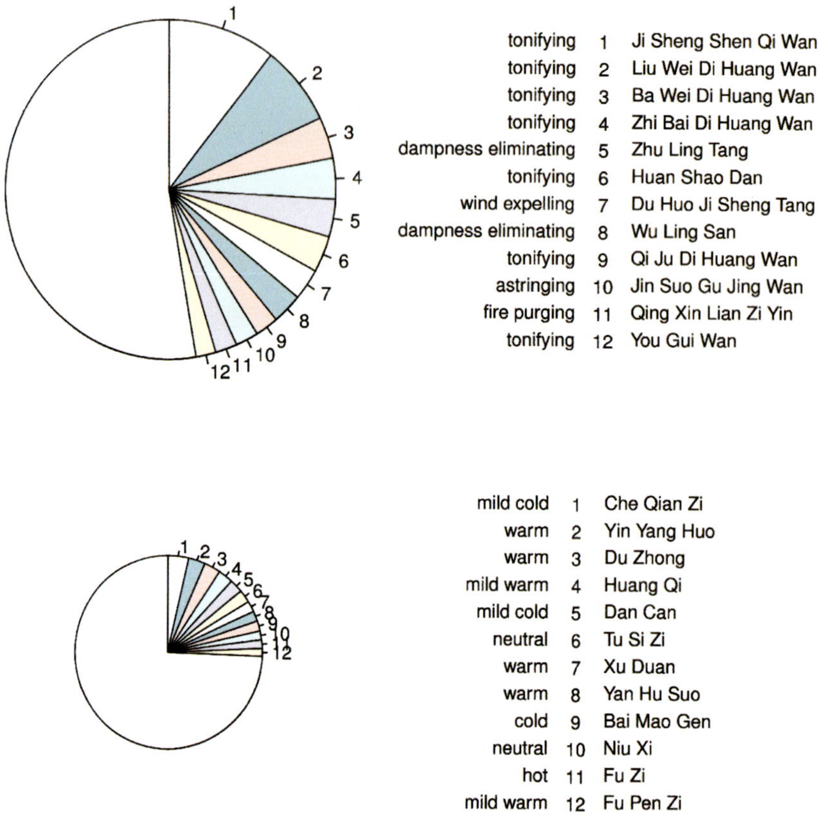

FIGURE 7.11a

Nephritis, nephrotic syndrome and nephrosis (ICD-9 = 580–589) are treated by TCM tonifying formulas ($p = 0.0002$). The top 12 ingredients are shown. The areas of the pies indicate the relative weights of the formulas and herbs in the prescription for the condition. *P* values are from overrepresentation tests.

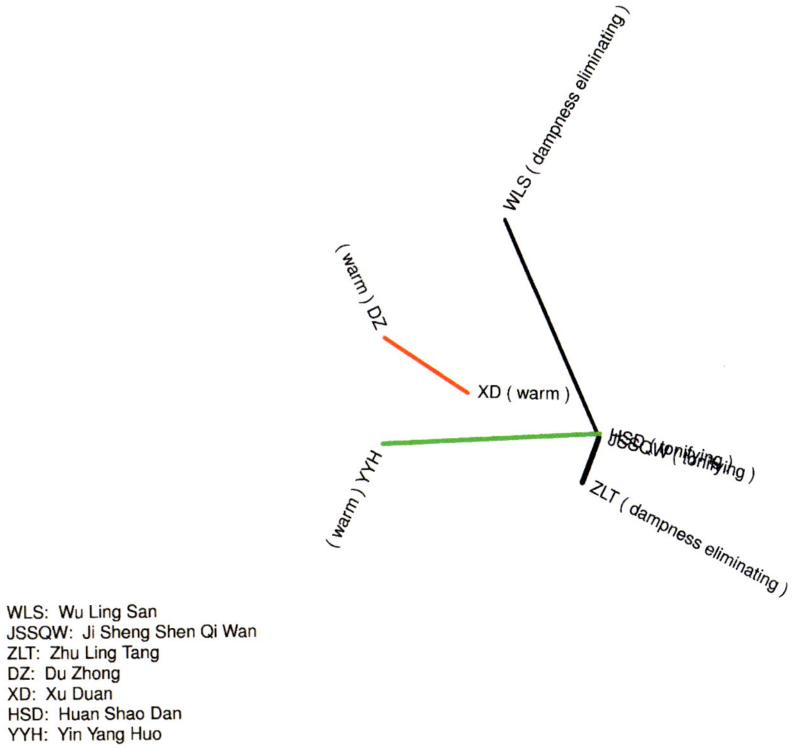

FIGURE 7.11b

The commonest TCM formula pair is JSSQW–ZLT, the commonest formula–herb pair is HSD–YYH and the commonest herb pair is DZ–XD for the treatment of kidney diseases (nephritis, nephrotic syndrome and nephrosis). The thickness of the line indicates the prevalence of the pair. Formula pairs are in black, formula–herb pairs in green and herb pairs in red. The TCM pharmacotherapeutic categories of the formulas and the TCM natures of the herbs are shown in parentheses.

7.16 Chronic Obstructive Pulmonary Disease: *Ma Xing Gan Shi Tang* and *Bei Mu*

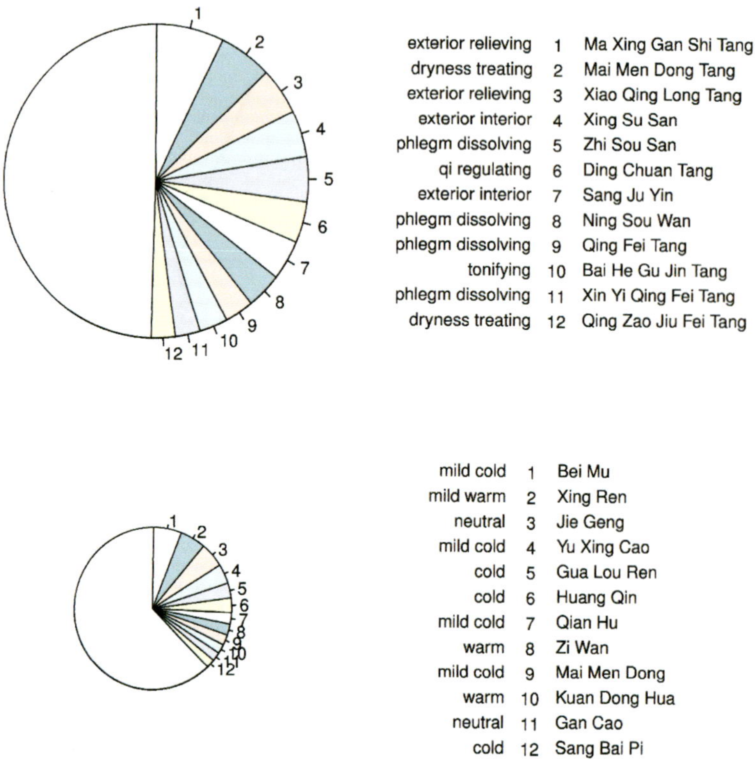

FIGURE 7.12a

Chronic obstructive pulmonary disease (ICD-9 = 490–492, 494–496) is treated by TCM phlegm-dissolving formulas ($p = 0.002$). The top 12 ingredients are shown. The areas of the pies indicate the relative weights of the formulas and herbs in the prescription for the condition. *P* values are from overrepresentation tests.

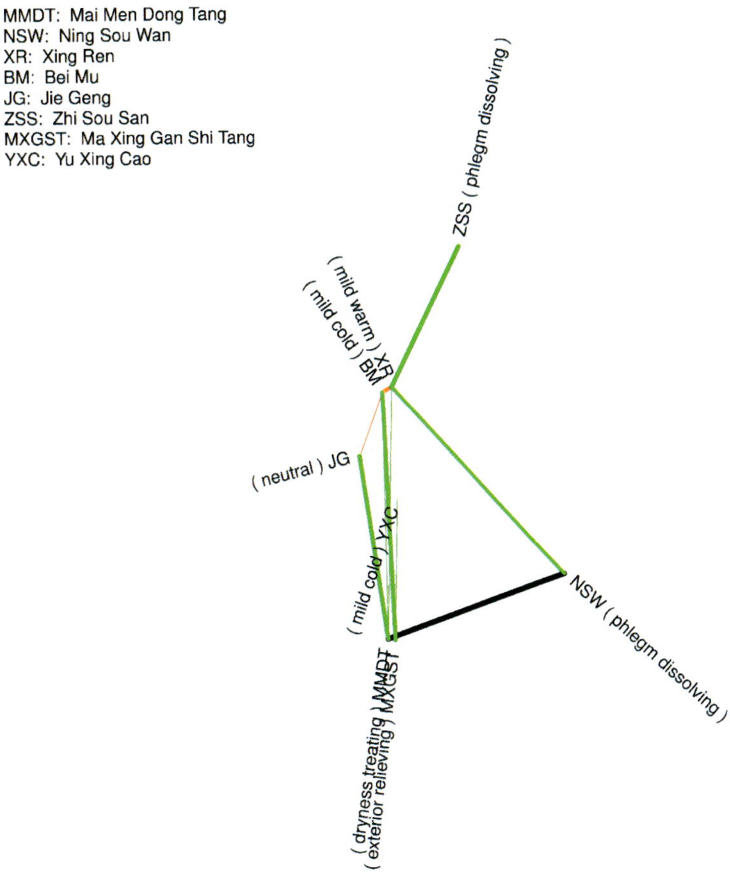

FIGURE 7.12b

The commonest TCM formula pair is MMDT–NSW, the commonest formula–herb pair is ZSS–XR, followed by MMDT–JG, MXGST–BM and NSW–XR, and the commonest herb pair is XR–BM for the treatment of COPD. The thickness of the line indicates the prevalence of the pair. Formula pairs are in black, formula–herb pairs in green and herb pairs in red. The TCM pharmacotherapeutic categories of the formulas and the TCM natures of the herbs are shown in parentheses.

7.17 Acute Bronchitis and Bronchiolitis: *Ma Xing Gan Shi Tang* and *Xing Ren*

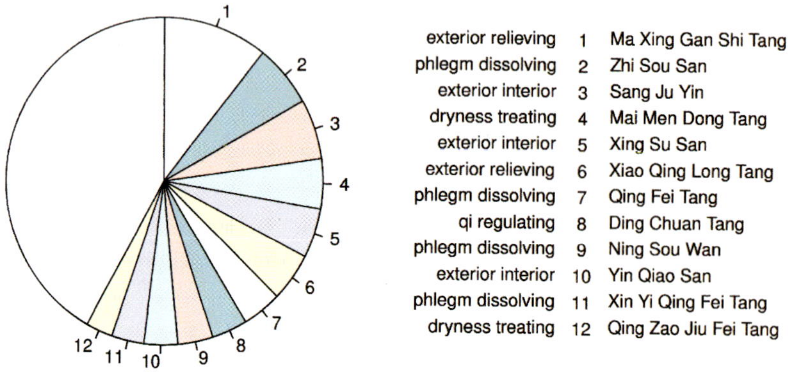

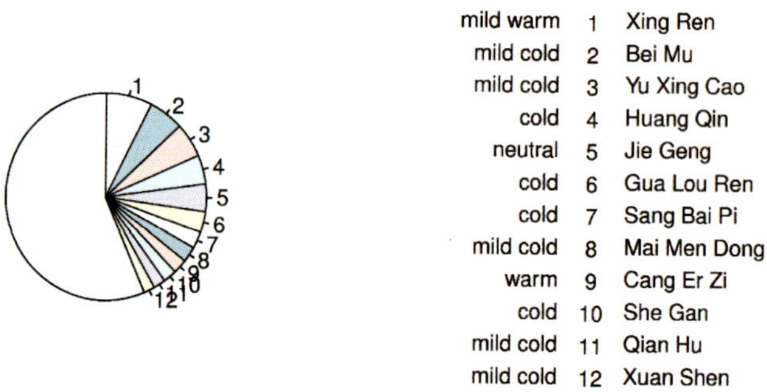

FIGURE 7.13a

Acute bronchitis and bronchiolitis (ICD-9 = 466) are treated by TCM phlegm-dissolving ($p = 0.002$) and exterior–interior ($p = 0.03$) formulas and TCM mild–cold ($p = 0.02$) herbs. The top 12 ingredients are shown. The areas of the pies indicate the relative weights of the formulas and herbs in the prescription for the condition. *P* values are from overrepresentation tests.

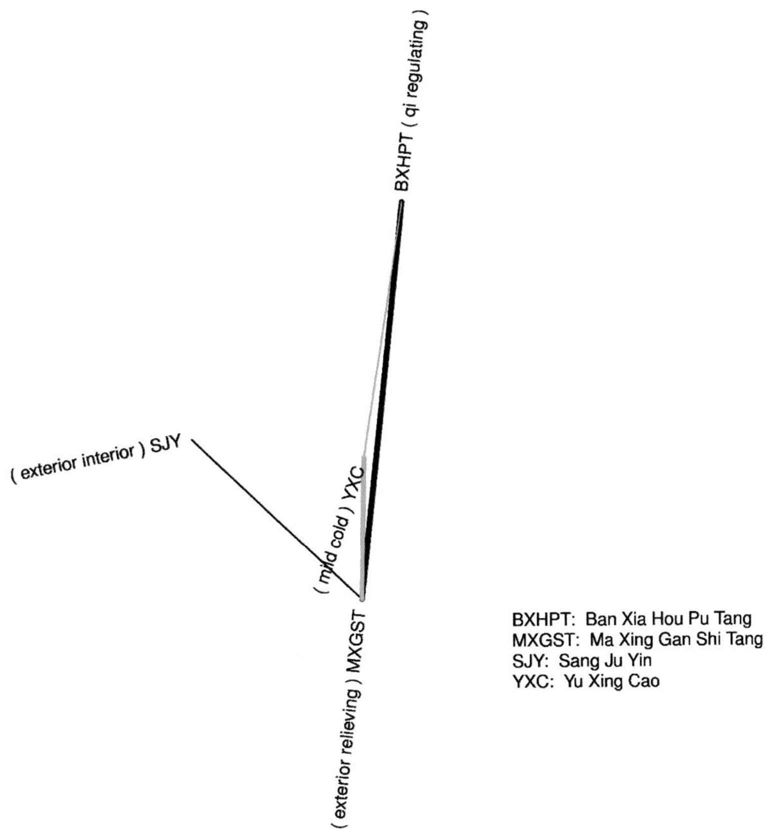

FIGURE 7.13b

The commonest TCM formula pair is MXGST–BXHPT and the commonest formula–herb pair is MXGST–YXC for the treatment of acute bronchitis and bronchiolitis. The thickness of the line indicates the prevalence of the pair. Formula pairs are in black and formula–herb pairs in green. The TCM pharmacotherapeutic categories of the formulas and the TCM natures of the herbs are shown in parentheses.

7.18 Tuberculosis: *Bai He Gu Jin Tang* and *Yu Xing Cao*

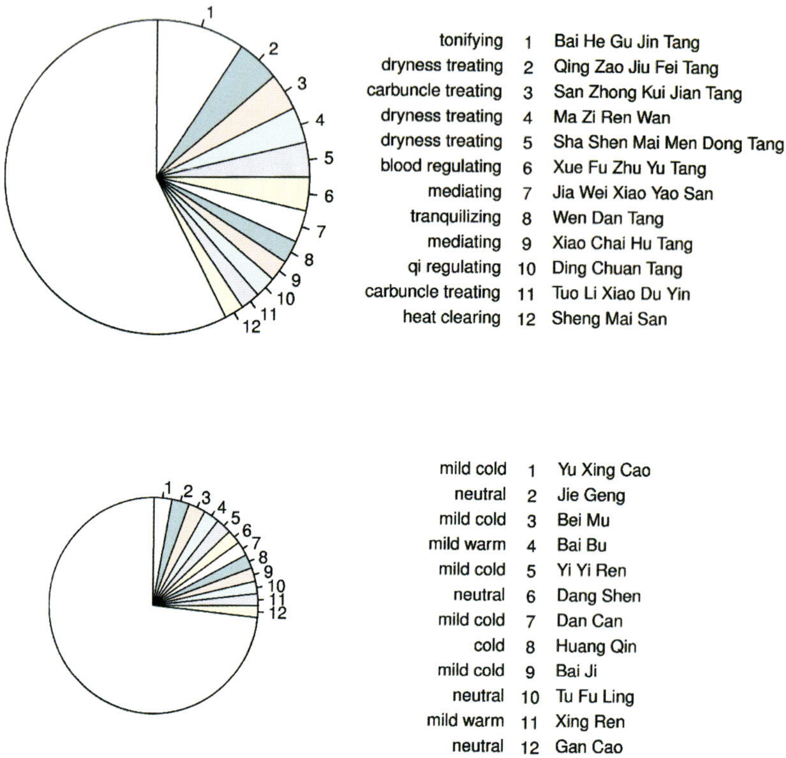

FIGURE 7.14a

Tuberculosis (ICD-9 = 10–18) is treated by TCM dryness-treating formulas ($p = 0.006$). The top 12 ingredients are shown. The areas of the pies indicate the relative weights of the formulas and herbs in the prescription for the condition. *P* values are from overrepresentation tests.

SLWLQY: Shi Liu Wei Liu Qi Yin
SZKJT: San Zhong Kui Jian Tang
XS: Xuan Shen
BM: Bei Mu
XR: Xing Ren
BZR: Bai Zi Ren
QH: Qiang Huo
GG: Ge Gen
SR: Sha Ren
SZR: Suan Zao Ren
HH: Hai Ha
FHS: Fu Hai Shi

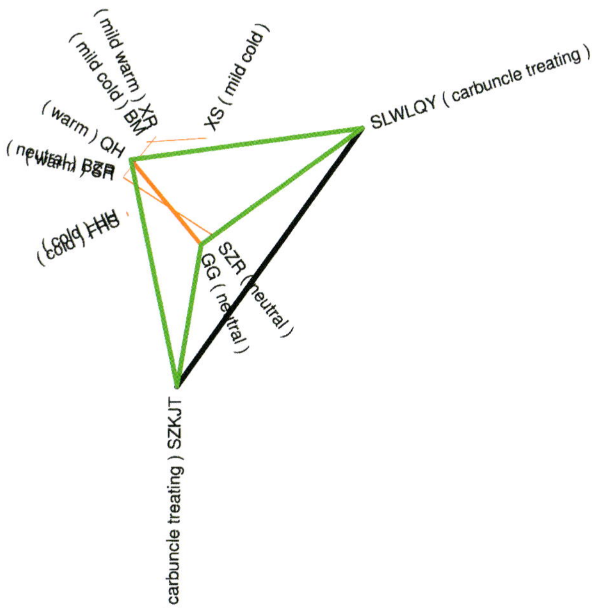

FIGURE 7.14b

The commonest TCM formula pair is SLWLQY–SZKJT, the commonest formula–herb pair is SZKJT–GG and the commonest herb pair is GG–QH, followed by SZR–SR, HH–FHS and BM–XS, for the treatment of tuberculosis. The thickness of the line indicates the prevalence of the pair. Formula pairs are in black, formula–herb pairs in green and herb pairs in red. The TCM pharmacotherapeutic categories of the formulas and the TCM natures of the herbs are shown in parentheses.

7.19 Pneumonia: *Yin Qiao San* and *Yu Xing Cao*

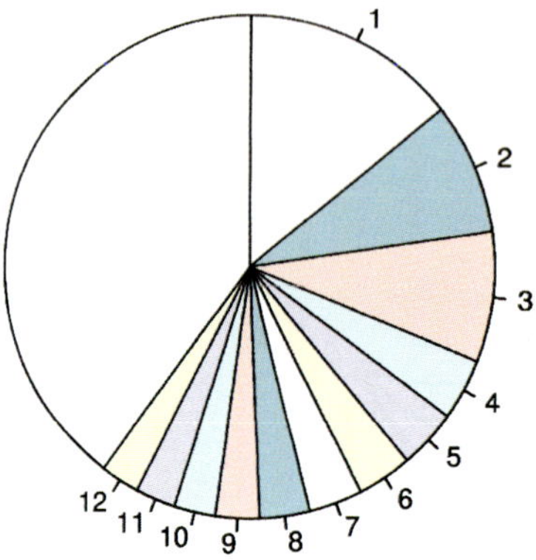

exterior interior	1	Yin Qiao San
exterior relieving	2	Ma Xing Gan Shi Tang
exterior interior	3	Sang Ju Yin
exterior relieving	4	Jing Fang Bai Du San
dampness eliminating	5	Ling Gui Zhu Gan Tang
dryness treating	6	Mai Men Dong Tang
exterior interior	7	Xing Su San
exterior relieving	8	Ge Gen Tang
exterior relieving	9	Chuan Xiong Cha Diao San
phlegm dissolving	10	Xin Yi Qing Fei Tang
dampness eliminating	11	Qiang Huo Sheng Shi Tang
mediating	12	Xiao Chai Hu Tang

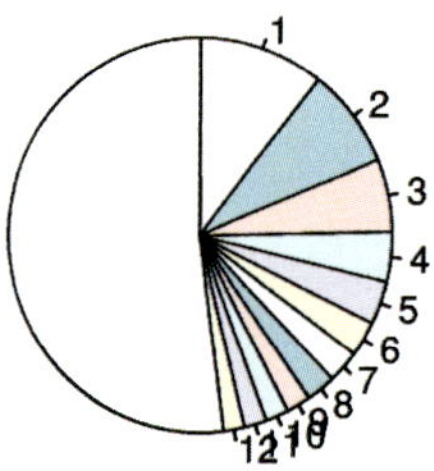

mild cold	1	Yu Xing Cao
neutral	2	Jie Geng
cold	3	Sang Bai Pi
cold	4	Niu Bang Zi
mild warm	5	Xing Ren
mild cold	6	Dong Gua Zi
cold	7	Pu Gong Ying
mild cold	8	Qian Hu
neutral	9	Gan Cao
warm	10	Bai Zhi
cold	11	Huang Qin
warm	12	Fang Feng

FIGURE 7.15a

Pneumonia (ICD-9 = 480–486) is treated by TCM exterior-relieving ($p = 0.003$) and exterior–interior ($p = 0.03$) formulas. The top 12 ingredients are shown. The areas of the pies indicate the relative weights of the formulas and herbs in the prescription for the condition. *P* values are from overrepresentation tests.

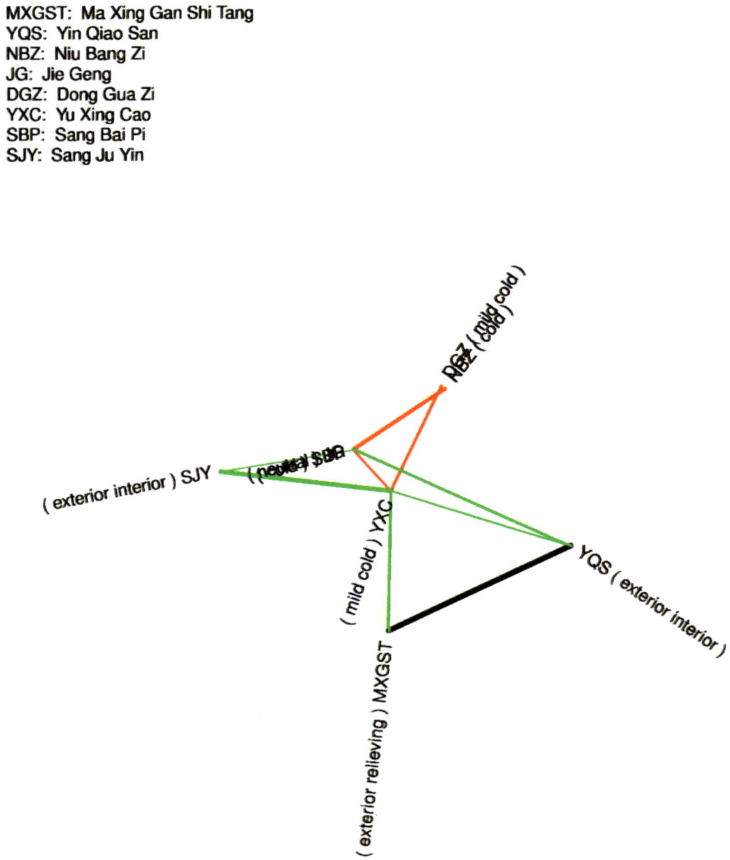

FIGURE 7.15b

The commonest TCM formula pair is MXGST–YQS, the commonest formula–herb pair is SJY–YXC, followed by MXGST–YXC and YQS–JG, and the commonest herb pair is JG–NBZ, followed by DGZ–YXC, for the treatment of pneumonia. The thickness of the line indicates the prevalence of the pair. Formula pairs are in black, formula–herb pairs in green and herb pairs in red. The TCM pharmacotherapeutic categories of the formulas and the TCM natures of the herbs are shown in parentheses.

7.20 Chronic Liver Disease and Cirrhosis: *Jia Wei Xiao Yao San* and *Yin Chen Hao*

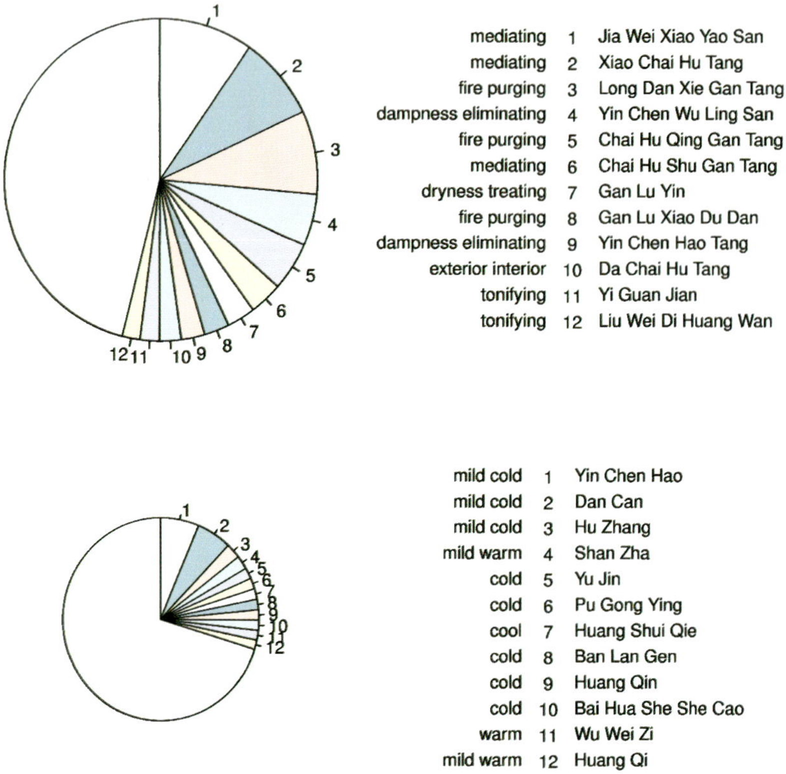

FIGURE 7.16a

Chronic liver disease and cirrhosis (ICD-9 = 571) are treated by TCM mediating formulas ($p = 0.03$) and TCM cold herbs ($p = 0.04$). The top 12 ingredients are shown. The areas of the pies indicate the relative weights of the formulas and herbs in the prescription for the condition. P values are from overrepresentation tests.

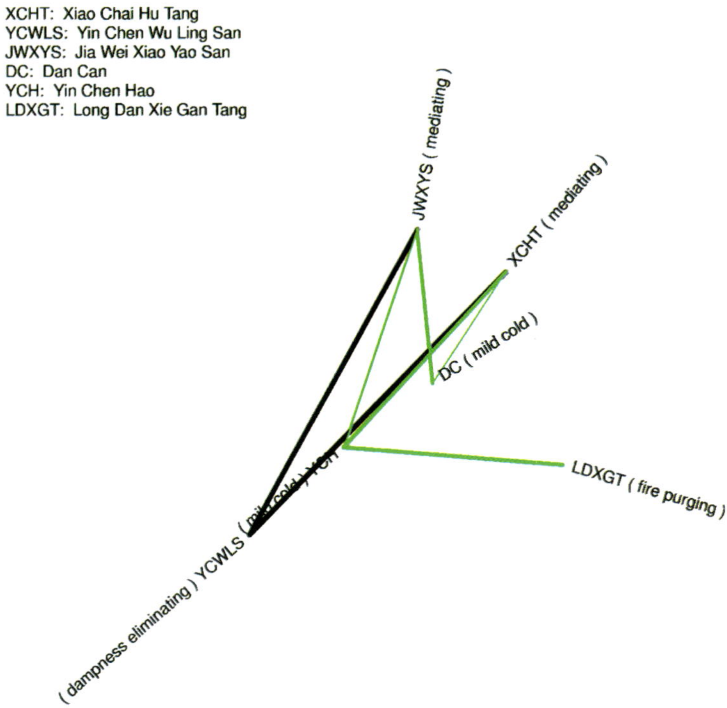

FIGURE 7.16b

The commonest TCM formula pair is XCHT–YCWLS and the commonest formula–herb pair is XCHT–YCH, followed by LDXGT–YCH and JWXYS–DC, for the treatment of chronic liver disease and cirrhosis. The thickness of the line indicates the prevalence of the pair. Formula pairs are in black and formula–herb pairs in green. The TCM pharmacotherapeutic categories of the formulas and the TCM natures of the herbs are shown in parentheses.

7.21 Obesity and Other Hyperalimentation: *Fang Feng Tong Sheng San* and *Shan Zha*

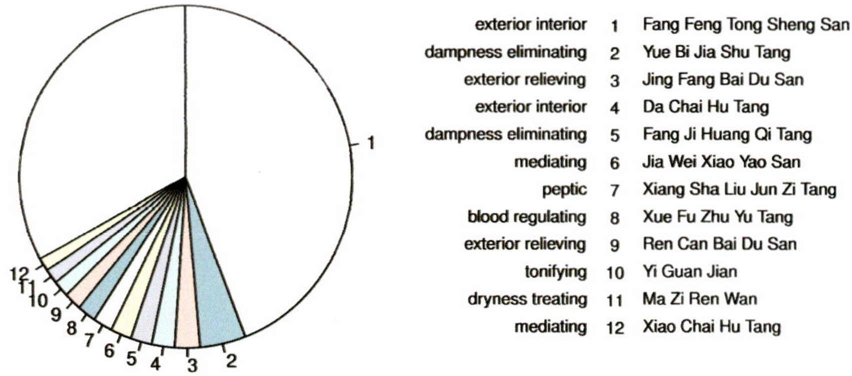

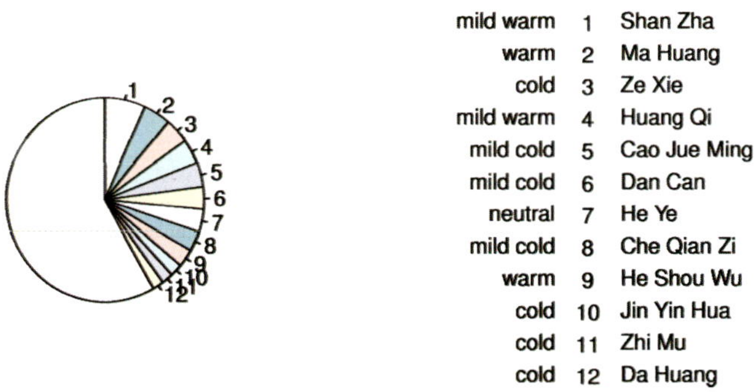

FIGURE 7.17a

Obesity (ICD-9 = 278) is predominantly treated by *fang feng tong sheng san*. The top 12 ingredients are shown. The areas of the pies indicate the relative weights of the formulas and herbs in the prescription for the condition.

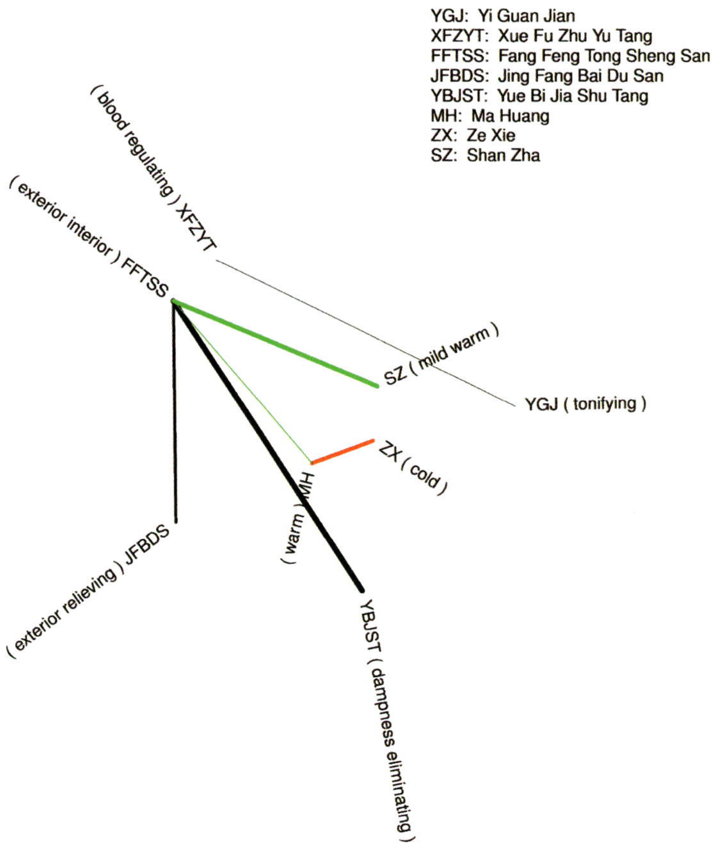

FIGURE 7.17b

The commonest TCM formula pair is FFTSS–YBJST, the commonest formula–herb pair is FFTSS–SZ and the commonest herb pair is MH–ZX for the treatment of obesity. The thickness of the line indicates the prevalence of the pair. Formula pairs are in black, formula–herb pairs in green and herb pairs in red. The TCM pharmacotherapeutic categories of the formulas and the TCM natures of the herbs are shown in parentheses.

7.22 Diarrhea: *Huo Xiang Zheng Qi San* and *Ge Gen*

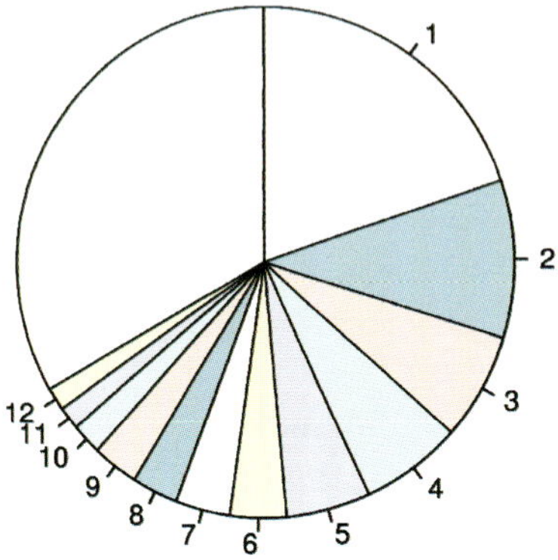

mediating	1	Huo Xiang Zheng Qi San
exterior interior	2	Ge Gen Huang Lian Huang Qin Tang
tonifying	3	Shen Ling Bai Zhu San
peptic	4	Wei Ling Tang
fire purging	5	Ban Xia Xie Xin Tang
peptic	6	Ping Wei San
peptic	7	Xiang Sha Liu Jun Zi Tang
cold dispersing	8	Li Zhong Tang
dampness eliminating	9	Wu Ling San
peptic	10	Bao He Wan
peptic	11	An Zhong San
tonifying	12	Bu Zhong Yi Qi Tang

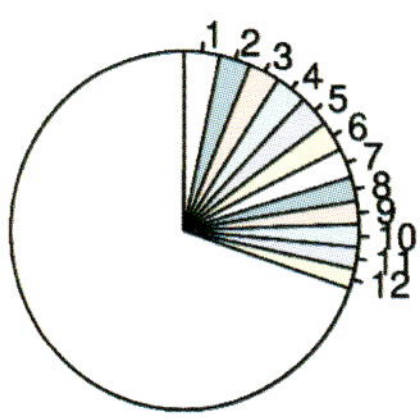

neutral	1	Ge Gen
warm	2	Hai Piao Shao
mild cold	3	Bai Shao
warm	4	Yan Hu Suo
warm	5	Mu Xiang
warm	6	Fang Feng
warm	7	Bai Shu
warm	8	Shen Qu
cold	9	Huang Qin
cold	10	Hua Shi
neutral	11	Fu Ling
warm	12	Chen Pi

FIGURE 7.18a

Diarrhea (ICD-9 = 787.91) is treated by TCM peptic formulas ($p = 0.00003$) and TCM warm herbs ($p = 0.02$). The top 12 ingredients are shown. The areas of the pies indicate the relative weights of the formulas and herbs in the prescription for the condition. *P* values are from overrepresentation tests.

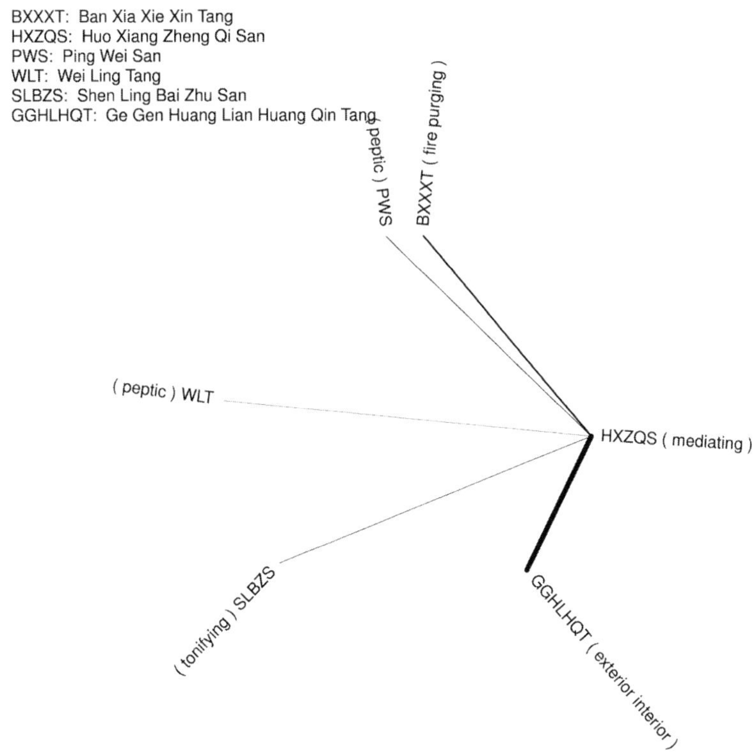

FIGURE 7.18b

The commonest TCM formula pair is HXZQS–GGHLHQT, followed by HXZQS–BXXXT and HXZQS–PWS, for the treatment of diarrhea. The thickness of the line indicates the prevalence of the pair. The TCM pharmacotherapeutic categories of the formulas are shown in parentheses.

8

Common Nonfatal Diseases

Big data is transforming not only information technology but also biotechnology. Biomedical studies are becoming data-driven and hypothesis-generating, in contrast to the hypothesis- or intuition-based approaches of conventional biomedical research. A year's worth of TCM prescription data offers an opportunity for quantitative TCM research. With 13.1 million TCM prescriptions for common nonfatal diseases and conditions, a statistically averaged prescription for each disease or condition is obtained. Although TCM, like other complementary and alternative medicines, advocates personalized medication, the average prescription serves as a reference prescription for a typical patient with the specific disease/condition. Personalized medicine can be achieved by adding/subtracting ingredients to/from the reference prescription. Different combinations of the identified top ingredients also help meet the demand for individualized prescription.

Analysis of large volumes of TCM prescriptions reveals that doses of the ingredients follow Zipf's law (discovered by linguist George Kingsley Zipf in 1935), which governs the frequencies of words in text corpora. If we liken TCM herbs to words and TCM formulas to phrases, TCM prescriptions can be thought of as a dialect used by TCM doctors in communications with the human body. Just as bilingualism or multilingualism is beneficial to cognitive development and is a norm in modern cultures, integration of TCM herbalism and conventional medicine can enrich human healthcare.

8.1 Common Cold, Cough, Allergic/Chronic Rhinitis

Acute viral nasopharyngitis is best known as the common cold. It is an acute viral infection of the upper respiratory tract, including the nose and throat. The number of viruses causing the common cold is over 200, rhinoviruses accounting for over a quarter of them. Symptoms of the common cold, ranging from sore throat, runny nose, cough, fever, muscle ache to headache, arise from the immune response to the infection. The illness shows a seasonal trend, with a high incidence in winter and early spring. People stay indoors in cold weather; common cold viruses stay longer and disperse farther when the humidity is low. The two factors raise transmissibility and explain the prevalence of the common cold in winter and spring although the infection is perennial.

Cough is a protective mechanism of the body to remove foreign materials or excessive secretions from the respiratory system. It is activated by the pulmonary irritant receptors in the epithelium of the upper respiratory tract in response to stimuli, which can be mechanical (foreign particles), chemical (irritants) or biological (microbes). Cough is one of the common reactions of the respiratory system to common cold infection.

Rhinitis is the inflammation of the mucous membranes in the nose in response to viruses, bacteria, irritants or allergens. Causes of chronic rhinitis can be of allergic or nonallergic origins. Allergic rhinitis results from parasitic immune response (i.e. immunoglobulin E) of the nasal membranes in atopic individuals to nonparasitic antigens. Nonparasitic antigens, or allergens, include pollen, dust, chemical irritants, animal dander and some food proteins. When the allergen is grass pollen, the allergy is known as hay fever. For nonallergic chronic rhinitis, vasomotor rhinitis is the commonest. It is induced by smells, fumes, smoke or temperature changes causing swelling and then drainage of the blood vessels in the lining of the nose. The incidence of chronic rhinitis can be seasonal or perennial, depending on the cause.

8.2 Sleep Disturbance, Headache, Palpitations, Dizziness

Sleep disturbances include insomnia, hypersomnia, circadian rhythm sleep disorder, night terrors, obstructive sleep apnea, tooth-grinding, sleepwalking and bedwetting. A sleep disturbance can be a primary sleep disorder not attributable to other causes. It can also be comorbid with or secondary to other conditions. Sleep disturbance has been associated with cognitive decline and other morbidity/mortality. For example, an age-independent phase advance of the sleep–wake cycle has been associated with lower cognitive function [Auyeung *et al.*, 2012]. Cognitive deficit was also associated with prolonged nocturnal sleep duration and daytime napping. Note, however, that observational studies do not differentiate between cause and effect. Further studies will help elucidate the role of sleep disturbances in pathogenesis including aging.

Functional elements of the brain lack pain receptors (or nociceptors). However, other parts of the brain including the meninges, blood vessels, cranial nerves, sinuses, and head and neck muscles are endowed with pain receptors. Problems, such as traction or inflammation, of the pain-sensitive (or pain-insensitive) parts can directly (or indirectly) trigger headache. Common primary headaches include migraine, cluster headache and tension headache. Migraine and cluster headache are unilateral, while tension headache is bilateral, affecting both sides of the head. The exact causes of the primary headaches are not known.

Normal heart rates are between 60 and 100 beats per minute, and people are not aware of their own heart beating. Palpitations are the sensation of abnormalities in the heartbeat, including rapid, irregular or forceful heartbeats. Causes of palpitations can be sympathetic overdrive or cardiac dysrhythmia. Examples of causes are overexertion, exercise, stress, anxiety, panic, adrenaline, alcohol, nicotine, caffeine, hyperthyroidism, hypoxia and low blood potassium.

Dizziness can be: (1) a spinning sensation known as vertigo; (2) an off-balance sensation called disequilibrium; or (3) a fainting sensation, i.e. light-headedness. Vertigo is caused by injury or aging of the inner ear or the balance center of the central nervous system. In particular, an underlying cause of episodic vertigo is diabetic neuropathy. Inadequate blood supply to the brain because of low blood pressure, low blood oxygen, low blood sugar and anemia can give rise to light-headedness. Hormonal changes during menstruation, depression and anxiety also contribute to the feeling of dizziness.

8.3 Arthralgia, Cervicalgia, Backache, Lumbago, Myalgia, Fibromyalgia, Neuralgia

Arthralgia, or joint pain, is a result of injury, disease or infection of a joint. Common causes of joint pain include rheumatoid arthritis, osteoarthritis and gout. Cervicalgia, or neck pain, is pain in the rear or side of cervical vertebrae including the neck, shoulders and upper back. It can also occur when the head rotates or twists. The causes of cervicalgia include muscle tightness, neck joint inflammation, bulging/degenerating intervertebral disks, pinched nerves, whiplash, overuse or posture.

Lumbago is pain in the region lateral to the lower spine including the lower back and buttocks. It can result from herniation of the intervertebral disks due to injury or overactivity. Poor posture due to a sagging mattress may cause lumbago. Degeneration of the intervertebral disks through aging or smoking can also cause it.

Myalgia, or muscle pain, stems from overuse, injury/trauma or chronic tension of the skeletal muscle. Torn muscles called strains can cause muscle pain, and so can torn ligaments called sprains. Fibromyalgia is a widespread pain not only in skeletal muscles, but also in soft tissues known as tender points. The causes of fibromyalgia are unknown and it is theorized that people with it have an increased sensitivity in the brain to pain because of repeated nerve stimulation. Myositis is inflammation of the skeletal muscle caused by injury, infection or autoimmune disease.

Neuralgia is intermittent but frequent sharp, shocking pain along the paths of nerves which have been damaged by injury, trauma or disease. Degeneration or improper regeneration of the damaged neurons sends non-nociceptive pain signals to the brain, causing sensations of intense burning or stabbing pains. The two commonest examples of neuralgia are postherpetic neuralgia and trigeminal neuralgia. The former is caused by neurons infected by shingles or herpes zoster and the latter by pressure on the trigeminal nerve, which is the largest nerve in the skull. Wearing ill-fitting shoes such as high-heeled ones can damage and subsequently inflame the nerves to the toes, causing numbness and pain in the affected toes. Inflammation of the peripheral nervous system is called neuritis. Diabetes and cancer can be underlying conditions causing neuritis.

8.4 Constipation, Dyspepsia, Bloating, Acute Gastritis

Constipation is harder or less passage of stools than normal due to obstructive defecation or colonic hypomotility. Improper coordination of bowel muscles can cause constipation. Absence of intestinal ganglion cells is also a cause. Dietary factors, including inadequate fiber or fluid intake, contribute to constipation. Endocrinal factors, such as hypothyroidism, are known risks for it. Some medications, such as painkillers, entail constipation as a side effect. Disturbance in gut microbial flora has also been linked to constipation. Probiotics, such as yogurt, which restore intestinal microbial balance, are potentially a cost-effective remedy for metabolic syndrome including constipation and obesity. Insoluble fiber in foods is metabolically inert. While moving through the digestive system, it absorbs water and pushes waste along with it to make the stools bulky yet soft, easing defecation. Sources of insoluble fiber include whole grains, wheat bran, celery and the skin of fruits such as tomatoes.

Dyspepsia is difficult digestion. Various symptoms of dyspepsia in the upper abdomen are early satiety, fullness, discomfort, bloating, belching, pain, and nausea with or without vomiting. The mechanisms underlying nonulcer or functional dyspepsia, excluding structural and metabolic ones, include gastric neuromuscular impairment resulting from autonomic nerve system–central nerve system dysregulation. Nonulcer dyspepsia is associated with gastritis and gastric reflux disease.

Bloating means a distended or swollen abdomen. Abdominal bloating can cause pain anywhere in the abdominal region due to stomach cramps. Bloating can be caused by overeating, food allergy or gas-producing foods, and is associated with constipation and menstruation. Soluble fiber in foods is readily fermented by the bacteria in the colon, producing gases and short-chain fatty acids (SCFAs). Foods rich in soluble fiber and low in fluid can cause bloating or constipation. On the other hand, SCFAs are known to suppress liver cholesterol synthesis and lower blood LDL cholesterol, promoting a healthy effect against atherosclerosis. Sources of soluble fiber include oats, almonds, bananas and carrots. Fresh plant foods that contain both soluble and insoluble fibers plus plenty of water promote healthy digestion.

Acute gastritis is inflammation of the mucosal lining of the stomach. The symptoms of acute gastritis are epigastric discomforts, including nausea, vomiting, belching, bloating and loss of appetite. Patients can occasionally present pains in the upper central abdomen or upper left abdomen. Excessive consumption of alcohol or prolonged use of nonsteroidal anti-inflammatory drugs (NSAIDs) such as aspirin can cause acute gastritis.

8.5 Chronic Hepatitis, Contact Dermatitis

Hepatitis is inflammation of the liver. Common causes of hepatitis are viral infection and alcohol abuse. In the case of viral hepatitis, infected individuals may present flu-like symptoms or show no symptoms at all. Most adults recover and develop antibodies against future infection. However, a small number of the infected, including most infants and children, fail to eliminate the virus six months after infection, becoming chronically infected. The symptoms of chronic hepatitis are nonspecific ranging from malaise, tiredness, weakness, liver enlargement to jaundice. Chronic hepatitis can lead to liver cancer or cirrhosis. The major hepatitis viruses are HBV and HAV. Both of them can be contracted through blood-to-blood contact. HBV can spread through other body fluids, including saliva, semen and vaginal fluid. While there is a vaccine against HBV, there is none against HAV.

Contact dermatitis is inflammation of the epidermis, i.e. the outer layer of the skin, after its direct contact with a substance. It is of two types: irritant and allergic. Irritant contact dermatitis is caused by contact with acidic or alkaline materials such as detergents, soaps, fabric softeners, solvents, hair dyes, weedkillers and rubber gloves. The reaction of the skin to the irritant is immediate, with patchy red rashes over the region of contact. The rashes can present widespread pain. Allergic contact dermatitis is due to cell-mediated allergic response to an agent to which one becomes hypersensitive. Common allergens are found in fabrics, clothing, perfumes, cosmetics, metals and poison ivy. Skin reaction to allergens can be delayed (by about one day), with red itchy rashes confined to the area of contact.

8.6 Pharmacokinetics of TCM Prescription by Relative Weighting of the Ingredients

Airborne pathogens and irritants inflict the nasopharynx, causing such conditions as the common cold, cough and allergic/chronic rhinitis. Physical work by muscles and bones of the body can cause pain in joints, (low) back, neck and muscles. Binge eating and *Helicobacter pylori* can cause bloating, dyspepsia or gastritis. We find that TCM prescribes: (1) exterior-relieving ($p = 0.0006$) and phlegm-dissolving ($p = 0.006$) formulas for the respiratory diseases; (2) blood-regulating ($p = 0.00002$) and wind-expelling ($p = 0.002$) formulas and warm ($p = 0.006$) herbs for musculoskeletal pain; and (3) peptic ($p = 0.0009$) and fire-purging ($p = 0.02$) formulas and warm ($p = 0.0001$) herbs for digestive dysfunctions. If the fraction of exterior-relieving formulas in the pool of all the prescribable formulas is x, a p value gives the chance that, when one randomly selects a number of formulas from the pool, one would get exterior-relieving formulas at a fraction of no less than x in the randomly selected formulas. A small p value indicates the existence of non-random factors, such as TCM herbalism, behind the prescriptions.

TCM exterior-relieving formulas relieve fever by sweating. In TCM, phlegm can be caused by not only chills but also overeating, alcohol and spleen deficiency. The early symptoms of phlegm *zheng* include fever and headache — akin to exopathic infection. One way

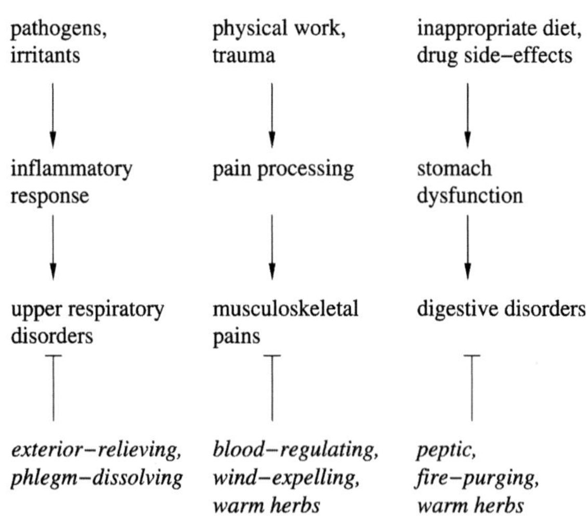

FIGURE 8.1

Common nonfatal diseases and conditions, and the prescribed TCM formulas and herbs. Upper respiratory disorders include the common cold, cough and allergic/chronic rhinitis. Musculoskeletal pains include neck pain, joint pain, backache, low back pain, neuralgia, neuritis, radiculitis, myalgia, myositis and fibromyositis. Digestive disorders include functional dyspepsia, gas/bloating and acute gastritis. Pointed arrows indicate promotion; blunt arrows indicate suppression.

of dissolving phlegm is to strengthen the spleen. TCM blood-regulating formulas alleviate pain by encouraging blood flow, which is supported by the gate control theory of pain [Melzack and Wall, 1965]. In TCM, joint and muscle pains are thought to be caused mainly by such exogenous factors as wind and dampness. Successful intrusion of either or both of the factors into a *qi*-deficient (i.e. immunodeficient) individual blocks his or her meridians, inducing pain. TCM peptic formulas treat indigestion by helping empty the stomach. One of the western equivalents of TCM fire is metabolism, whose excess can elevate oxidative stress. TCM fire-purging formulas are therefore theorized to be antioxidant and anti-inflammatory. TCM warm herbs relieve stasis and dampness by promoting blood flow.

TCM prescriptions for the common nonfatal diseases and conditions are specific to the pathologies, which in turn are dependent on the organ and tissue systems of the body. For example, prescriptions for musculoskeletal pains are distinct from those for other conditions. Moreover, prescriptions for digestive morbidities differ from those for other morbidities. The common cold, cough, allergic/chronic rhinitis, headache and dizziness all affect the head. TCM prescriptions for these conditions are therefore similar in terms of formula and herbal ingredients. On the other hand, conditions such as sleep disturbance, constipation, contact dermatitis, chronic hepatitis and palpitations are prescribed ingredients that distinguish one condition from another, suggesting that in TCM these conditions are considered to be related (or secondary) to yet other independent conditions not considered in this chapter. Furthermore, clustering of the musculoskeletal pain prescriptions indicates that different anatomical sites need to be exposed to different weighting of the prominent ingredients for pain. That is to say, TCM herbalism changes the pharmacokinetics of a TCM prescription by varying the weights of the ingredients. Therefore, if the disease mechanism is the same (e.g. pain) but the disease sites are different (e.g. neck versus shoulder), then the TCM prescription for shoulder pain, which is not included in the current edition of this book, can be obtained from linear imputation of the ones for neck pain and backache, both of which are included in this chapter. The average number of formulas in the prescriptions for nonfatal diseases/conditions is found to be between two and three; so is the average number of herbs. Formulas are invariantly heavier than herbs in the prescription. The doses of the ingredients are found to follow the 100:65:50:42:36 ratios. Compared with the less steep drop of the ingredient doses in the prescriptions for fatal diseases and malignant neoplasms, TCM relies on the top few ingredients for the treatment of nonfatal diseases

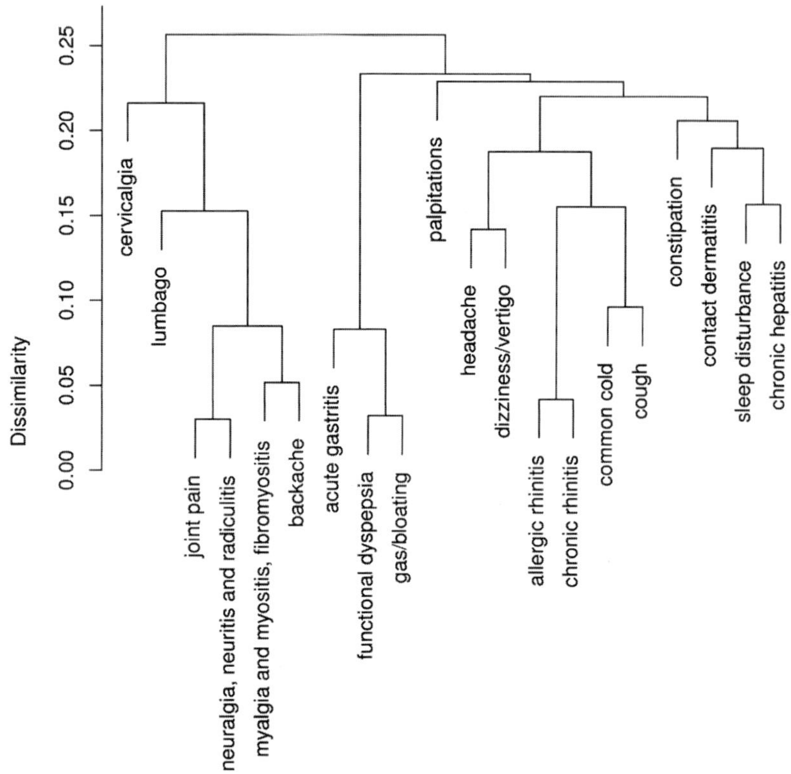

FIGURE 8.2

Clustering of TCM prescriptions for common nonfatal diseases and conditions. Prescriptions which are similar, in terms of the ingredients and the relative weights of the ingredients in the prescription, fall within a branch of the tree in the hierarchical clustering analysis. Prescriptions for musculoskeletal pains, digestive conditions and upper respiratory diseases cluster within separate branches. The vertical axis measures pairwise distance or dissimilarity between prescriptions.

and conditions. In a linguistic analogy, more frequent use of fewer lexicons is practiced in the dialogue between the TCM doctor and the body suffering from nonfatal conditions.

8.7 The Common Cold: *Yin Qiao San* and *Jie Geng*

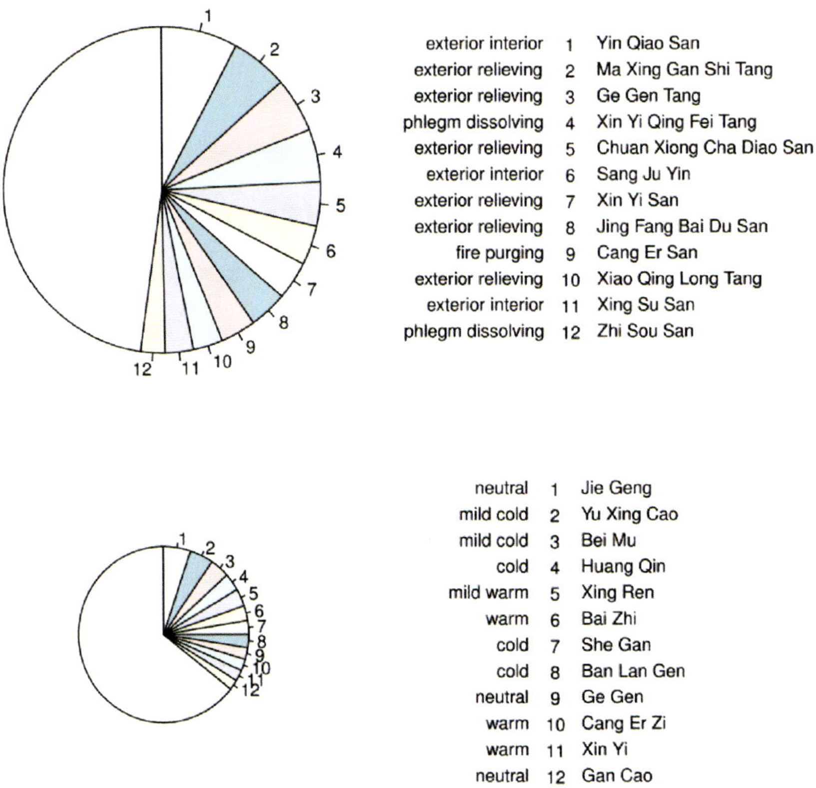

FIGURE 8.3a

The common cold (ICD-9 = 460) is treated by TCM exterior-relieving ($p = 0.00002$) and exterior–interior ($p = 0.03$) formulas. The top 12 ingredients are shown. The areas of the pies indicate the relative weights of the formulas and herbs in the prescription for the condition. *P* values are from overrepresentation tests.

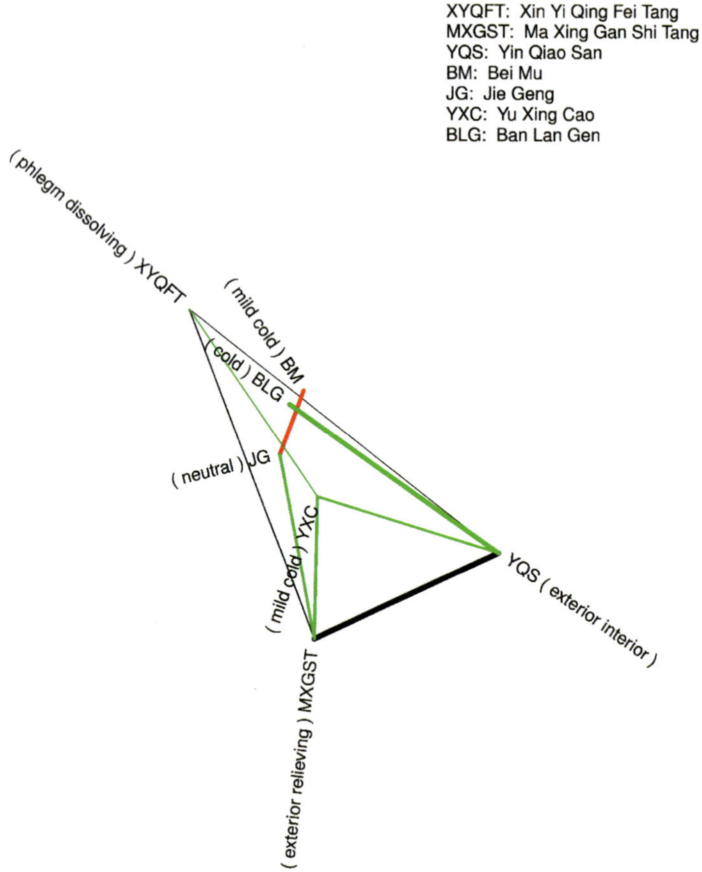

FIGURE 8.3b

The commonest TCM formula pair is YQS–MXGST, the commonest formula–herb pair is YQS–BLG, followed by MXGST–YXC and MXGST–JG, and the commonest herb pair is JG–BM for the treatment of the common cold. The thickness of the line indicates the prevalence of the pair. Formula pairs are in black, formula–herb pairs in green and herb pairs in red. The TCM pharmacotherapeutic categories of the formulas and the TCM the natures of the herbs are shown in parentheses.

8.8 Cough: *Ma Xing Gan Shi Tang* and *Jie Geng*

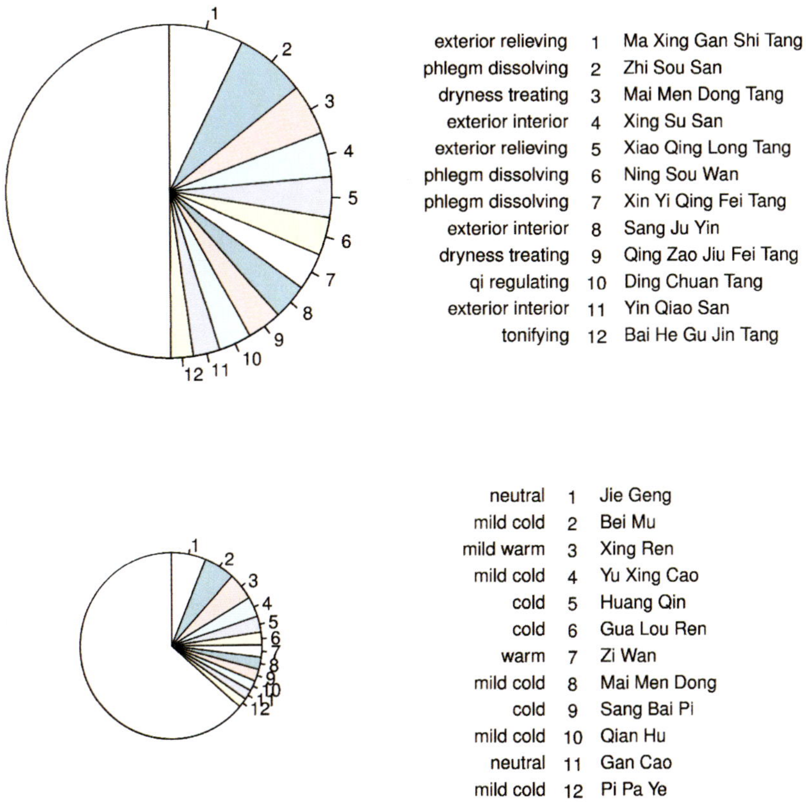

FIGURE 8.4a

Cough (ICD-9 = 7862) is treated by TCM phlegm-dissolving ($p = 0.02$) and exterior–interior ($p = 0.03$) formulas and TCM mild–cold ($p = 0.02$) herbs. The top 12 ingredients are shown. The areas of the pies indicate the relative weights of the formulas and herbs in the prescription for the condition. *P* values are from over-representation tests.

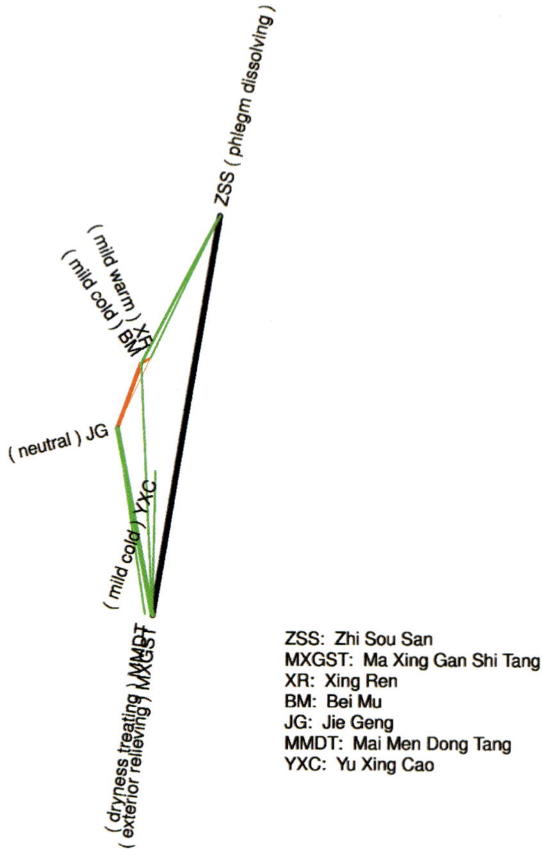

FIGURE 8.4b

The commonest TCM formula pair is MXGST–ZSS, the commonest formula–herb pair is MXGST–JG, followed by ZSS–BM, MXGST–BM and MXGST–YXC, and the commonest herb pair is BM–JG, followed by BM–XR, for the treatment of cough. The thickness of the line indicates the prevalence of the pair. Formula pairs are in black, formula–herb pairs in green and herb pairs in red. The TCM pharmacotherapeutic categories of the formulas and the TCM natures of the herbs are shown in parentheses.

8.9 Allergic Rhinitis: *Xin Yi Qing Fei Tang* and *Chan Tui*

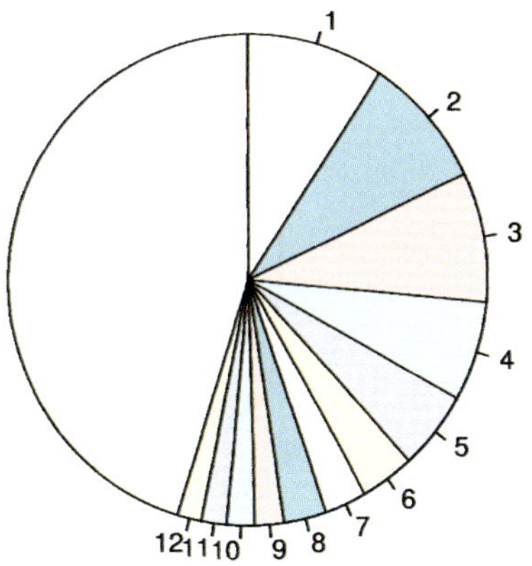

phlegm dissolving	1	Xin Yi Qing Fei Tang
exterior relieving	2	Xin Yi San
exterior relieving	3	Xiao Qing Long Tang
fire purging	4	Cang Er San
exterior relieving	5	Ge Gen Tang
tonifying	6	Bu Zhong Yi Qi Tang
exterior relieving	7	Gui Zhi Tang
astringing	8	Yu Ping Feng San
exterior relieving	9	Xiao Qing Long San
dampness eliminating	10	Ling Gui Zhu Gan Tang
exterior relieving	11	Chuan Xiong Cha Diao San
exterior relieving	12	Ma Xing Gan Shi Tang

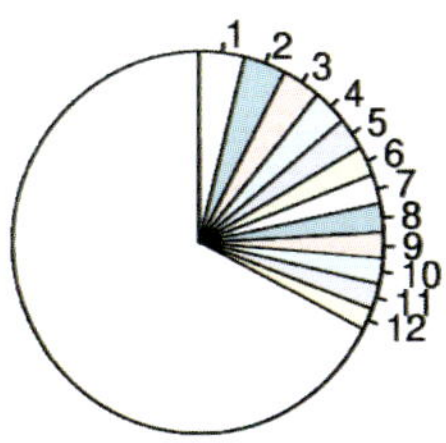

cool	1	Chan Tui
warm	2	Bai Zhi
warm	3	Cang Er Zi
mild cold	4	Yu Xing Cao
warm	5	Xin Yi
warm	6	Fang Feng
neutral	7	Jie Geng
mild warm	8	Jing Jie
neutral	9	Gan Cao
cold	10	Huang Qin
warm	11	E Bu Shi Cao
mild cold	12	Bei Mu

FIGURE 8.5a

Allergic rhinitis (ICD-9 = 4779) is treated by TCM exterior-relieving formulas ($p = 0.0000006$). The top 12 ingredients are shown. The areas of the pies indicate the relative weights of the formulas and herbs in the prescription for the conditions. *P* values are from overrepresentation tests.

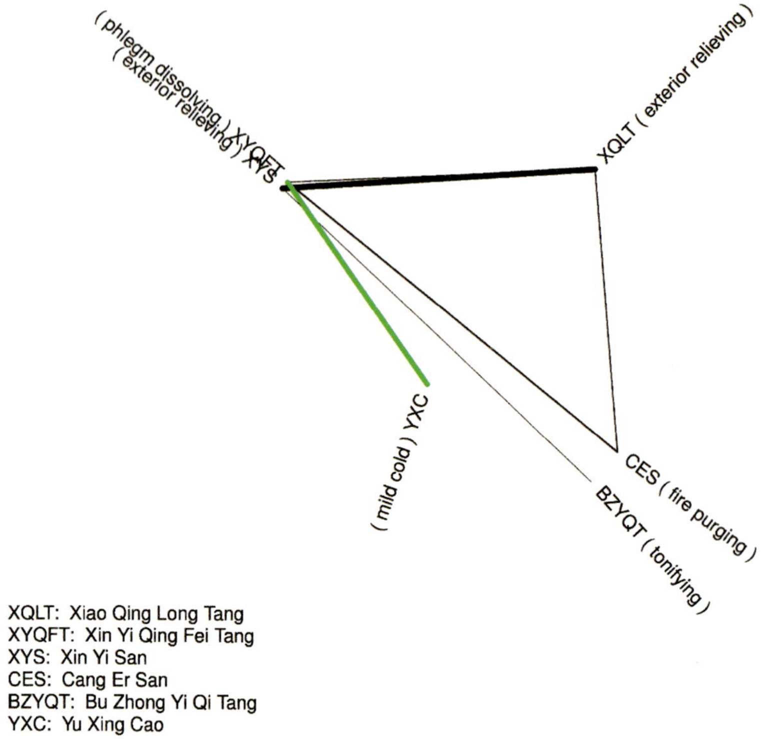

FIGURE 8.5b

The commonest TCM formula pair is XYS–XQLT and the commonest formula–herb pair is XYQFT–YXC for the treatment of allergic rhinitis. The thickness of the line indicates the prevalence of the pair. Formula pairs are in black and formula–herb pairs in green. The TCM pharmacotherapeutic categories of the formulas and the TCM natures of the herbs are shown in parentheses.

8.10 Chronic Rhinitis: *Xin Yi Qing Fei Tang* and *Yu Xing Cao*

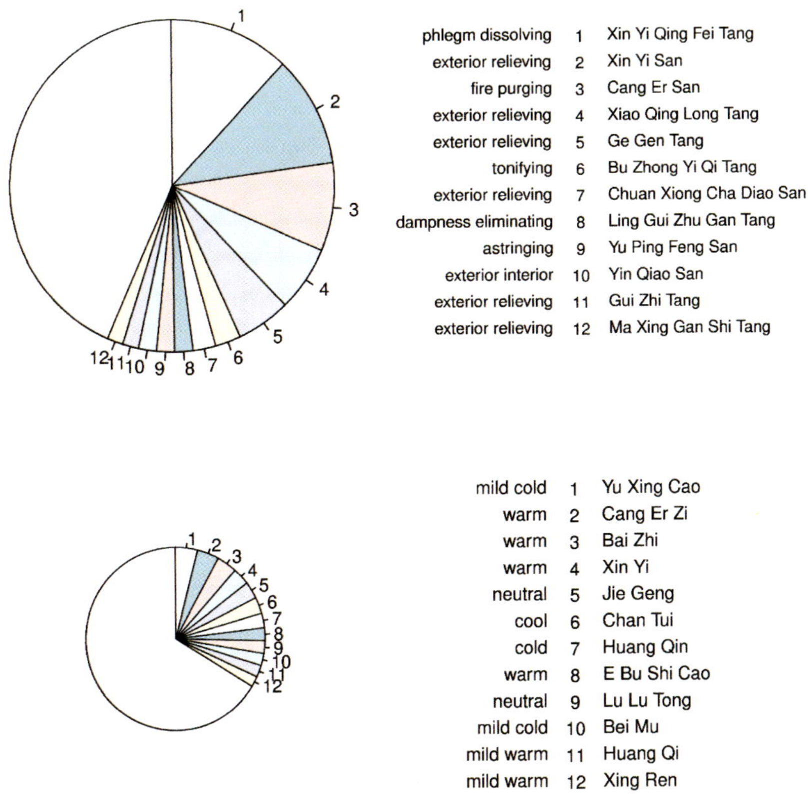

FIGURE 8.6a

Chronic rhinitis (ICD-9 = 4720) is treated by TCM exterior-relieving formulas ($p = 0.00002$). The top 12 ingredients are shown. The areas of the pies indicate the relative weights of the formulas and herbs in the prescription for the condition. *P* values are from overrepresentation tests.

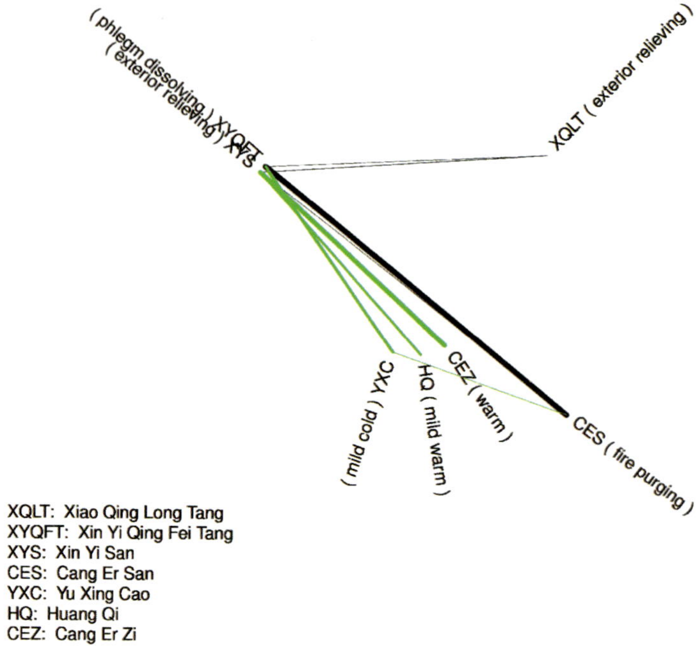

FIGURE 8.6b

The commonest TCM formula pair is XYQFT–CES and the commonest formula–herb pair is XYS–CEZ, followed by XYQFT–YXC, for the treatment of chronic rhinitis. The thickness of the line indicates the prevalence of the pair. Formula pairs are in black and formula–herb pairs in green. The TCM pharmacotherapeutic categories of the formulas and the TCM natures of the herbs are shown in parentheses.

8.11 Joint Pain: *Shu Jing Huo Xue Tang* and *Yan Hu Suo*

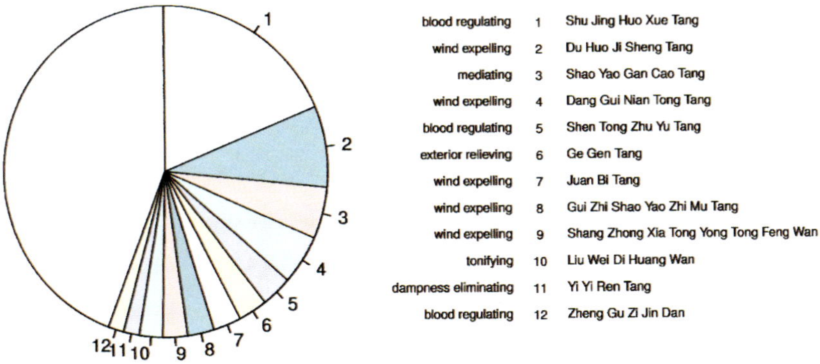

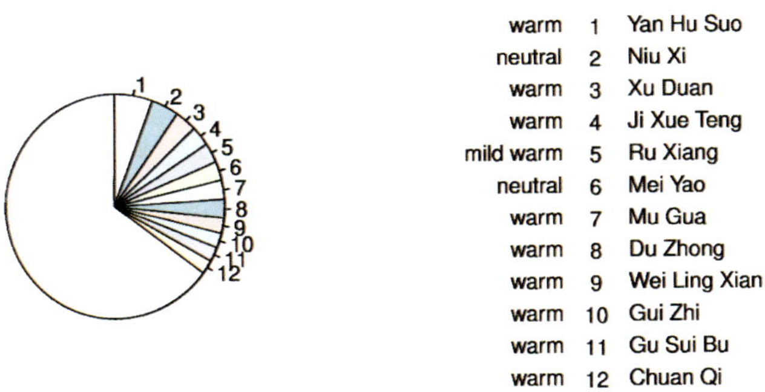

FIGURE 8.7a

Joint pain (ICD-9 = 7194) is treated by TCM wind-expelling (p = 0.0001) and blood-regulating (p = 0.04) formulas and TCM warm (p = 0.0005) herbs. The top 12 ingredients are shown. The areas of the pies indicate the relative weights of the formulas and herbs in the prescription for the condition. P values are from over-representation tests.

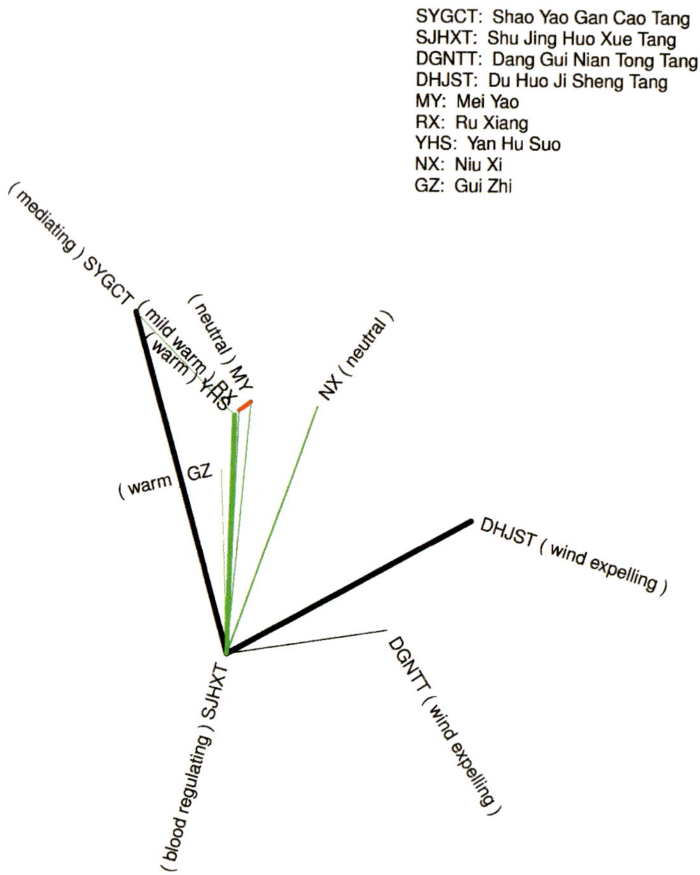

FIGURE 8.7b

The commonest TCM formula pair is SJHXT–DHJST, the commonest formula–herb pair is SJHXT–YHS, followed by SJHXT–NX, and the commonest herb pair is MY–RX for the treatment of joint pain. The thickness of the line indicates the prevalence of the pair. Formula pairs are in black, formula–herb pairs in green and herb pairs in red. The TCM pharmacotherapeutic categories of the formulas and the TCM natures of the herbs are shown in parentheses.

8.12 Lumbago: *Du Huo Ji Sheng Tang* and *Du Zhong*

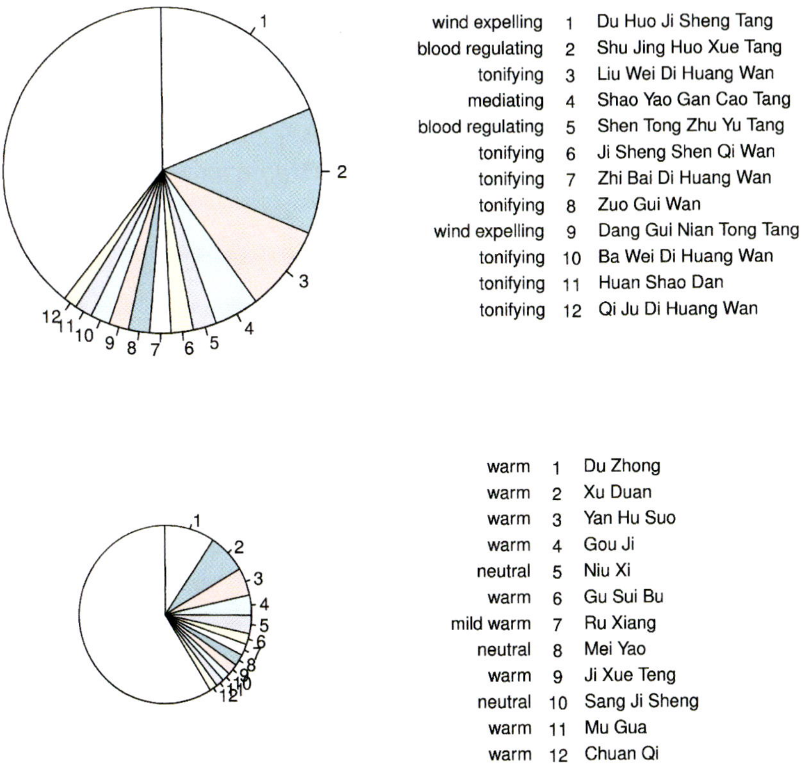

FIGURE 8.8a

Lumbago (ICD-9 = 7242) is treated by TCM tonifying formulas (p = 0.0002) and TCM warm herbs (p = 0.003). The top 12 ingredients are shown. The areas of the pies indicate the relative weights of the formulas and herbs in the prescription for the condition. P values are from overrepresentation tests.

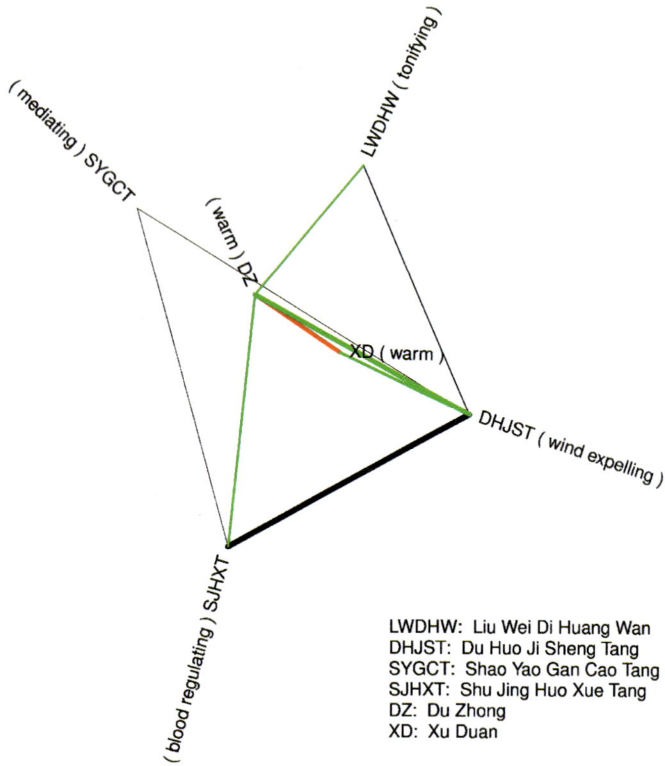

FIGURE 8.8b

The commonest TCM formula pair is DHJST–SJHXT, the commonest formula–herb pair is DHJST–DZ and the commonest herb pair is DZ–XD for the treatment of lumbago. The thickness of the line indicates the prevalence of the pair. Formula pairs are in black, formula–herb pairs in green and herb pairs in red. The TCM pharmacotherapeutic categories of the formulas and the TCM natures of the herbs are shown in parentheses.

8.13 Myalgia and Myositis, Fibromyositis: *Shu Jing Huo Xue Tang* and *Yan Hu Suo*

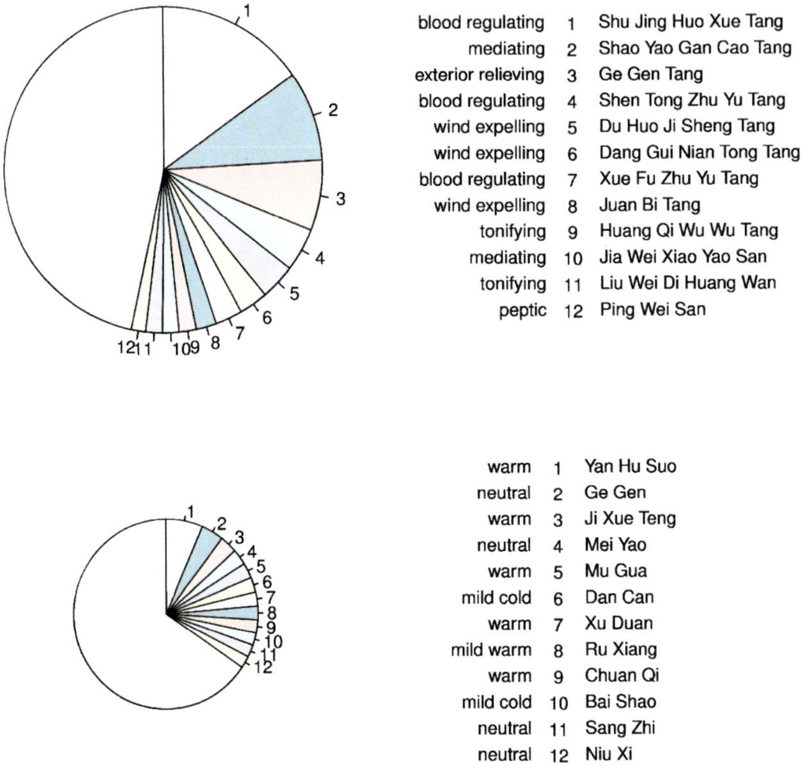

FIGURE 8.9a

Myalgia and myositis, fibromyositis (ICD-9 = 7291) are treated by TCM wind-expelling ($p = 0.02$) and blood-regulating ($p = 0.04$) formulas. The top 12 ingredients are shown. The areas of the pies indicate the relative weights of the formulas and herbs in the prescription for the condition. *P* values are from overrepresentation tests.

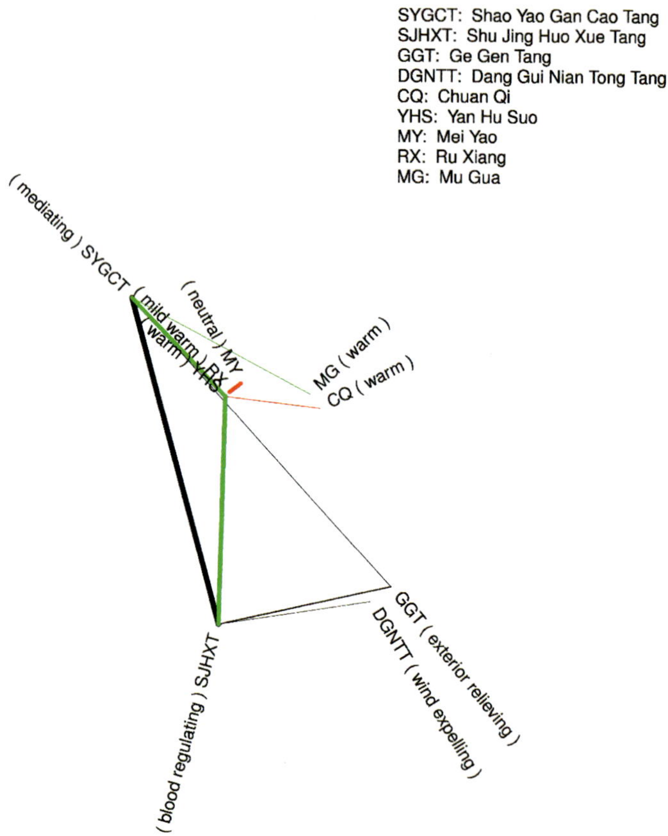

FIGURE 8.9b

The commonest TCM formula pair is SJHXT–SYGCT, the commonest formula–herb pair is SJHXT–YHS and the commonest herb pair is MY–RX for the treatment of myalgia and myositis, fibromyositis. The thickness of the line indicates the prevalence of the pair. Formula pairs are in black, formula–herb pairs in green and herb pairs in red. The TCM pharmacotherapeutic categories of the formulas and the TCM natures of the herbs are shown in parentheses.

8.14 Neuralgia, Neuritis and Radiculitis: *Shu Jing Huo Xue Tang* and *Yan Hu Suo*

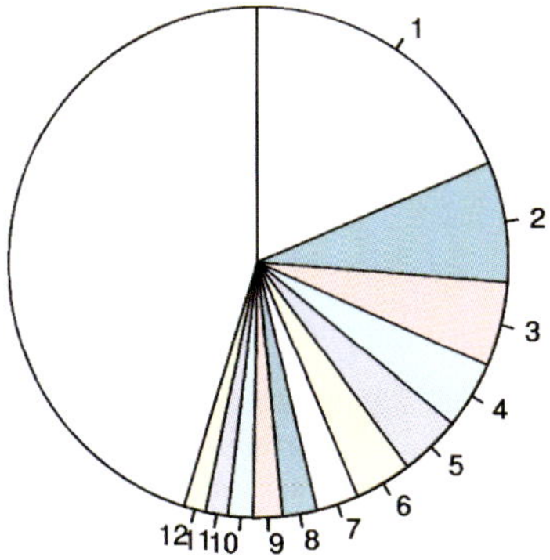

blood regulating	1	Shu Jing Huo Xue Tang
wind expelling	2	Du Huo Ji Sheng Tang
mediating	3	Shao Yao Gan Cao Tang
wind expelling	4	Dang Gui Nian Tong Tang
exterior relieving	5	Ge Gen Tang
blood regulating	6	Shen Tong Zhu Yu Tang
tonifying	7	Liu Wei Di Huang Wan
blood regulating	8	Xue Fu Zhu Yu Tang
tonifying	9	Huang Qi Wu Wu Tang
wind expelling	10	Juan Bi Tang
dampness eliminating	11	Qiang Huo Sheng Shi Tang
mediating	12	Jia Wei Xiao Yao San

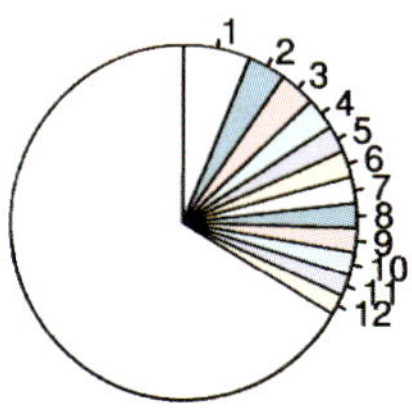

warm	1	Yan Hu Suo
neutral	2	Niu Xi
warm	3	Ji Xue Teng
warm	4	Xu Duan
warm	5	Mu Gua
warm	6	Du Zhong
mild warm	7	Ru Xiang
warm	8	Wei Ling Xian
neutral	9	Mei Yao
warm	10	Chuan Qi
neutral	11	Ge Gen
mild cold	12	Dan Can

FIGURE 8.10a

Neuralgia, neuritis and radiculitis (ICD-9 = 7292) are treated by TCM wind-expelling ($p = 0.02$) and blood-regulating ($p = 0.04$) formulas and TCM warm ($p = 0.02$) herbs. The top 12 ingredients are shown. The areas of the pies indicate the relative weights of the formulas and herbs in the prescription for the condition. *P* values are from overrepresentation tests.

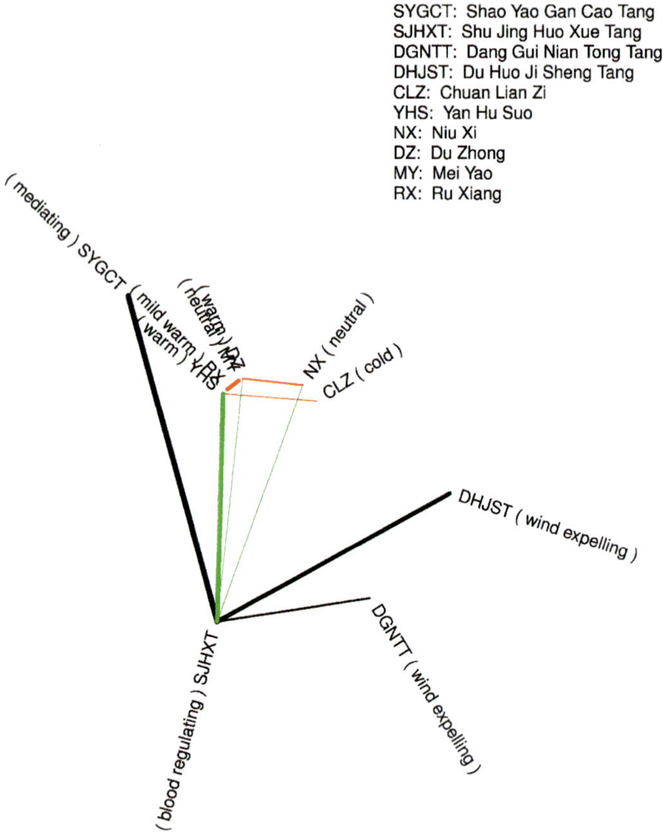

FIGURE 8.10b

The commonest TCM formula pair is SJHXT–SYGCT, the commonest formula–herb pair is SJHXT–YHS and the commonest herb pair is MY–RX, followed by DZ–NX, for the treatment of neuralgia, neuritis and radiculitis. The thickness of the line indicates the prevalence of the pair. Formula pairs are in black, formula–herb pairs in green and herb pairs in red. The TCM pharmacotherapeutic categories of the formulas and the TCM natures of the herbs are shown in parentheses.

8.15 Backache: *Shu Jing Huo Xue Tang* and *Yan Hu Suo*

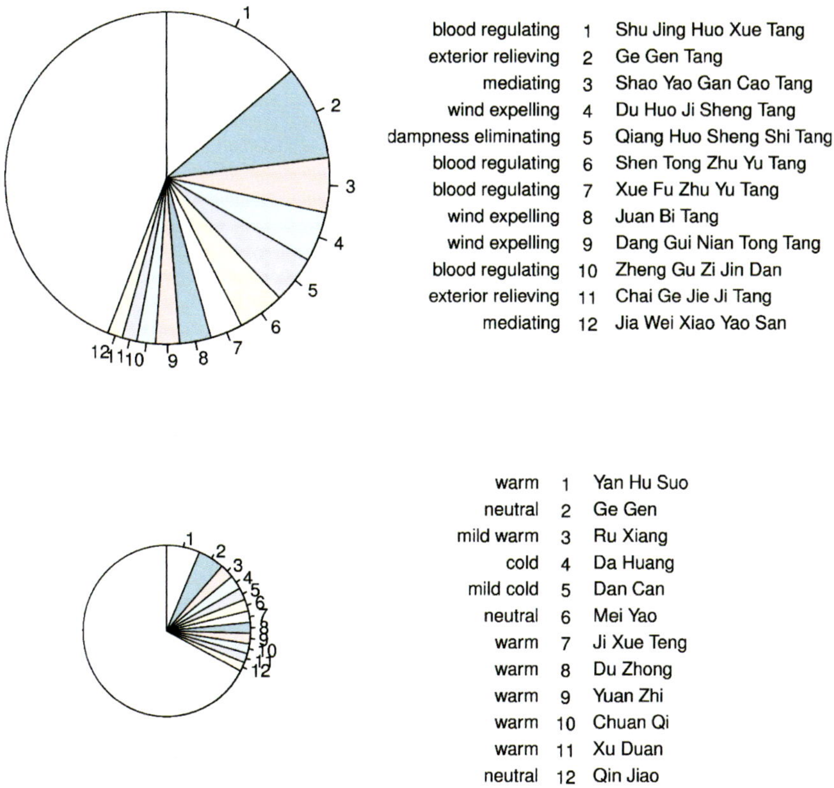

FIGURE 8.11a

Backache (ICD-9 = 7245) is treated by TCM blood-regulating ($p = 0.006$) and wind-expelling ($p = 0.02$) formulas. The top 12 ingredients are shown. The areas of the pies indicate the relative weights of the formulas and herbs in the prescription for the condition. *P* values are from overrepresentation tests.

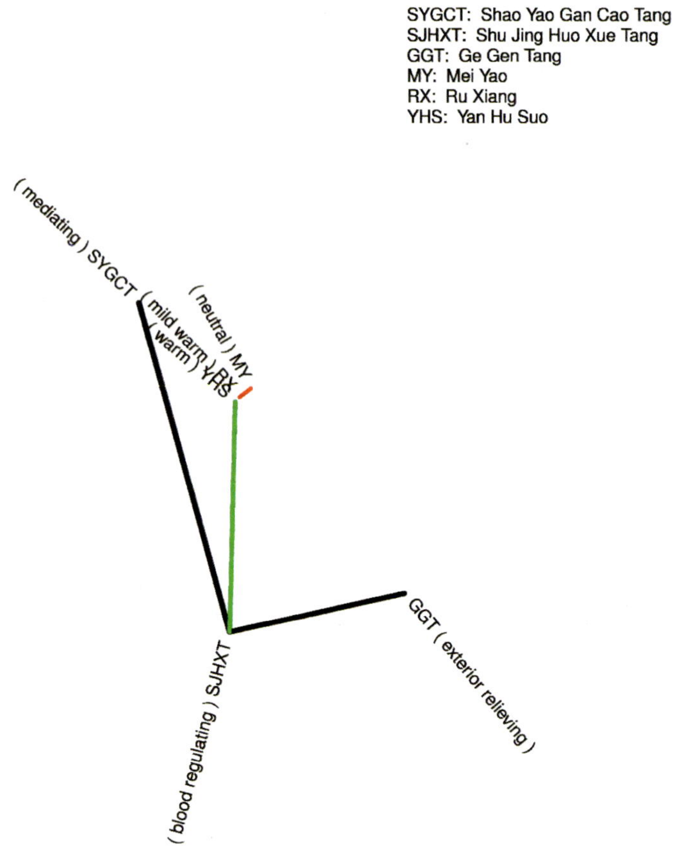

FIGURE 8.11b

The commonest TCM formula pair is SJHXT–SYGCT, the commonest formula–herb pair is SJHXT–YHS and the commonest herb pair is MY–RX for the treatment of backache. The thickness of the line indicates the prevalence of the pair. Formula pairs are in black, formula–herb pairs in green and herb pairs in red. The TCM pharmacotherapeutic categories of the formulas and the TCM natures of the herbs are shown in parentheses.

8.16 Cervicalgia: *Ge Gen Tang* and *Ge Gen*

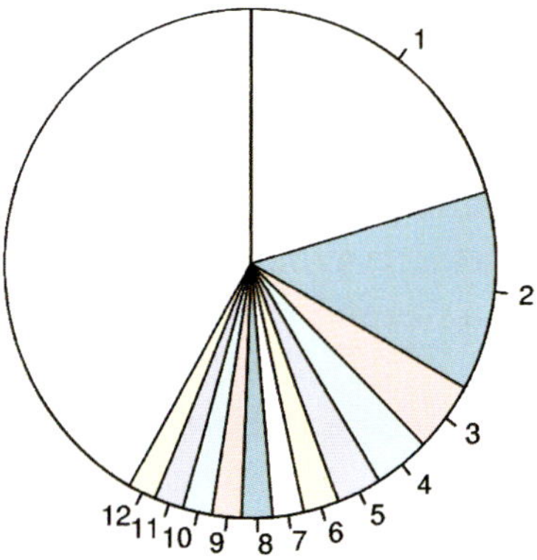

exterior relieving	1	Ge Gen Tang
blood regulating	2	Shu Jing Huo Xue Tang
mediating	3	Shao Yao Gan Cao Tang
dampness eliminating	4	Qiang Huo Sheng Shi Tang
blood regulating	5	Xue Fu Zhu Yu Tang
exterior relieving	6	Chai Ge Jie Ji Tang
wind expelling	7	Juan Bi Tang
wind expelling	8	Gou Teng San
exterior relieving	9	Chuan Xiong Cha Diao San
blood regulating	10	Shen Tong Zhu Yu Tang
mediating	11	Jia Wei Xiao Yao San
exterior relieving	12	Jiu Wei Qiang Huo Tang

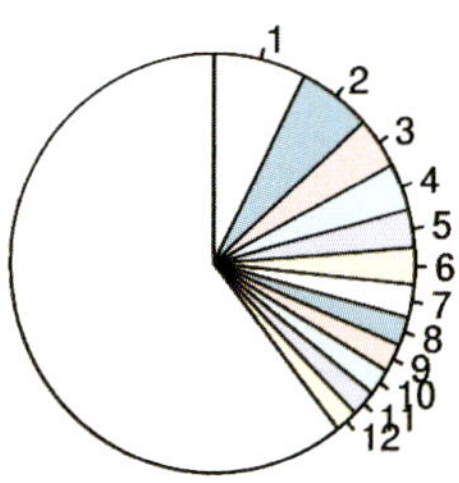

neutral	1	Ge Gen
neutral	2	Fu Shen
mild cold	3	Sha Can
warm	4	Yan Hu Suo
warm	5	Yi Tiao Gen
warm	6	Hao Ben
cool	7	Gou Teng
warm	8	Xu Duan
mild cold	9	Chi Shao
warm	10	Wei Ling Xian
warm	11	Qiang Huo
warm	12	Ji Xue Teng

FIGURE 8.12a

Cervicalgia (ICD-9 = 7231) is treated by TCM exterior-relieving ($p = 0.003$) and blood-regulating ($p = 0.006$) formulas and TCM warm ($p = 0.02$) herbs. The top 12 ingredients are shown. The areas of the pies indicate the relative weights of the formulas and herbs in the prescription for the condition. *P* values are from overrepresentation tests.

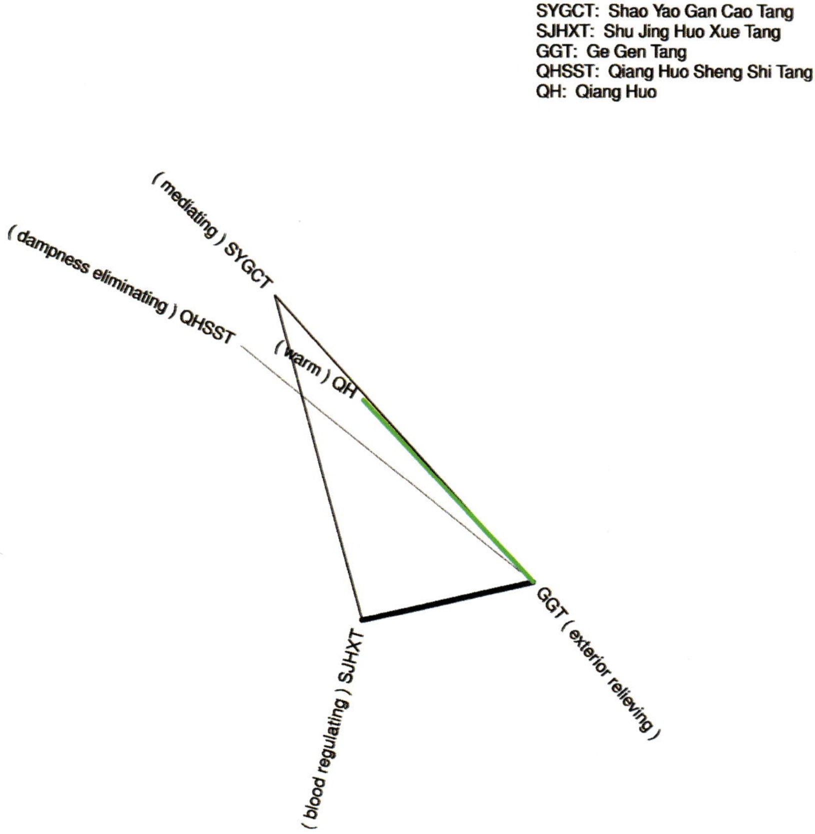

FIGURE 8.12b

The commonest TCM formula pair is GGT–SJHXT, followed by GGT–SYGCT, and the commonest formula–herb pair is GGT–QH for the treatment of cervicalgia. The thickness of the line indicates the prevalence of the pair. Formula pairs are in black and formula–herb pairs in green. The TCM pharmacotherapeutic categories of the formulas and the TCM natures of the herbs are shown in parentheses.

8.17 Sleep Disturbance: *Suan Zao Ren Tang* and *Ye Jiao Teng*

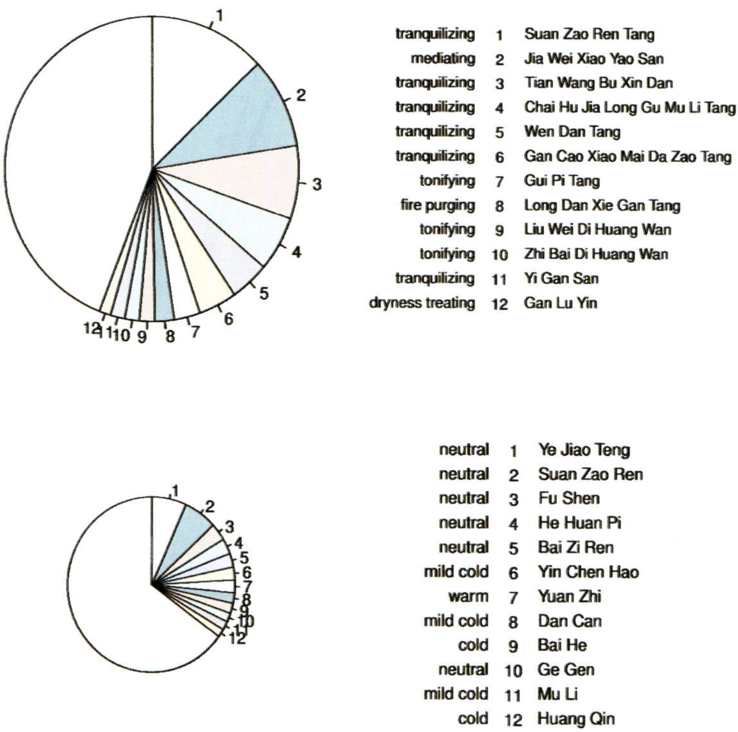

FIGURE 8.13a

Sleep disturbance (ICD-9 = 7805) is treated by TCM tranquilizing formulas (p = 0.0000001) and TCM neutral herbs (p = 0.02). The top 12 ingredients are shown. The areas of the pies indicate the relative weights of the formulas and herbs in the prescription for the condition. *P* values are from overrepresentation tests.

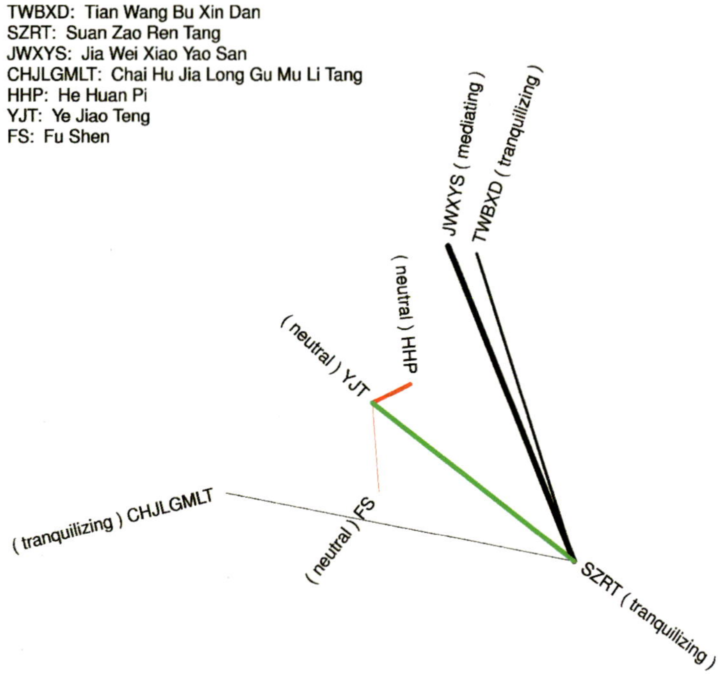

FIGURE 8.13b

The commonest TCM formula pair is SZRT–JWXYS, the commonest formula–herb pair is SZRT–YJT and the commonest herb pair is HHP–YJT for the treatment of sleep disturbance. The thickness of the line indicates the prevalence of the pair. Formula pairs are in black, formula–herb pairs in green and herb pairs in red. The TCM pharmacotherapeutic categories of the formulas and the TCM natures of the herbs are shown in parentheses.

8.18 Constipation: *Ma Zi Ren Wan* and *Da Huang*

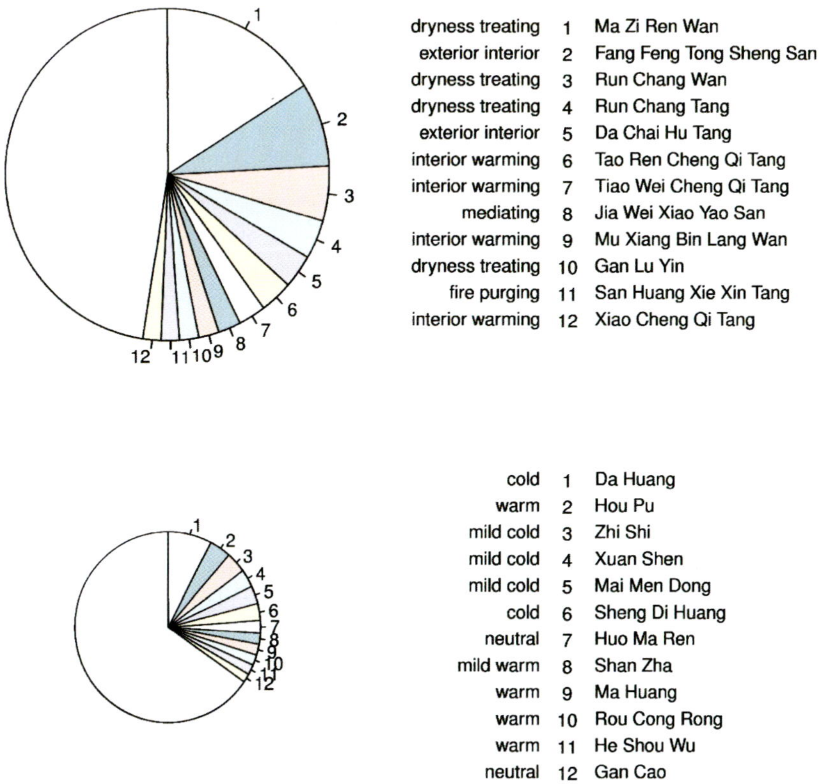

FIGURE 8.14a

Constipation (ICD-9 = 5640) is treated by TCM interior-warming ($p = 0.00001$) and dryness-treating ($p = 0.0004$) formulas. The top 12 ingredients are shown. The areas of the pies indicate the relative weights of the formulas and herbs in the prescription for the condition. *P* values are from overrepresentation tests.

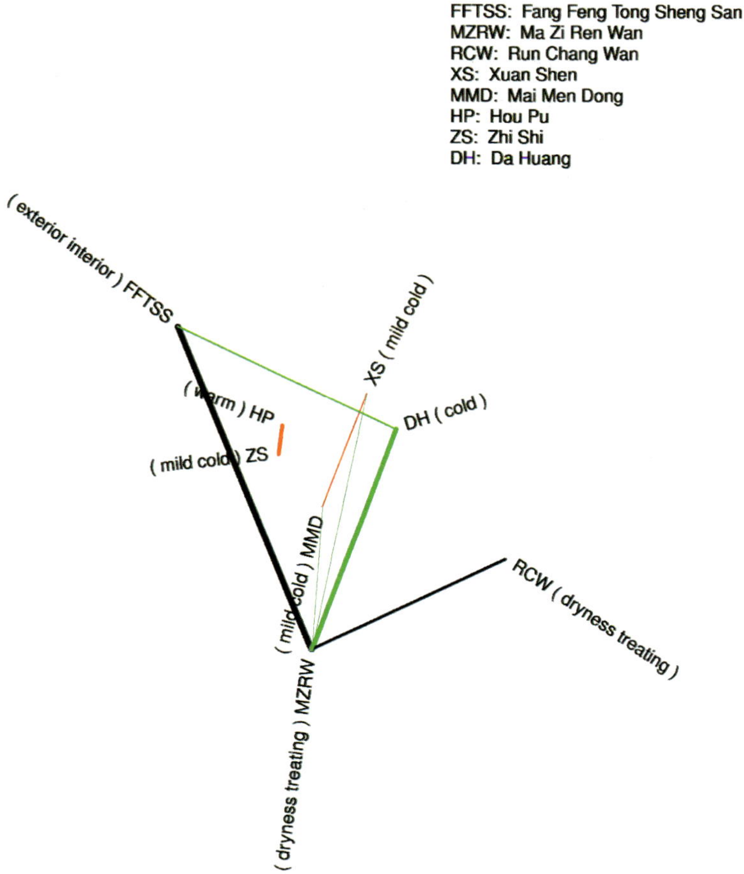

FIGURE 8.14b

The commonest TCM formula pair is MZRW–FFTSS, the commonest formula–herb pair is MZRW–DH and the commonest herb pair is HP–ZS for the treatment of constipation. The thickness of the line indicates the prevalence of the pair. Formula pairs are in black, formula–herb pairs in green and herb pairs in red. The TCM pharmacotherapeutic categories of the formulas and the TCM natures of the herbs are shown in parentheses.

8.19 Contact Dermatitis: *Xiao Feng San* and *Lian Qiao*

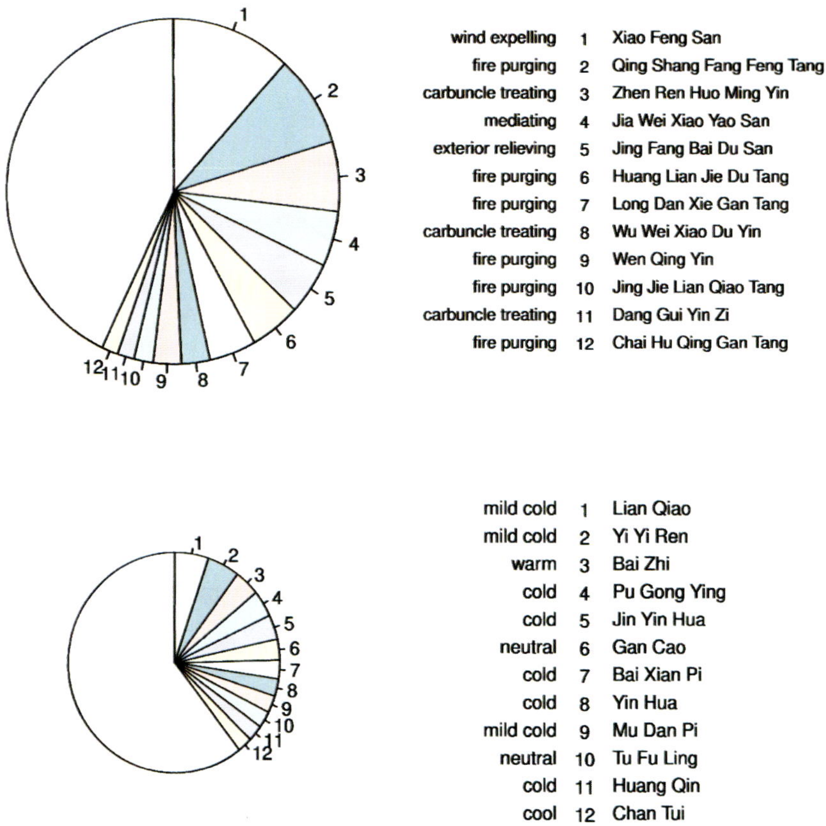

FIGURE 8.15a

Contact dermatitis (ICD-9 = 6929) is treated by TCM fire-purging ($p = 0.0008$) and carbuncle-treating ($p = 0.01$) formulas and TCM cold ($p = 0.04$) herbs. The top 12 ingredients are shown. The areas of the pies indicate the relative weights of the formulas and herbs in the prescription for the condition. *P* values are from over-representation tests.

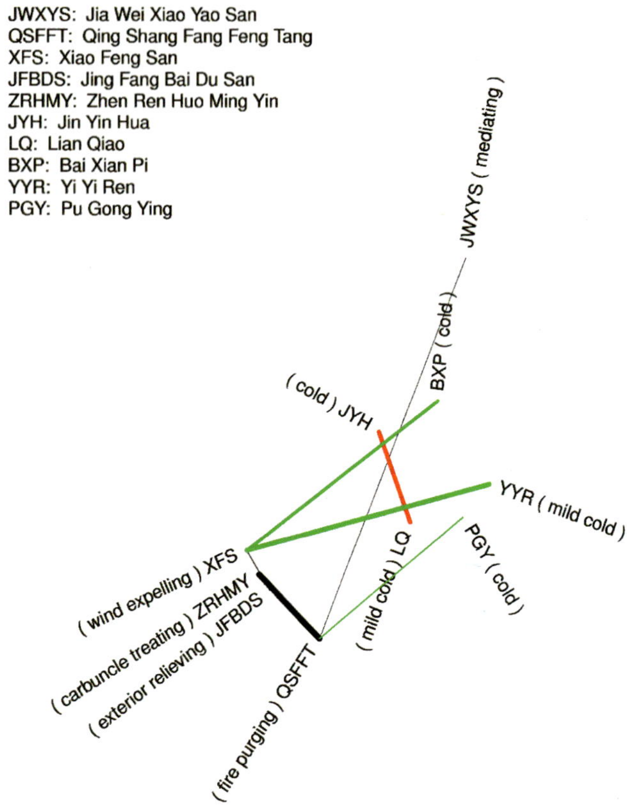

FIGURE 8.15b

The commonest TCM formula pair is QSFFT–ZRHMY, the commonest formula–herb pair is XFS–YYR and the commonest herb pair is LQ–JYH for the treatment of contact dermatitis. The thickness of the line indicates the prevalence of the pair. Formula pairs are in black, formula–herb pairs in green and herb pairs in red. The TCM pharmacotherapeutic categories of the formulas and the TCM natures of the herbs are shown in parentheses.

8.20 Chronic Hepatitis: *Jia Wei Xiao Yao San* and *Yin Chen Hao*

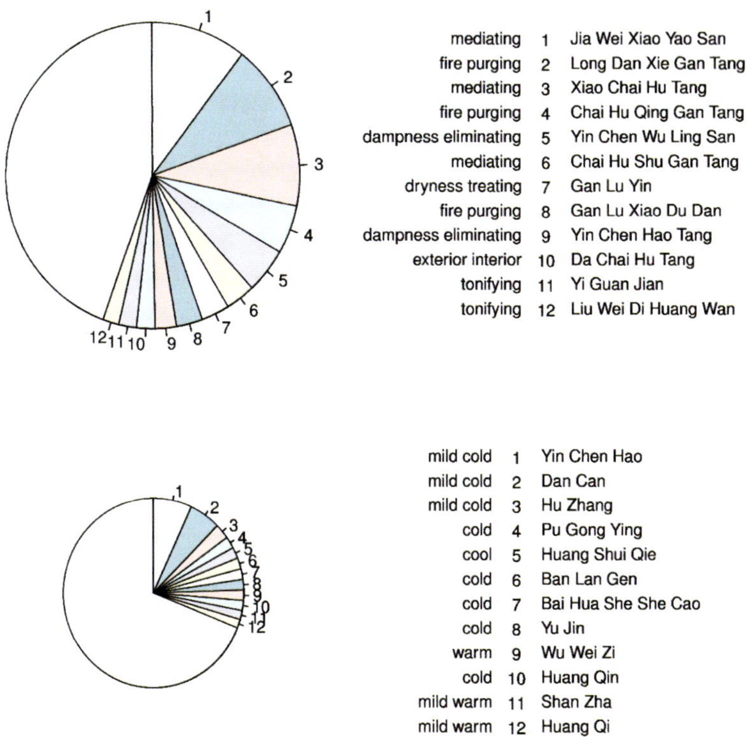

FIGURE 8.16a

Chronic hepatitis (ICD-9 = 5714) is treated by TCM mediating formulas ($p = 0.03$) and TCM cold herbs ($p = 0.04$). The top 12 ingredients are shown. The areas of the pies indicate the relative weights of the formulas and herbs in the prescription for the condition. *P* values are from overrepresentation tests.

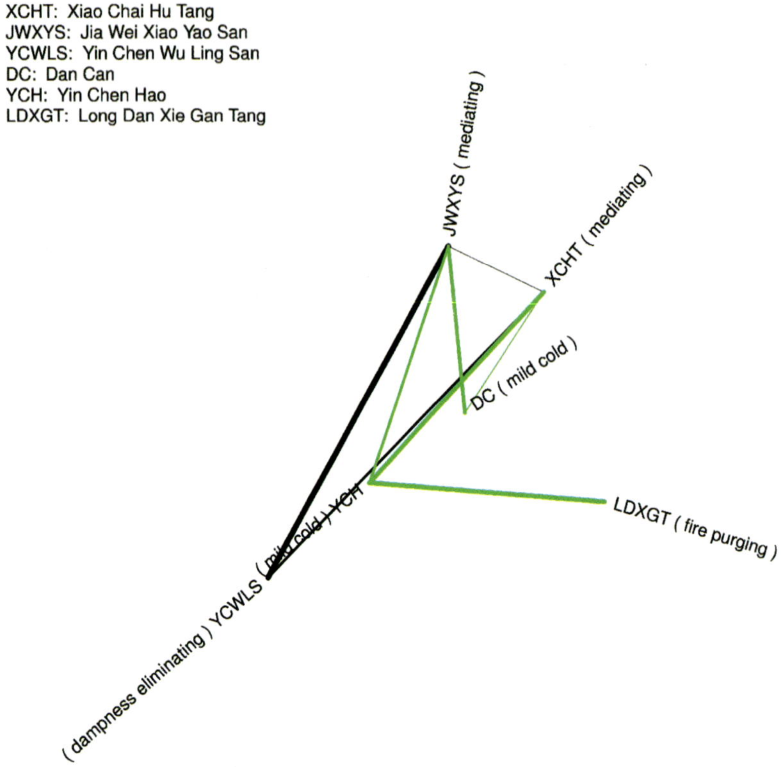

FIGURE 8.16b

The commonest TCM formula pair is JWXYS–YCWLS and the commonest formula–herb pair is LDXGT–YCH, followed by XCHT–YCH and JWXYS–DC, for the treatment of chronic hepatitis. The thickness of the line indicates the prevalence of the pair. Formula pairs are in black and formula–herb pairs in green. The TCM pharmacotherapeutic categories of the formulas and the TCM natures of the herbs are shown in parentheses.

8.21 Headache: *Chuan Xiong Cha Diao San* and *Ge Gen*

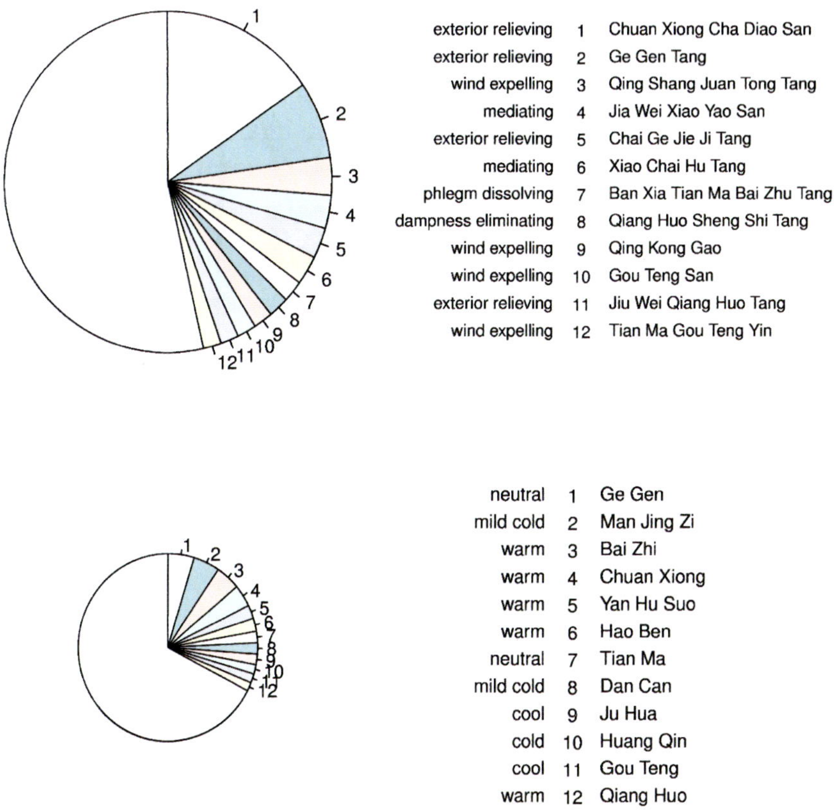

FIGURE 8.17a

Headache (ICD-9 = 7840) is treated by TCM wind-expelling ($p = 0.002$) and exterior-relieving ($p = 0.003$) formulas. The top 12 ingredients are shown. The areas of the pies indicate the relative weights of the formulas and herbs in the prescription for the condition.*P* values are from overrepresentation tests.

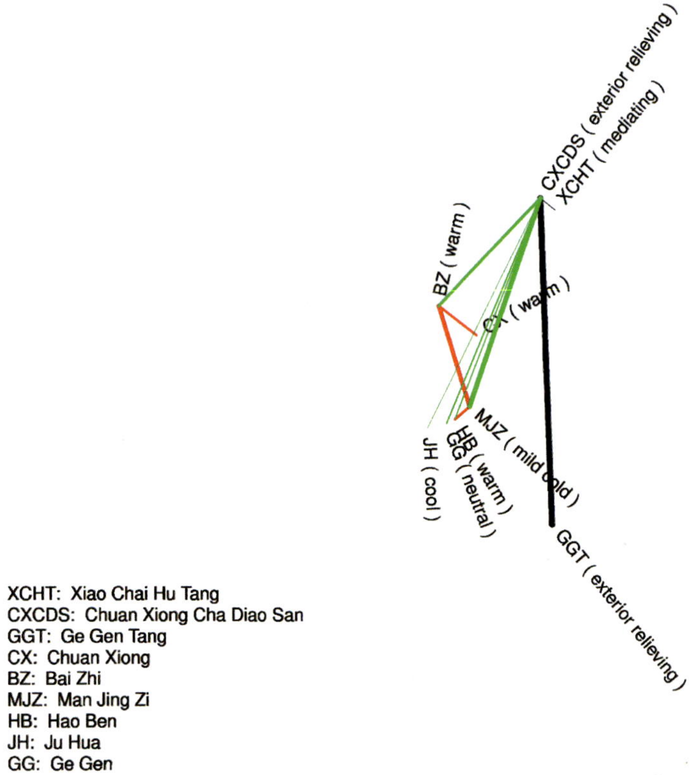

FIGURE 8.17b

The commonest TCM formula pair is CXCDS–GGT, the commonest formula–herb pair is CXCDS–MJZ and the commonest herb pair is MJZ–BZ, followed by MJZ–HB, for the treatment of headache. The thickness of the line indicates the prevalence of the pair. Formula pairs are in black, formula–herb pairs in green and herb pairs in red. The TCM pharmacotherapeutic categories of the formulas and the TCM natures of the herbs are shown in parentheses.

8.22 Palpitations: *Zhi Gan Cao Tang* and *Dan Can*

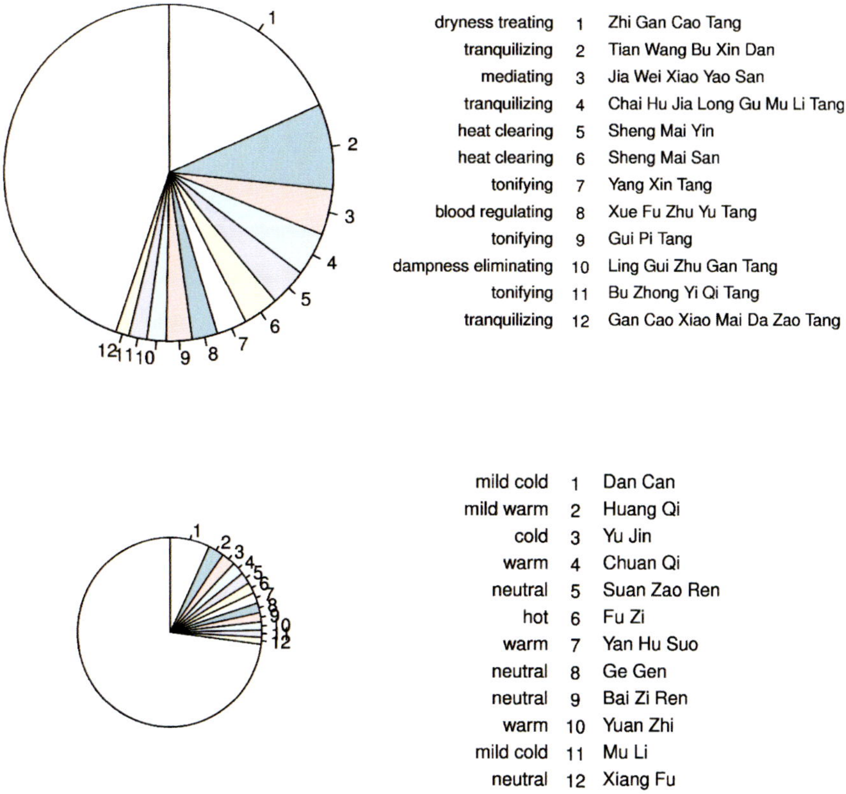

FIGURE 8.18a

Palpitations (ICD-9 = 7851) are treated by TCM tranquilizing ($p = 0.004$) and heat-clearing ($p = 0.04$) formulas. The top 12 ingredients are shown. The areas of the pies indicate the relative weights of the formulas and herbs in the prescription for the condition. *P* values are from overrepresentation tests.

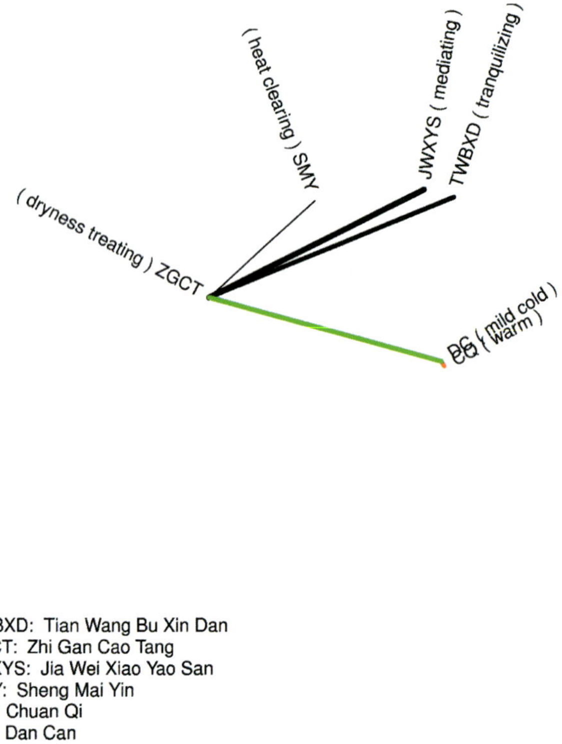

FIGURE 8.18b

The commonest TCM formula pair is ZGCT–JWXYS, the commonest formula–herb pair is ZGCT–DC and the commonest herb pair is DC–CQ for the treatment of palpitations. The thickness of the line indicates the prevalence of the pair. Formula pairs are in black, formula–herb pairs in green and herb pairs in red. The TCM pharmacotherapeutic categories of the formulas and the TCM nature of the herbs are shown in parentheses.

8.23 Dizziness/Vertigo: *Ling Gui Zhu Gan Tang* and *Dan Can*

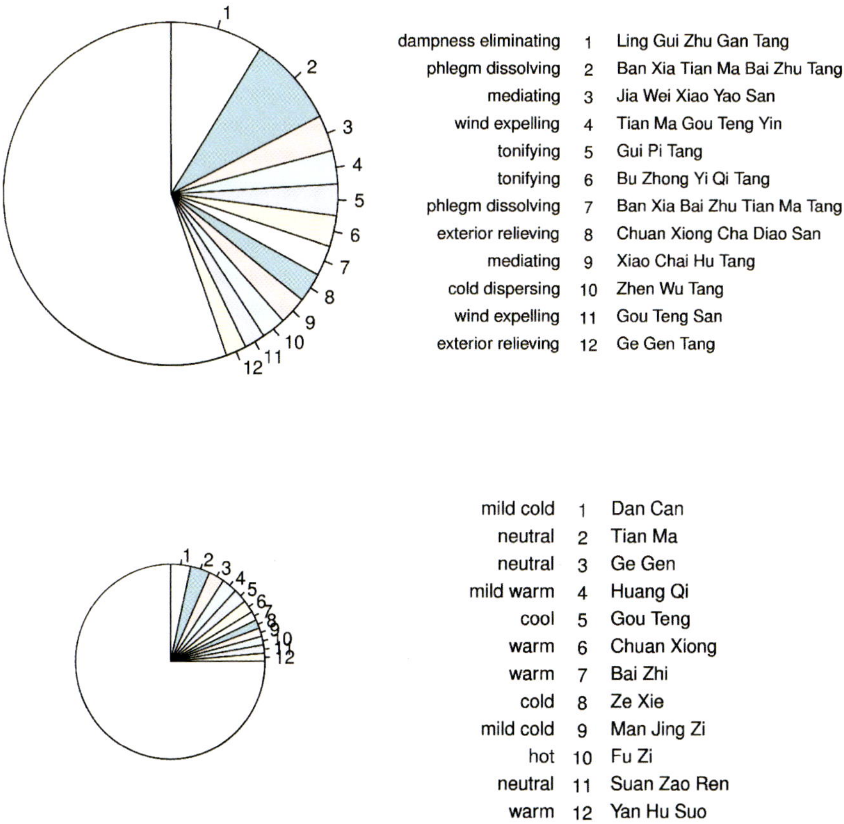

FIGURE 8.19a

Dizziness/vertigo (ICD-9 = 7804) might be treated by TCM wind-expelling (p = 0.12) or phlegm-dissolving (p = 0.13) formulas. The top 12 ingredients are shown. The areas of the pies indicate the relative weights of the formulas and herbs in the prescription for the condition. P values are from overrepresentation tests.

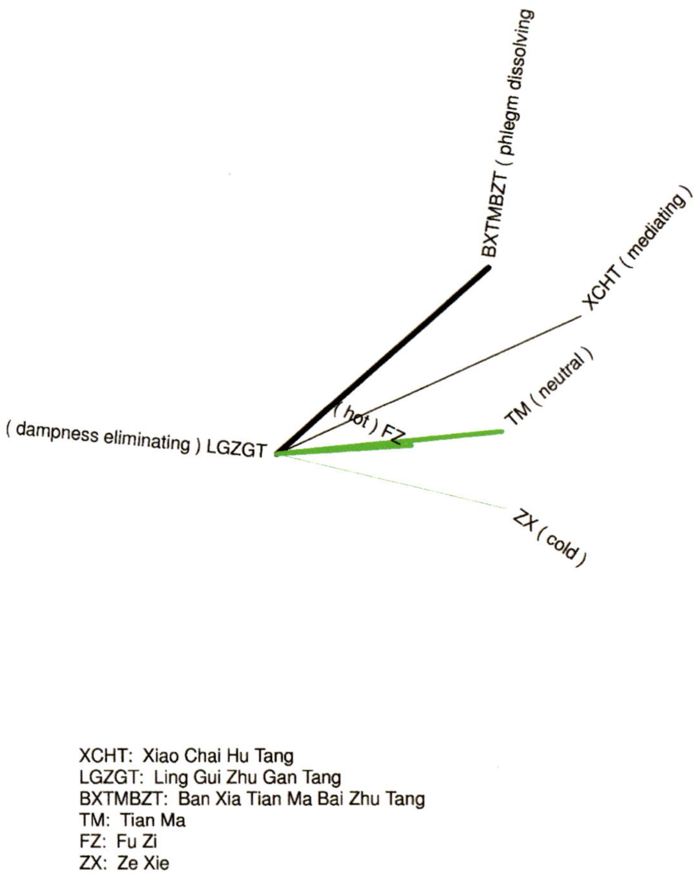

FIGURE 8.19b

The commonest TCM formula pair is LGZGT–BXTMBZT and the commonest formula–herb pair is LGZGT–TM for the treatment of dizziness/vertigo. The thickness of the line indicates the prevalence of the pair. Formula pairs are in black and formula–herb pairs in green. The TCM pharmacotherapeutic categories of the formulas and the TCM natures of the herbs are shown in parentheses.

8.24 Functional Dyspepsia: *Ban Xia Xie Xin Tang* and *Hai Piao Shao*

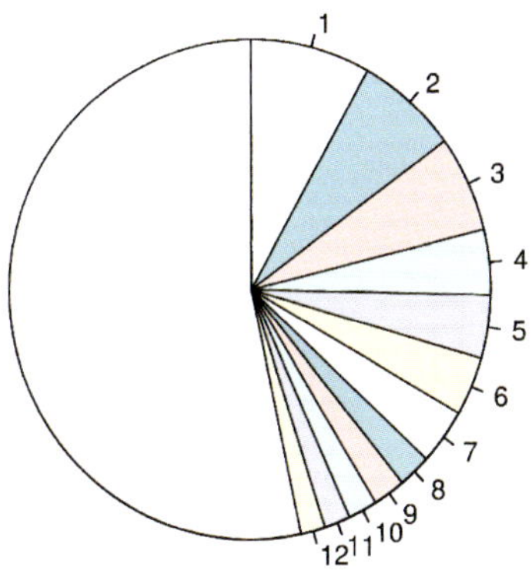

fire purging	1	Ban Xia Xie Xin Tang
peptic	2	Xiang Sha Liu Jun Zi Tang
peptic	3	Ping Wei San
tonifying	4	Shen Ling Bai Zhu San
peptic	5	Bao He Wan
mediating	6	Huo Xiang Zheng Qi San
peptic	7	An Zhong San
mediating	8	Jia Wei Xiao Yao San
mediating	9	Xiao Chai Hu Tang
mediating	10	Si Ni San
tonifying	11	Bu Zhong Yi Qi Tang
mediating	12	Chai Hu Shu Gan Tang

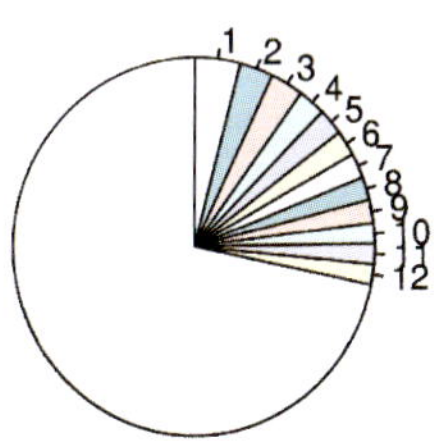

warm	1	Hai Piao Shao
warm	2	Yan Hu Suo
warm	3	Shen Qu
neutral	4	Mai Ya
warm	5	Hou Pu
mild cold	6	Bei Mu
warm	7	Mu Xiang
warm	8	Sha Ren
mild warm	9	Shan Zha
neutral	10	Fu Ling
mild cold	11	Zhi Shi
mild cold	12	Bai Ji

FIGURE 8.20a

Functional dyspepsia (ICD-9 = 5368, 5369) is treated by TCM mediating (p = 0.0002) and peptic (p = 0.0006) formulas. The top 12 ingredients are shown. The areas of the pies indicate the relative weights of the formulas and herbs in the prescription for the condition. P values are from overrepresentation tests.

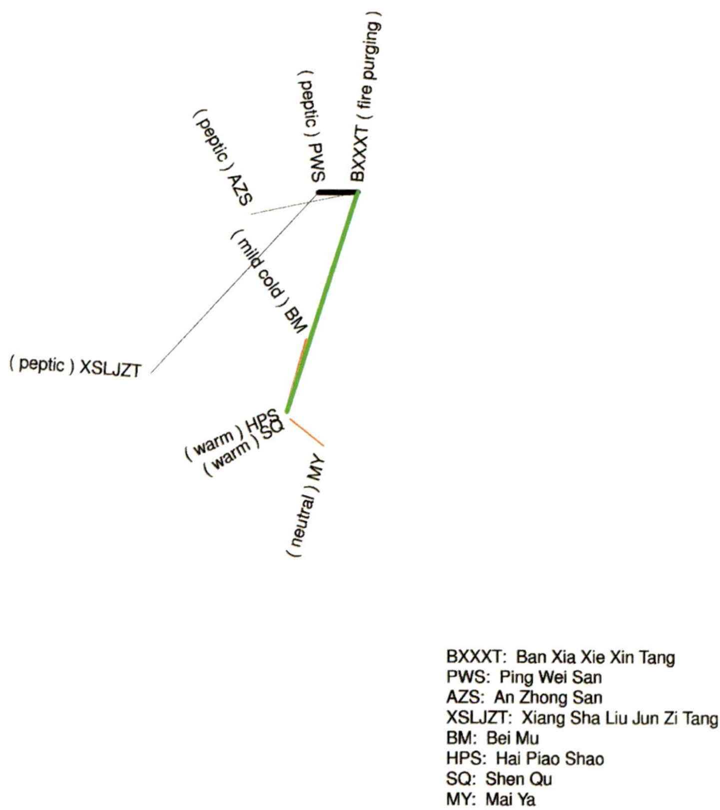

FIGURE 8.20b

The commonest TCM formula pair is BXXXT–PWS, the commonest formula–herb pair is BXXXT–HPS and the commonest herb pair is HPS–BM for the treatment of functional dyspepsia. The thickness of the line indicates the prevalence of the pair. Formula pairs are in black, formula–herb pairs in green and herb pairs in red. The TCM pharmacotherapeutic categories of the formulas and the TCM nature of the herbs are shown in parentheses.

8.25 Gas/Bloating: *Ban Xia Xie Xin Tang* and *Hai Piao Shao*

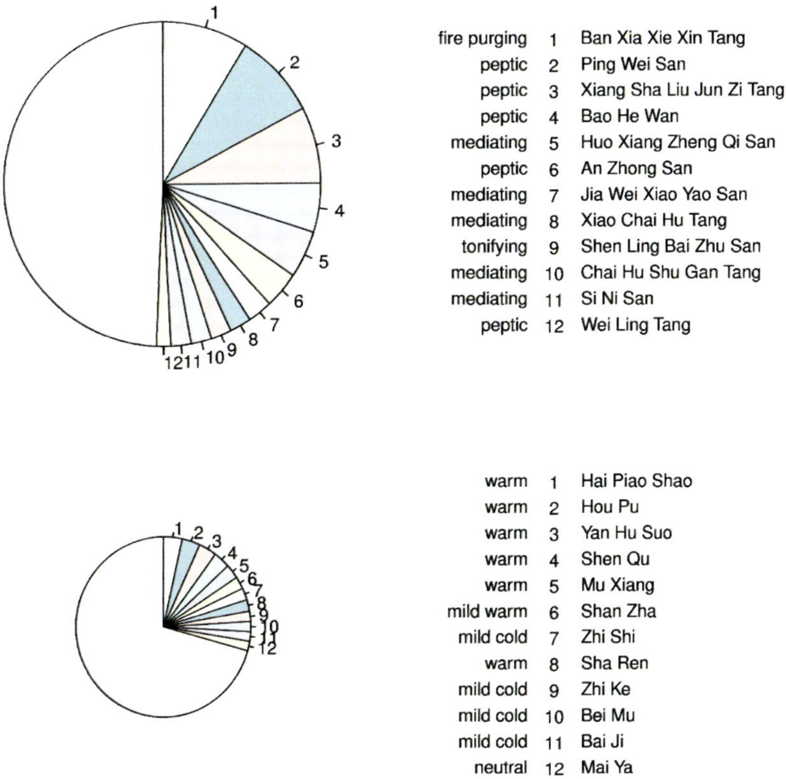

FIGURE 8.21a

Gas/bloating (ICD-9 = 7873) is treated by TCM peptic (p = 0.00003) and mediating (p = 0.0002) formulas. The top 12 ingredients are shown. The areas of the pies indicate the relative weights of the formulas and herbs in the prescription for the condition. P values are from overrepresentation tests.

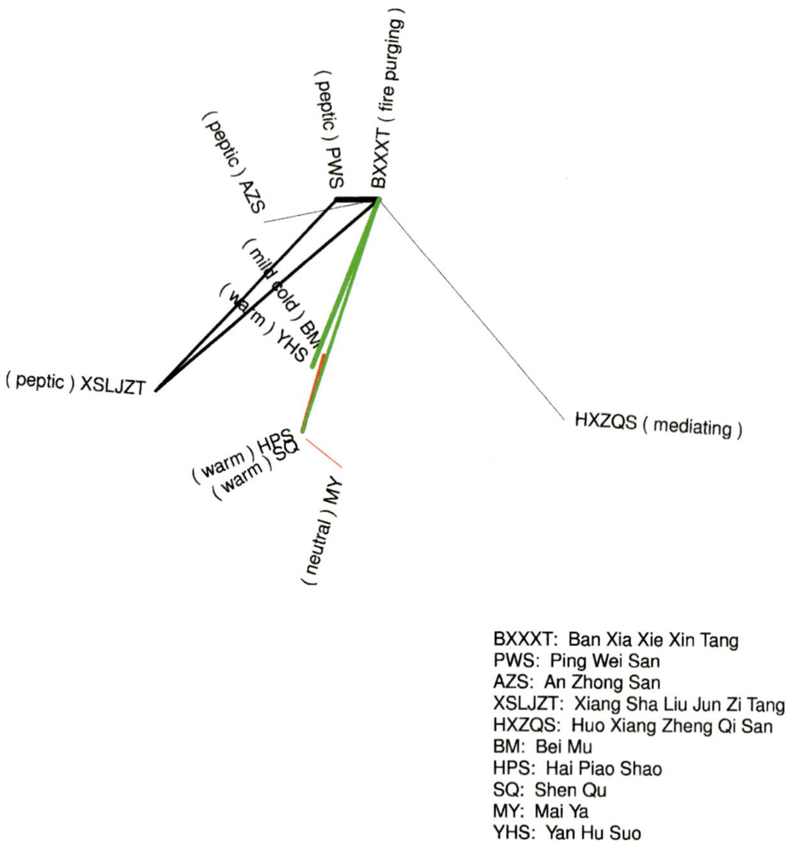

FIGURE 8.21b

The commonest TCM formula pair is BXXXT–PWS, followed by BXXXT–XSLJZT, the commonest formula–herb pair is BXXXT–YHS and the commonest herb pair is BM–HPS for the treatment of gas/bloating. The thickness of the line indicates the prevalence of the pair. Formula pairs are in black, formula–herb pairs in green and herb pairs in red. The TCM pharmacotherapeutic categories of the formulas and the TCM nature of the herbs are shown in parentheses.

8.26 Acute Gastritis: *Ban Xia Xie Xin Tang* and *Hai Piao Shao*

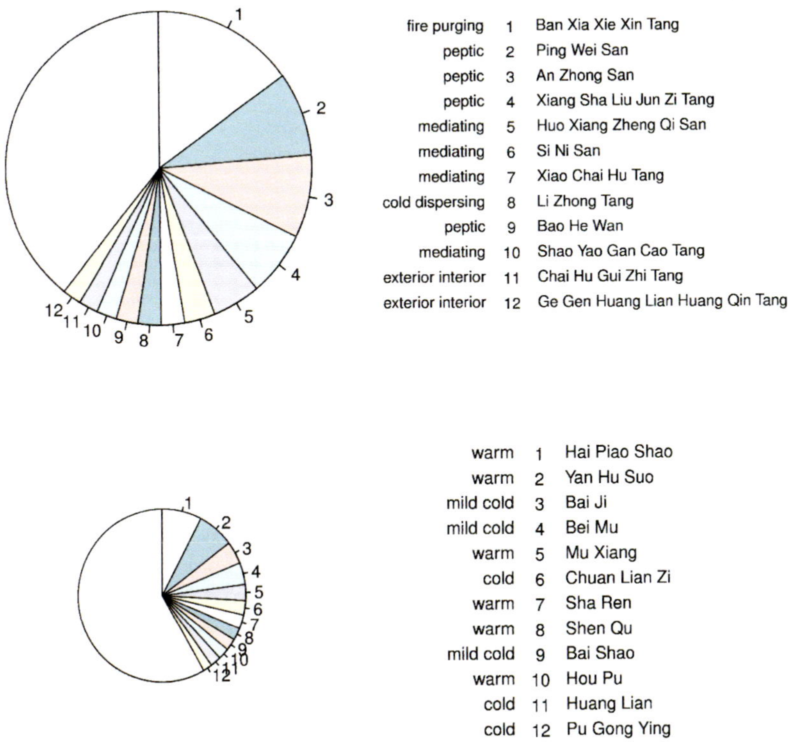

FIGURE 8.22a

Acute gastritis (ICD-9 = 5350) is treated by TCM peptic ($p = 0.0006$) and mediating ($p = 0.003$) formulas. The top 12 ingredients are shown. The areas of the pies indicate the relative weights of the formulas and herbs in the prescription for the condition. *P* values are from overrepresentation tests.

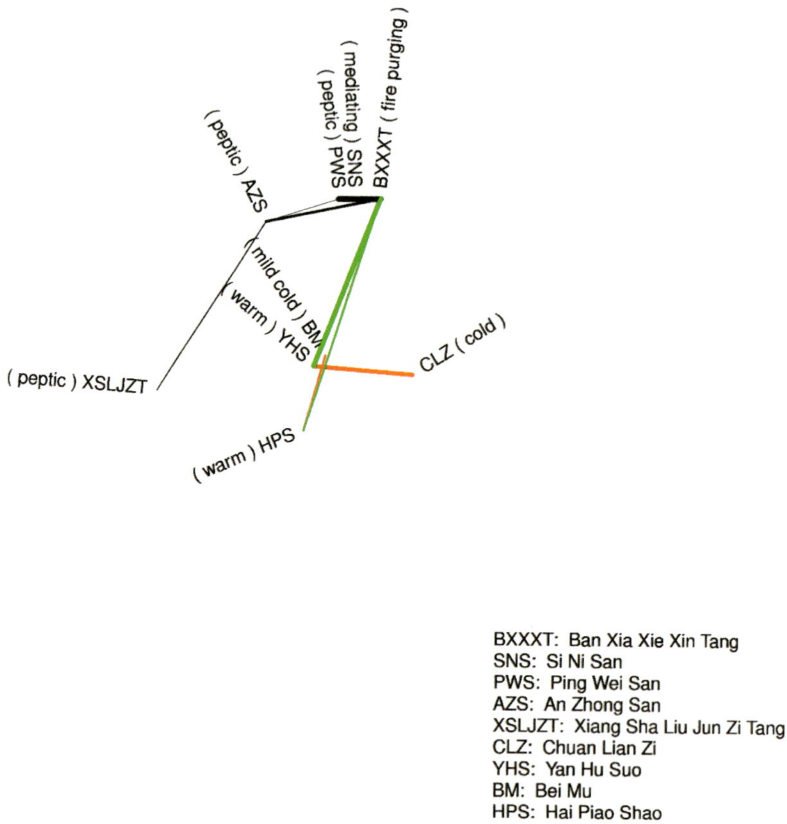

FIGURE 8.22b

The commonest TCM formula pair is BXXXT–PWS, the commonest formula–herb pair is BXXXT–YHS and the commonest herb pair is YHS–CLZ for the treatment of acute gastritis. The thickness of the line indicates the prevalence of the pair. Formula pairs are in black, formula–herb pairs in green and herb pairs in red. The TCM pharmacotherapeutic categories of the formulas and the TCM nature of the herbs are shown in parentheses.

9

Condition of the Reproductive System

The conventional treatment for erectile dysfunction is by Viagra, which works by inhibiting the PDE5 enzyme in the smooth muscle cells that line the blood vessels supplying the erectile tissue of the penis. Sexual life with PDE5 inhibitors is, however, not without imperfections. By contrast, TCM is found to treat erectile dysfunction by combining tonifying formulas, astringing formulas and warm herbs. Tonifying formulas invigorate *qi* to improve physical fitness; astringing formulas retain bodily fluids including semen, preventing premature ejaculation; TCM warm herbs activate the kidney, which regulates sex hormones, increasing the sex drive. For impotence of psychogenic causes, TCM is found to additionally prescribe tranquilizing formulas which help regularize normal mental activities, including eroticism. A regimen that includes TCM prescription between Viagra intakes can therefore be considered an example of integrative therapy.

In addition to holism, personalized medicine is the other feature of TCM therapy. Customized prescriptions follow TCM *zheng* differentiations. TCM *zheng* is a profile of signs and symptoms of the patient through the TCM doctor's observation, olfaction, interrogation and palpation. It is therefore macroscopic diagnosis in comparison with the microscopically histological examination of modern western medicine. A disease can develop different *zhengs*, depending on the patient's psychosomatic condition. *Zheng* differentiation therefore helps determine the subtype of the disease which the patient is having. Factors that prevent one from incorporating *zheng* into conventional diagnosis are: (1) nonstandardization of *zheng* terminology and (2) subjectivity of *zheng* differentiation. The second hurdle stems in part from the nonquantitative nature of *zheng* differentiation. Since TCM *zheng* and TCM prescription have a one-to-one correspondence, the identified prescriptions for a disease reveal the dominant *zhengs* of the disease. With 1.8 million TCM prescriptions for prevalent gynecologic and andrologic conditions, not only are the commonest prescriptions identified but representative *zhengs* are also understood. As TCM *zhengs* are macroscopic, they are more easily self-comprehended. Knowledge of one's own *zheng* is hoped to help prevent disease, which in the long run lowers the healthcare burden of the society.

9.1 Menstruation, Premenstrual Syndrome, Menopause, Osteoporosis

Fertile women undergo cyclic changes in psychophysiology in preparation for pregnancy. The egg-containing ovarian follicles grow and the uterine lining thickens, following increasing secretion of ovarian estrogen, which is stimulated by FSH and LH hormones released from the pituitary gland in the brain. At the time when the estrogen level peaks and the FSH and LH levels spike, one of the follicles in one of the ovaries matures and ruptures to release an egg in a process called ovulation. The ovaries then start secreting progesterone and the uterine lining turns from a proliferative lining into a secretory lining in preparation for embryogenesis. Meanwhile, the released egg travels via the oviduct toward the uterus, awaiting fertilization. If conception and implantation occurs and succeeds, the blood-vessel- and gland-rich uterine lining becomes the placenta. If not, the ovaries stop producing estrogen and progesterone and the uterine lining breaks down. The disintegrated uterine lining, together with some blood, secretion and mucus, is shed from the body through the cervix and vagina, giving rise to menses. Reproductive hormone secretion and uterine lining regeneration repeat every 28 ± 7 days. A menstrual flow lasts for 3–5 days and the average volume of the menstrual fluid is 35 ml.

Shedding of the uterine lining is accomplished by uterine muscles. Contractions of uterine muscles cut off the blood supply, reduce blood loss and push the menstrual fluid into the vagina. They can cause sharp or dull pain in the pelvis or lower abdomen in some women. Severe uterine pain during menstruation that interferes with daily activities is called dysmenorrhea. In addition to uterine pain, breast swelling/pain, nausea, vomiting, bloating, acne, headache, faints, fatigue, constipation and diarrhea are some of the discomforts of menstruation.

The intervals between menstruations vary in a woman. If the difference between the longest and shortest intervals is more than 8 days, the menstruation is considered irregular. If the longest is longer than 35 days, it is oligomenorrhea. If the shortest is shorter than 21 days, it is polymenorrhea. If the volume of menstrual fluid is over 80 ml (i.e. more than 10 tampons or sanitary towels per day), it is menorrhagia. If menses is absent for more than three months, it is amenorrhea. The causes of amenorrhea include excessive exercise, anorexia, weight loss, pregnancy and lactation; the causes of menorrhagia and polymenorrhea include hormone deregulation, fibroids, endometriosis, pelvic infections, polyps and blood clotting; the causes of oligomenorrhea and irregular menstruation include stress, dietary change, hormonal imbalance and contraceptives.

Menstruation not only causes physical discomforts but may also induce changes in the sense of well-being before its onset. Examples of mood changes are anxiety, depression, emotional hypersensitivity, food cravings and changes in libido. Although the exact symptoms vary from woman to woman and from cycle to cycle in a woman, the chief complaints are irritability, tension and unhappiness. If the mood changes occur predictably in the postovulatory part of the cycle and vanish before/upon menstrual flow, with the mood changes severe enough to interrupt daily life, the condition is called premenstrual syndrome (PMS). A thick, whitish/yellowish fluid which may be contained within or expelled from the vagina is called leukorrhea. The causes of leucorrhea are (1) estrogen stimulation and (2) inflammatory response of the vagina or cervix to bacterial infection.

Once the stock of ova becomes depleted, the ovary stops producing estrogen and progesterone, and menstruation ceases permanently as a result. When a woman has not had the menses for a year, she is one year into menopause. The median age at which menopause occurs is 51. The transition from regular menstruation to menopause is gradual and can go from irregular menstruation, through infrequent menstruation, toward menopause over a course of years. Psychophysiological symptoms during the transition are due to hormone changes and can have the following categories of symptoms: (1) vasomotor changes, including hot flashes, night sweats, migraine, palpitations and heart disease; (2) urogenital changes such as genitourinary tissue atrophy and vaginal dryness; (3) skeletal changes such as back pain, lack of energy and osteoporosis; (4) skin and soft tissue changes such as dry skin and breast atrophy; (5) psychological changes such as depression, anxiety, forgetfulness, lack of concentration and increased stress; and (6) sexual changes such as a lowered sex drive. As time goes on, the distresses of menopause fade. However, because of estrogen deficiency, postmenopausal women are at higher risk of osteoporosis and cardiovascular disease.

Osteoporosis is the thinning and weakening of bone tissues due to loss of bone mineral density over time. It is the commonest type of bone disease. Bones undergo resorption and formation, called bone remodeling, every moment throughout life. The resorption process by osteoclasts transfers calcium from the bone into the blood, and the formation process by osteoblasts does the opposite. A breakdown in the dynamic balance between resorption and formation in favor of resorption leads to osteoporosis. Bones become brittle in osteoporosis. The symptoms of osteoporosis include fractures without trauma, loss of height, low back pain, neck pain and a stooped or hunchback posture resulting from wedging together several vertebrae in a row. Estrogen is known to downregulate osteoclasts and upregulate osteoblasts. Women over 50 after menopause and men over 70 with declining testosterone are at high risk of osteoporosis. Patients with chronic kidney disease which fails to maintain calcium and phosphorus in the blood are also prone to osteoporosis.

9.2 Male/Female Infertility, Male Organic/ Psychogenic Impotence

Infertility is the inability to conceive after at least one year of regular unprotected sexual intercourse. About one-third of infertile cases are attributable to men, one-third to women, and the rest to both sexes and unknown factors. The causes of infertility can be genetic, medical, metabolic, environmental or, most often, a combination of the foregoing. The causes of female infertility include: (1) anovulation due to excessive exercise, starvation/malnutrition or underweight; (2) failure of fertilized egg transportation due, for example, to fallopian tube occlusion; (3) failure of fertilized egg implantation due to uterine disorders such as fibrosis and endometriosis; (4) damage to the reproductive system due to pelvic inflammatory disease; and (5) advanced maternal age (over 35). The causes of male infertility are low quantity, poor quality and low motility of sperm due to arduous bicycle or horseback training, prostatitis, impotence and age over 40. Obesity, tobacco smoking, radio- and chemotherapy are also known to cause infertility in both men and women. In addition, environmental chemicals such as pesticides and cosmetics have been linked to infertility.

Male impotence or erectile dysfunction is the inability of a man to develop and sustain a firm-enough penile erection for mutually satisfactory intercourse with his partner. Erection is the result of blood entering and remaining in the spongelike bodies in the penis. The brain, in response to visual, auditory, tactile or imagined stimuli, sends signals through the spinal cord down to the penile nerves. Neurotransmitters from the nerve endings control penile smooth muscles to dilate arteries and compress veins, allowing the erection body to be filled with blood. After ejaculation, neurotransmitters are no longer released and the veins open to drain the blood, whereby the erection subsides. As the phenomenon of erection involves a complex interplay among neuroendocrinal, vascular and psychological systems, the causes of erectile dysfunction can be organic and/or psychogenic. Organic impotence can be due to: (1) spinal cord or nerve injuries through diabetic peripheral neuropathy or prostate cancer surgery; (2) vascular diseases such as hypertension or atherosclerosis; (3) hormone imbalances such as decreased testosterone and/or increased prolactin; and (4) side effects of antidepressants, antihypertensive drugs or radio/chemotherapy. Psychogenic impotence is absence of or reduced interest in sexual activities with current or other partners, causing marked distress and interpersonal difficulty. The causes of psychogenic impotence include stress, depression, performance anxiety and relationship problems.

9.3 TCM Gynecologic and TCM Tonifying Formulas for Menstrual Disorders and Male Impotence

Stressful events and improper diets can disrupt the menstrual cycle. Hormonal changes give rise to menopausal conditions. Aging and medication can cause male impotence. In the prescription data is unraveled a preponderance of TCM gynecologic (p = 0.000002) and mediating (p = 0.00003) formulas and TCM mild–cold (p = 0.001) herbs for the menstrual conditions, including dysmenorrhea, PMS, amenorrhea, oligomenorrhea, excess or frequent menstruation, irregular menstruation and other/unspecified disorders of menstruation and abnormal bleeding from the female genital tract. On the other hand, TCM mediating formulas (p = 0.02) are prescribed for the menopausal state and postmenopausal

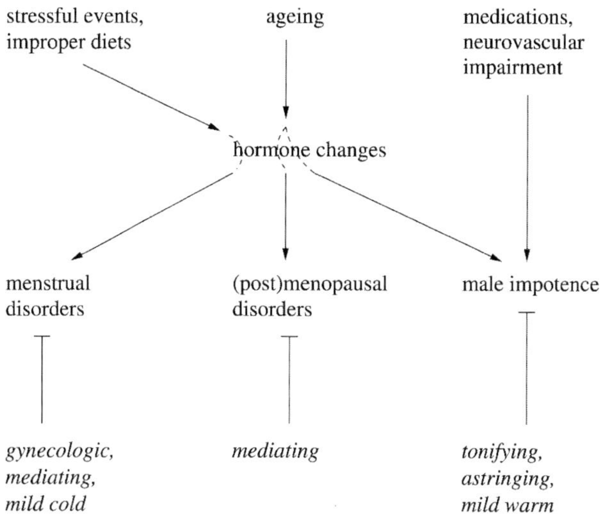

FIGURE 9.1

Reproductive system conditions and the prescribed TCM formulas and herbs. Menstrual disorders include dysmenorrhea, amenorrhea, oligomenorrhea, polymenorrhea, irregular menstruation, premenstrual tension syndrome and other/unspecified disorders of menstruation and abnormal bleeding from the female genital tract. Male impotence includes organic and psychogenic causes. Pointed arrows indicate promotion; blunt arrows indicate suppression. Note the short dashed lines that connect the arrows.

disorder, while TCM tonifying ($p = 0.004$) and astringing ($p = 0.009$) formulas and mild–warm ($p = 0.01$) herbs are prescribed for male impotence and infertility.

TCM has developed gynecologic formulas for the healthcare of female reproduction with regard to menstruation, pregnancy, gestation and lactation. It treats exterior syndromes by sweating, and interior syndromes by draining and purging. For conditions which are intermediate, TCM is said to mediate between exterior and interior by: (1) antagonizing pathogenesis; (2) bolstering defense; and (3) alternating (1) and (2), by the use of TCM mediating formulas. TCM mild–cold herbs remove TCM dampness and heat resulting from inflammation. TCM tonification aims to restore and rebalance *yin*, *yang*, *qi* and blood. TCM astringing formulas prevent loss of such bodily fluids as water, blood and semen. TCM mild–warm herbs can promote metabolism by, for example, enhancing mitochondrial activities, which may, through ATP-dependent chromatin modifiers, open chromatin. Since modified chromatin is heritable across cell generations, effects of TCM prescriptions can persist after the therapeutic course ends. Epigenetic mechanisms of TCM pharmacology, if proven, can be advantageous over

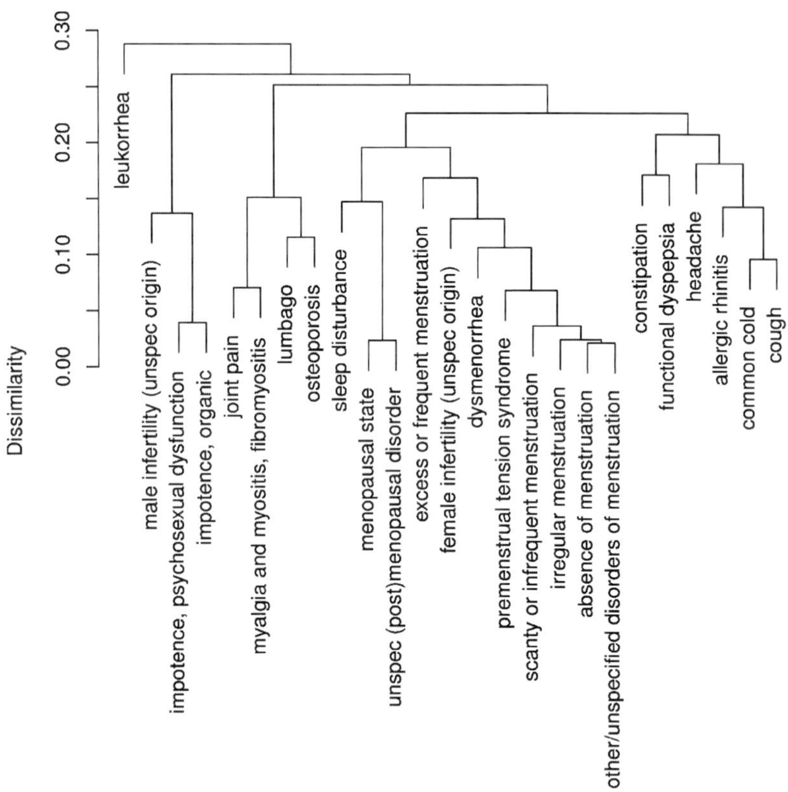

FIGURE 9.2

Clustering of TCM prescriptions for reproductive system conditions. Prescriptions which are similar, in terms of the ingredients and the relative weights of the ingredients in the prescription, fall within a branch of the tree in the hierarchical clustering analysis. Prescriptions for musculoskeletal pains, upper respiratory diseases and digestive problems are also shown for comparison. The vertical axis measures pairwise distance or dissimilarity between prescriptions.

receptor-based pharmaceuticals, such as Viagra, for the treatment of chronic and aging-associated disorders. The average numbers of formulas and herbs per prescription are between two and three. The relative doses of the ingredients in a typical five-ingredient prescription are 100:55:39:30:25.

9.4 Dysmenorrhea: *Dang Gui Shao Yao San* and *Yan Hu Suo*

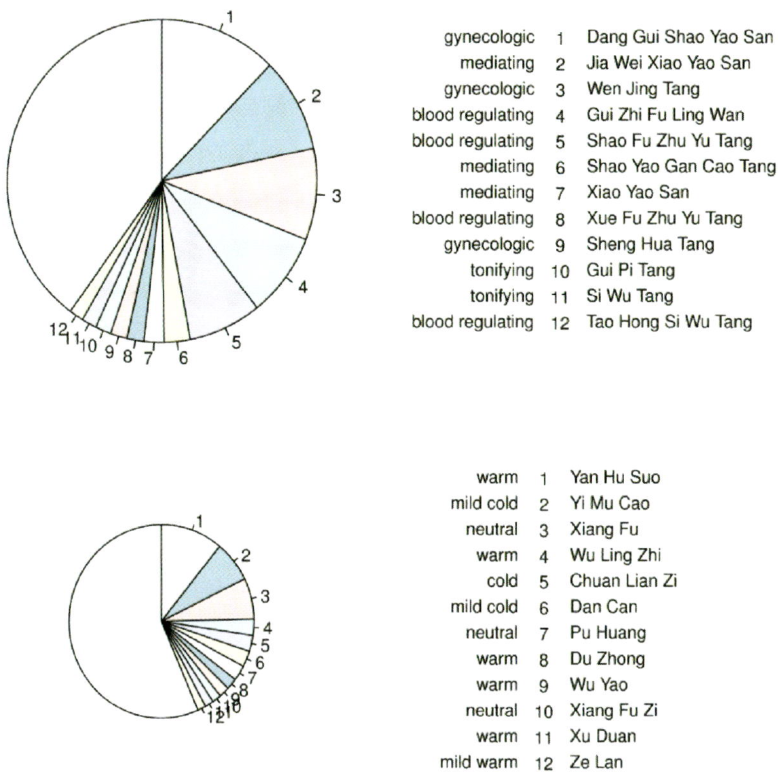

FIGURE 9.3a

Dysmenorrhea (ICD-9 = 6253) is treated by TCM blood-regulating ($p = 0.006$), gynecologic ($p = 0.008$) or mediating ($p = 0.03$) formulas. The top 12 ingredients are shown. The segments of the pies indicate the relative weights of the formulas and herbs in the prescription for the condition. *P* values are from overrepresentation tests.

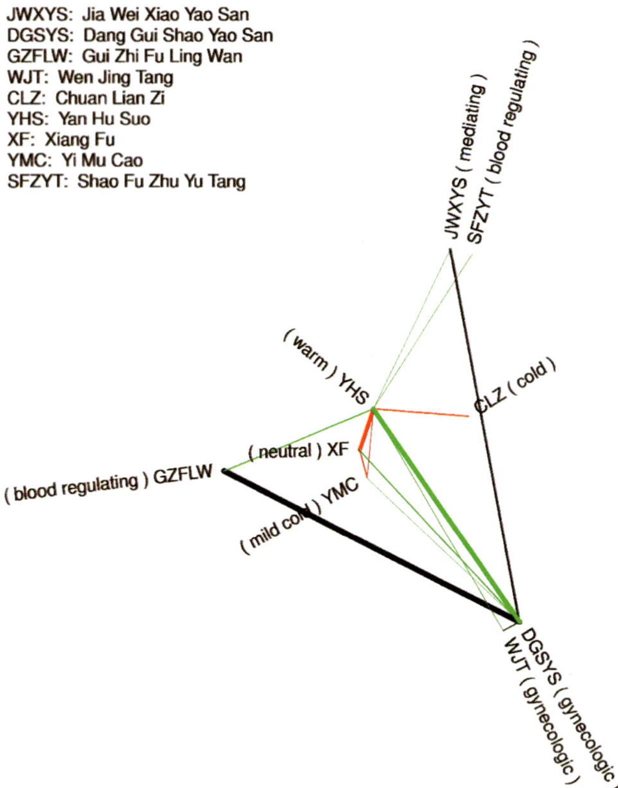

FIGURE 9.3b

The commonest TCM formula pair is DGSYS–GZFLW, the commonest formula–herb pair is DGSYS–YHS, followed by GZFLW–YHS, and the commonest herb pair is YHS–XF for the treatment of dysmenorrhea. The thickness of the line indicates the prevalence of the pair. Formula pairs are in black, formula–herb pairs in green and herb pairs in red. The TCM pharmacotherapeutic categories of the formulas and the TCM natures of the herbs are shown in parentheses.

9.5 Premenstrual Tension Syndrome: *Jia Wei Xiao Yao San* and *Yi Mu Cao*

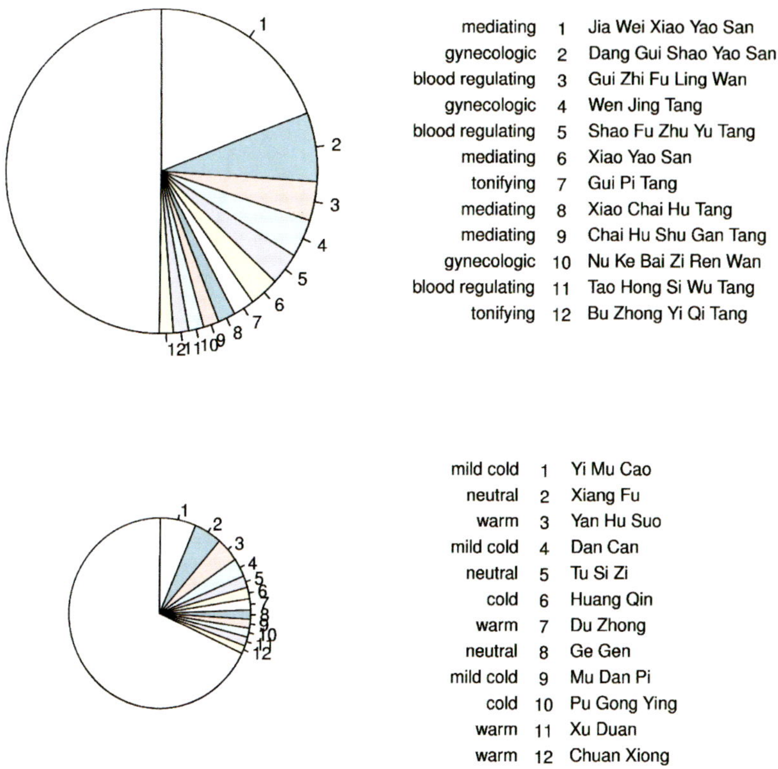

FIGURE 9.4a

Premenstrual tension syndrome (ICD-9 = 6254) is treated by TCM mediating ($p = 0.003$), gynecologic ($p = 0.008$) or blood-regulating ($p = 0.04$) formulas. The top 12 ingredients are shown. The areas of the pies indicate the relative weights of the formulas and herbs in the prescription for the condition. *P* values are from over-representation tests.

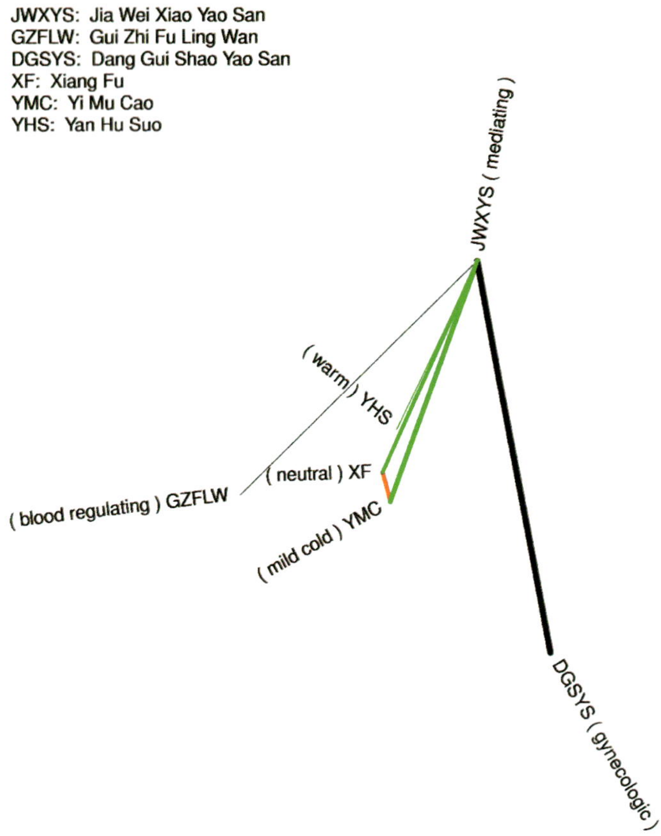

FIGURE 9.4b

The commonest TCM formula pair is JWXYS–DGSYS, the commonest formula–herb pair is JWXYS–YMC and the commonest herb pair is YMC–XF for the treatment of premenstrual tension syndrome. The thickness of the line indicates the prevalence of the pair. Formula pairs are in black, formula–herb pairs in green and herb pairs in red. The TCM pharmacotherapeutic categories of the formulas and the TCM natures of the herbs are shown in parentheses.

9.6 Absence of Menstruation: *Jia Wei Xiao Yao San* and *Yi Mu Cao*

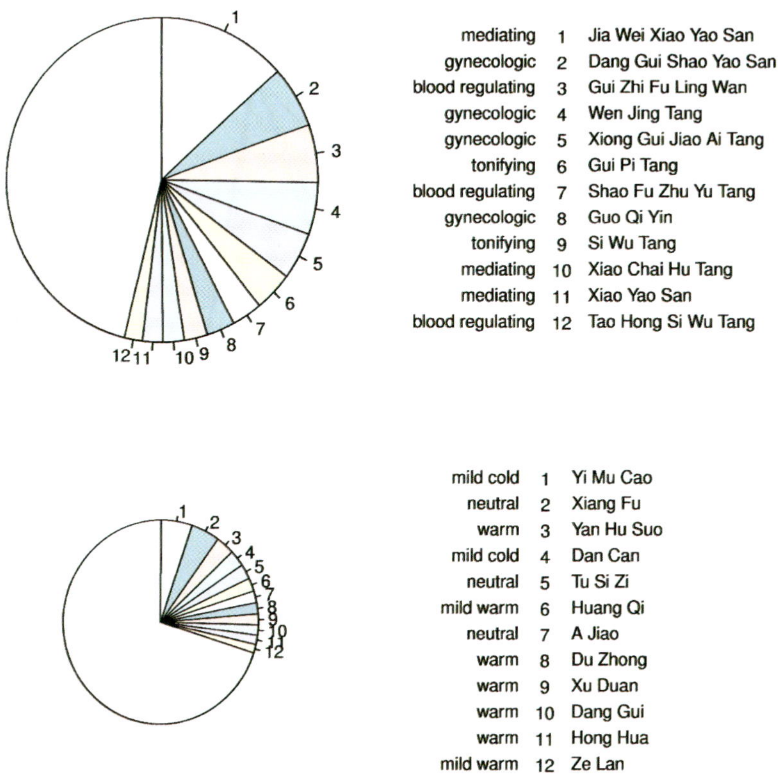

FIGURE 9.5a

Absence of menstruation (ICD-9 = 6260) is treated by TCM gynecologic ($p = 0.0006$), mediating ($p = 0.03$) or blood-regulating ($p = 0.04$) formulas. The top 12 ingredients are shown. The areas of the pies indicate the relative weights of the formulas and herbs in the prescription for the condition. *P* values are from over-representation tests.

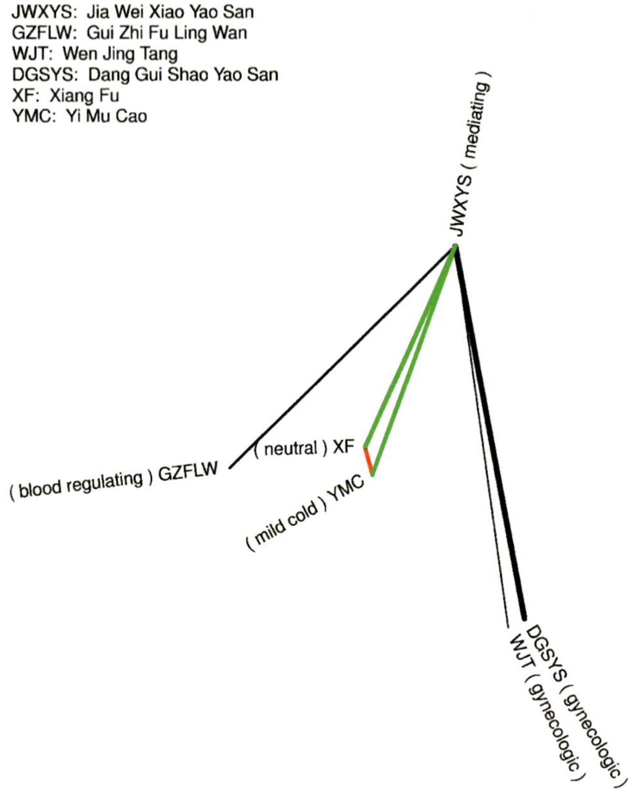

FIGURE 9.5b

The commonest TCM formula pair is JWXYS–DGSYS, the commonest formula–herb pair is JWXYS–XF and the commonest herb pair is XF–YMC for the treatment of absence of menstruation. The thickness of the line indicates the prevalence of the pair. Formula pairs are in black, formula–herb pairs in green and herb pairs in red. The TCM pharmacotherapeutic categories of the formulas and the TCM natures of the herbs are shown in parentheses.

9.7 Scanty or Infrequent Menstruation: *Jia Wei Xiao Yao San* and *Yi Mu Cao*

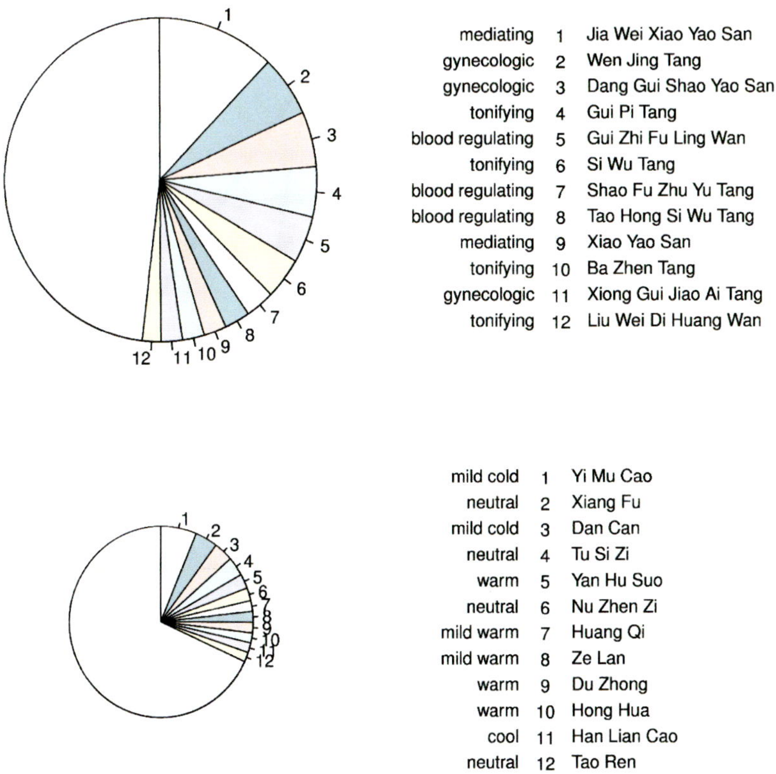

FIGURE 9.6a

Scanty or infrequent menstruation (ICD-9 = 6261) is treated by TCM gynecologic ($p = 0.008$) and blood-regulating ($p = 0.04$) formulas. The top 12 ingredients are shown. The areas of the pies indicate the relative weights of the formulas and herbs in the prescription for the condition. *P* values are from overrepresentation tests.

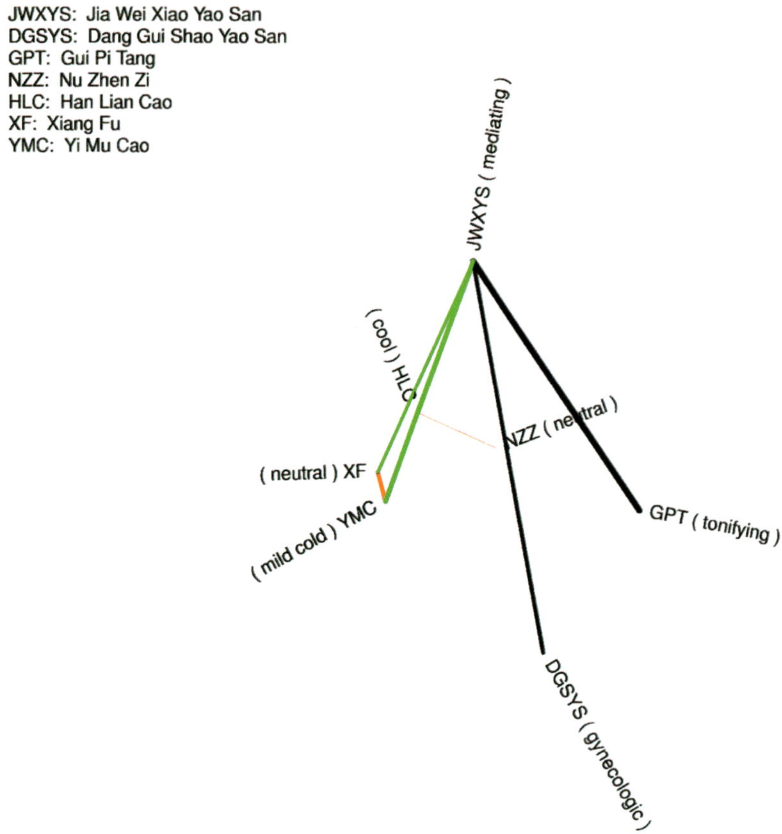

FIGURE 9.6b

The commonest TCM formula pair is JWXYS–GPT, the commonest formula–herb pair is JWXYS–YMC and the commonest herb pair is YMC–XF for the treatment of scanty or infrequent menstruation. The thickness of the line indicates the prevalence of the pair. Formula pairs are in black, formula–herb pairs in green and herb pairs in red. The TCM pharmacotherapeutic categories of the formulas and the TCM natures of the herbs are shown in parentheses.

9.8 Excessive or Frequent Menstruation: *Xiong Gui Jiao Ai Tang* and *Xian He Cao*

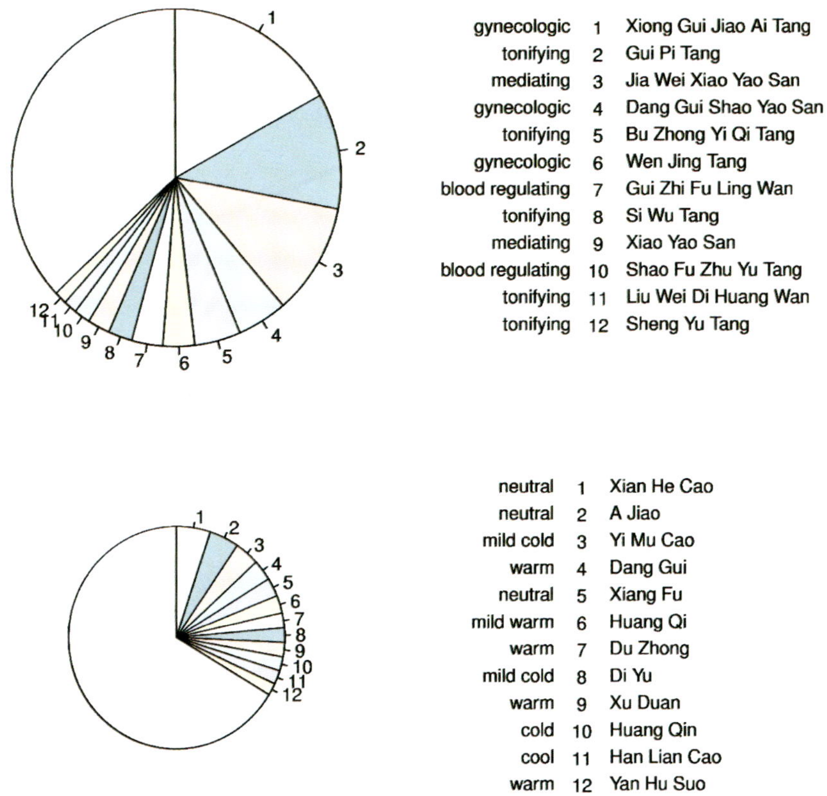

FIGURE 9.7a

Excess or frequent menstruation (ICD-9 = 6262) is treated by TCM gynecologic ($p = 0.008$) and tonifying ($p = 0.01$) formulas. The top 12 ingredients are shown. The areas of the pies indicate the relative weights of the formulas and herbs in the prescription for the condition. *P* values are from overrepresentation tests.

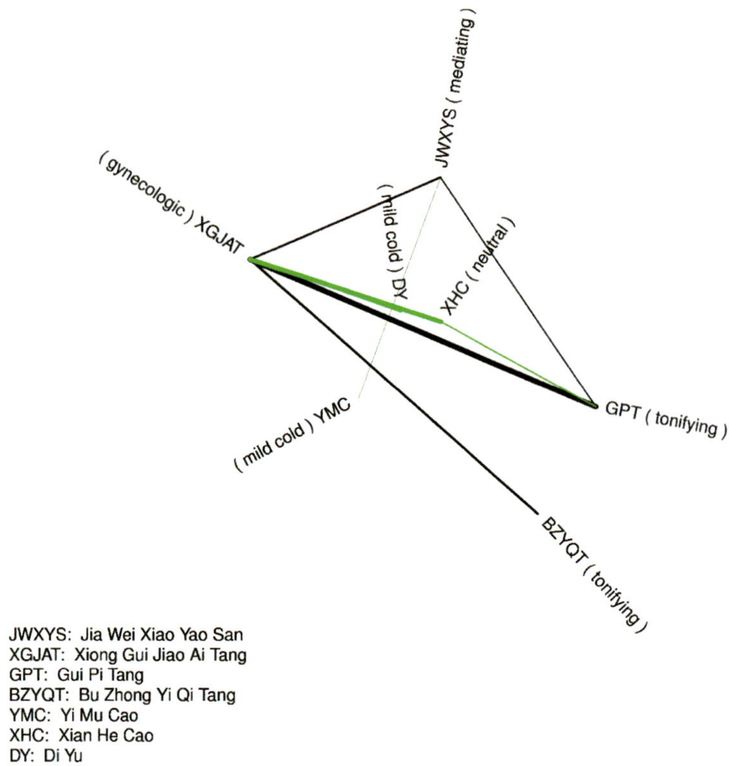

FIGURE 9.7b

The commonest TCM formula pair is XGJAT–GPT, followed by XGJAT–BZYQT, and the commonest formula–herb pair is XGJAT–XHC for the treatment of excess or frequent menstruation. The thickness of the line indicates the prevalence of the pair. Formula pairs are in black and formula–herb pairs in green. The TCM pharmacotherapeutic categories of the formulas and the TCM natures of the herbs are shown in parentheses.

9.9 Irregular Menstruation: *Jia Wei Xiao Yao San* and *Yi Mu Cao*

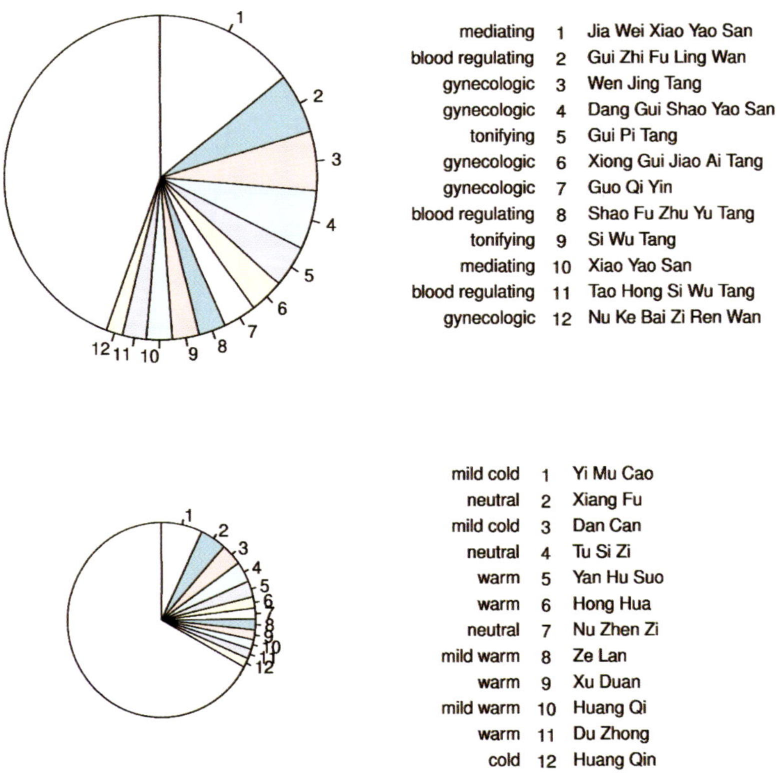

FIGURE 9.8a

Irregular menstruation (ICD-9 = 6264) is treated by TCM gynecologic ($p = 0.00003$) and blood-regulating ($p = 0.04$) formulas. The top 12 ingredients are shown. The areas of the pies indicate the relative weights of the formulas and herbs in the prescription for the condition. *P* values are from overrepresentation tests.

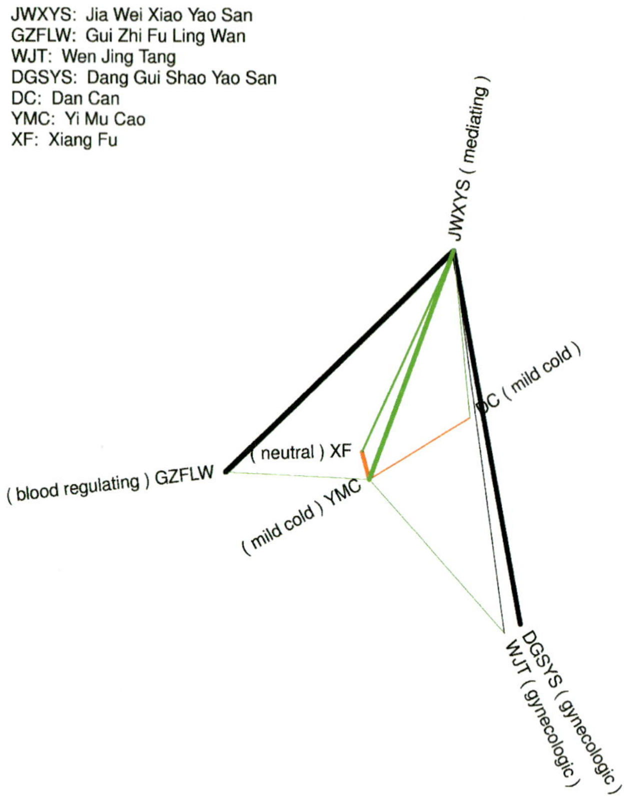

FIGURE 9.8b

The commonest TCM formula pair is JWXYS–GZFLW, the commonest formula–herb pair is JWXYS–YMC and the commonest herb pair is YMC–XF for the treatment of irregular menstruation. The thickness of the line indicates the prevalence of the pair. Formula pairs are in black, formula–herb pairs in green and herb pairs in red. The TCM pharmacotherapeutic categories of the formulas and the TCM natures of the herbs are shown in parentheses.

9.10 Other/Unspecified Disorders of Menstruation: *Jia Wei Xiao Yao San* and *Yi Mu Cao*

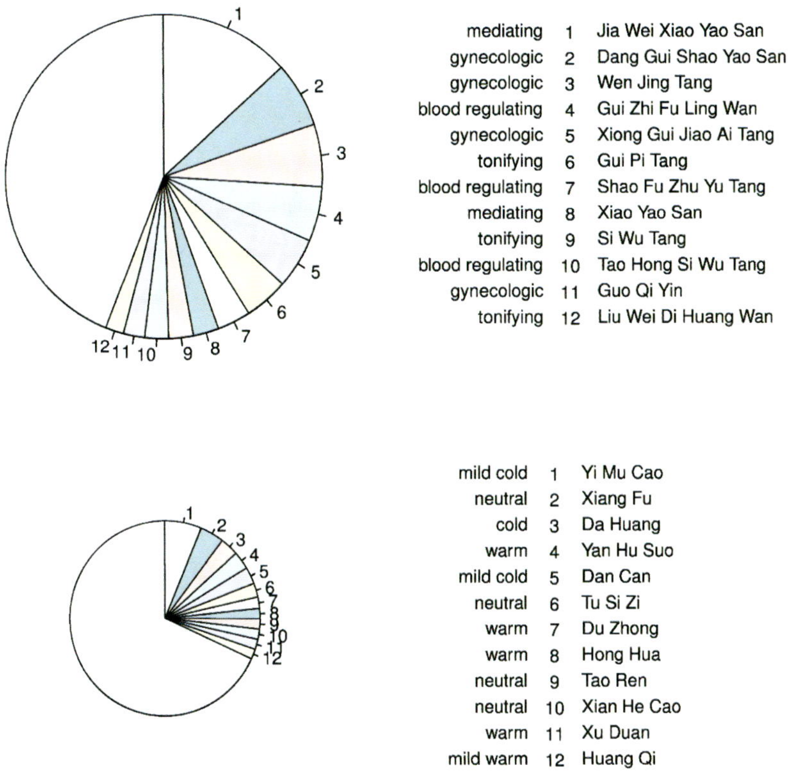

FIGURE 9.9a

Other/unspecified disorders of menstruation (ICD-9 = 6268, 6269) are treated by TCM gynecologic ($p = 0.0006$) and blood-regulating ($p = 0.04$) formulas. The top 12 ingredients are shown. The areas of the pies indicate the relative weights of the formulas and herbs in the prescription for the condition. *P* values are from over-representation tests.

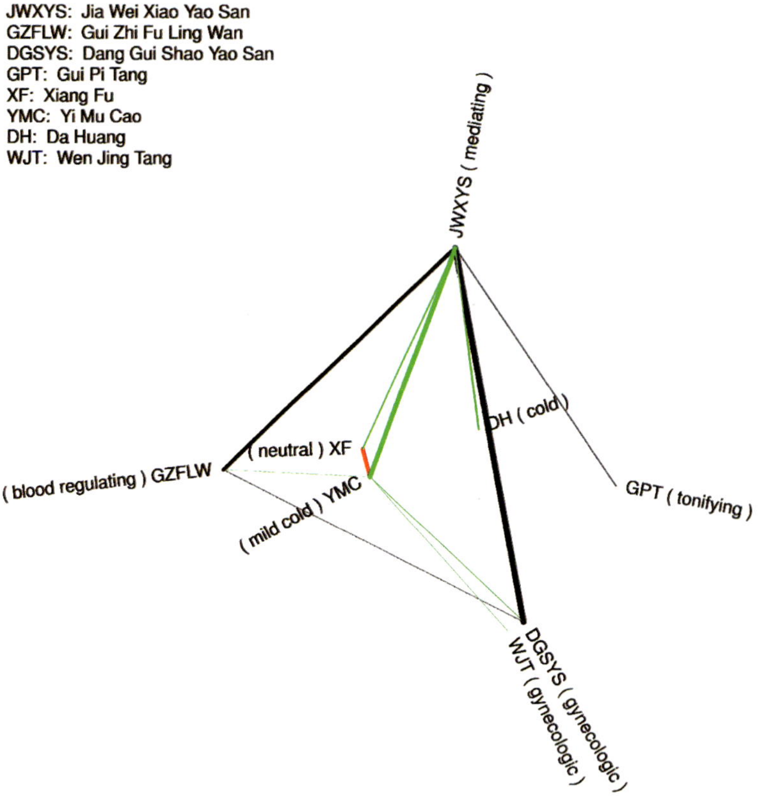

FIGURE 9.9b

The commonest TCM formula pair is JWXYS–DGSYS, the commonest formula–herb pair is JWXYS–YMC, followed by JWXYS–DH, and the commonest herb pair is YMC–XF for the treatment of other/unspecified disorders of menstruation. The thickness of the line indicates the prevalence of the pair. Formula pairs are in black, formula–herb pairs in green and herb pairs in red. The TCM pharmacotherapeutic categories of the formulas and the TCM natures of the herbs are shown in parentheses.

9.11 Menopausal State: *Jia Wei Xiao Yao San* and *Suan Zao Ren*

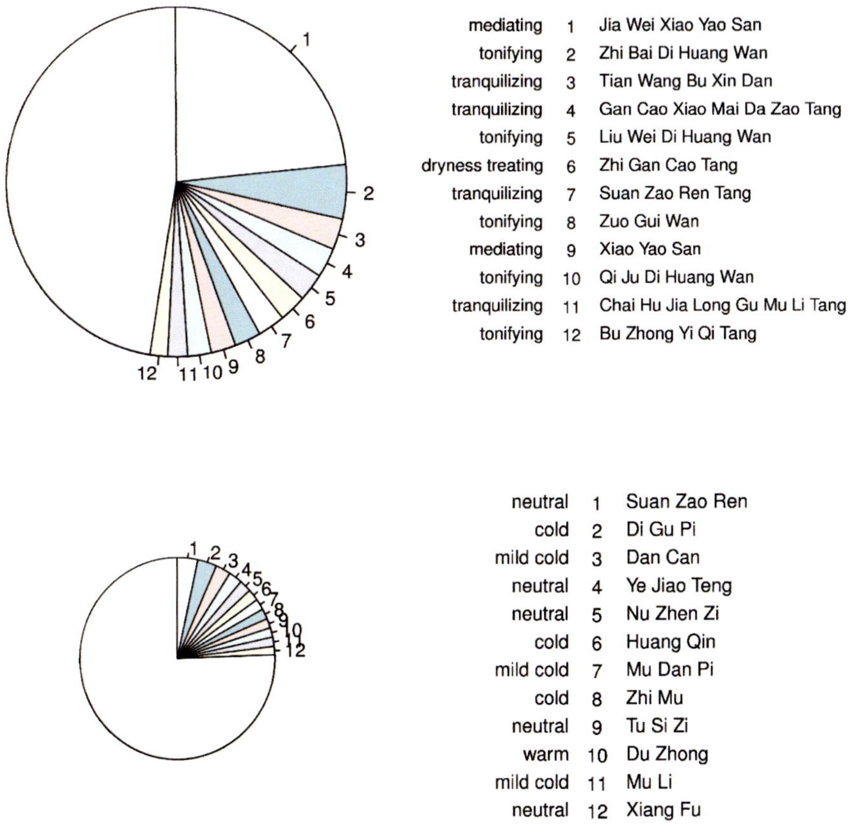

FIGURE 9.10a

The menopausal state (ICD-9 = 6272) is treated by TCM tranquilizing ($p = 0.0002$) and tonifying ($p = 0.01$) formulas. The top 12 ingredients are shown. The areas of the pies indicate the relative weights of the formulas and herbs in the prescription for the condition. P values are from overrepresentation tests.

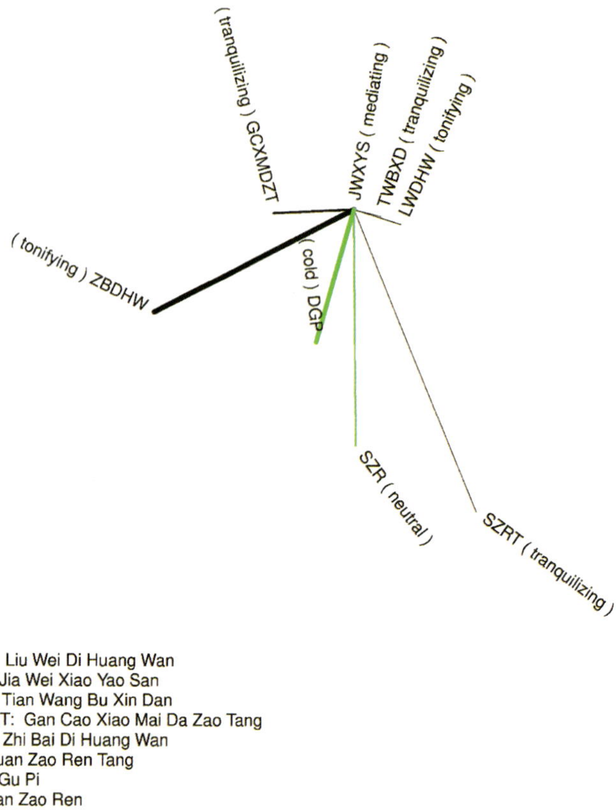

FIGURE 9.10b

The commonest TCM formula pair is JWXYS–ZBDHW and the commonest formula–herb pair is JWXYS–DGP for the treatment of the menopausal state. The thickness of the line indicates the prevalence of the pair. Formula pairs are in black and formula–herb pairs in green. The TCM pharmacotherapeutic categories of the formulas and the TCM natures of the herbs are shown in parentheses.

9.12 Unspecified (Post)Menopausal Disorder: *Jia Wei Xiao Yao San* and *Suan Zao Ren*

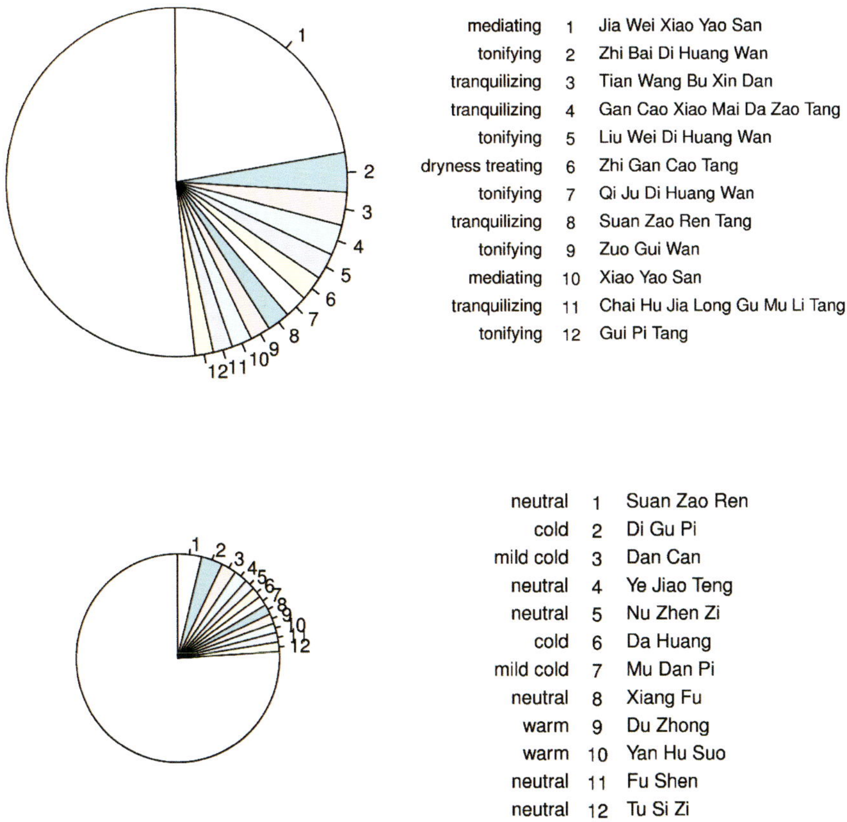

FIGURE 9.11a

Unspecified (post)menopausal disorder (ICD-9 = 6279) is treated by TCM tranquilizing ($p = 0.0002$) and tonifying ($p = 0.01$) formulas. The top 12 ingredients are shown. The areas of the pies indicate the relative weights of the formulas and herbs in the prescription for the condition. *P* values are from overrepresentation tests.

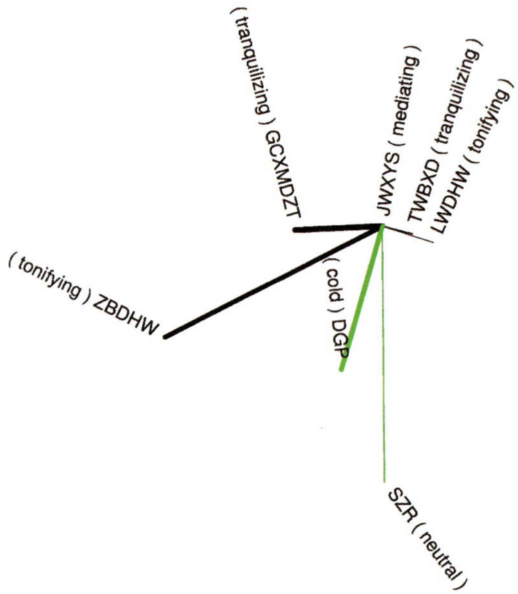

LWDHW: Liu Wei Di Huang Wan
JWXYS: Jia Wei Xiao Yao San
TWBXD: Tian Wang Bu Xin Dan
GCXMDZT: Gan Cao Xiao Mai Da Zao Tang
ZBDHW: Zhi Bai Di Huang Wan
DGP: Di Gu Pi
SZR: Suan Zao Ren

FIGURE 9.11b

The commonest TCM formula pair is JWXYS–GCXMDZT and the commonest formula–herb pair is JWXYS–DGP for the treatment of unspecified (post)menopausal disorder. The thickness of the line indicates the prevalence of the pair. Formula pairs are in black and formula–herb pairs in green. The TCM pharmacotherapeutic categories of the formulas and the TCM natures of the herbs are shown in parentheses.

9.13 Leukorrhea: *Wan Dai Tang* and *Tu Fu Ling*

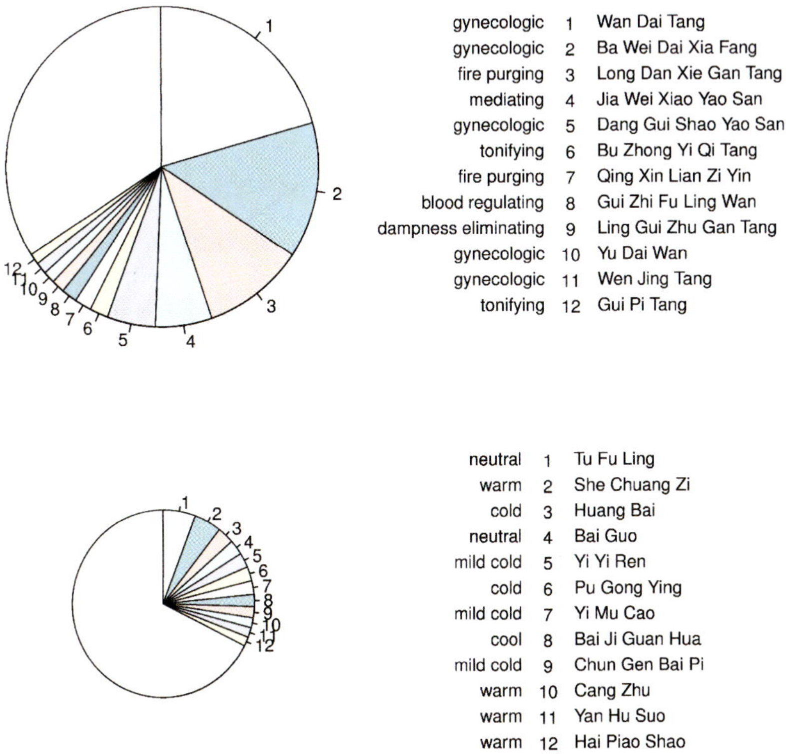

FIGURE 9.12a

Leukorrhea (ICD-9 = 6235) is treated by TCM gynecologic formulas ($p = 0.00003$). The top 12 ingredients are shown. The areas of the pies indicate the relative weights of the formulas and herbs in the prescription for the condition. *P* values are from overrepresentation tests.

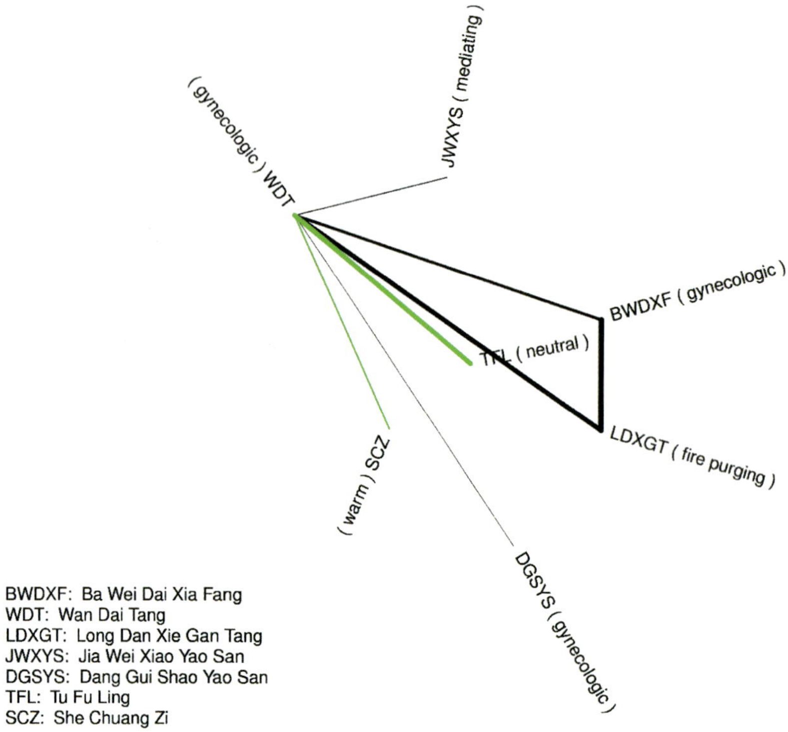

FIGURE 9.12b

The commonest TCM formula pair is LDXGT–BWDXF and the commonest formula–herb pair is WDT–TFL for the treatment of leukorrhea. The thickness of the line indicates the prevalence of the pair. Formula pairs are in black and formula–herb pairs in green. The TCM pharmacotherapeutic categories of the formulas and the TCM natures of the herbs are shown in parentheses.

9.14 Osteoporosis: *Du Huo Ji Sheng Tang* and *Du Zhong*

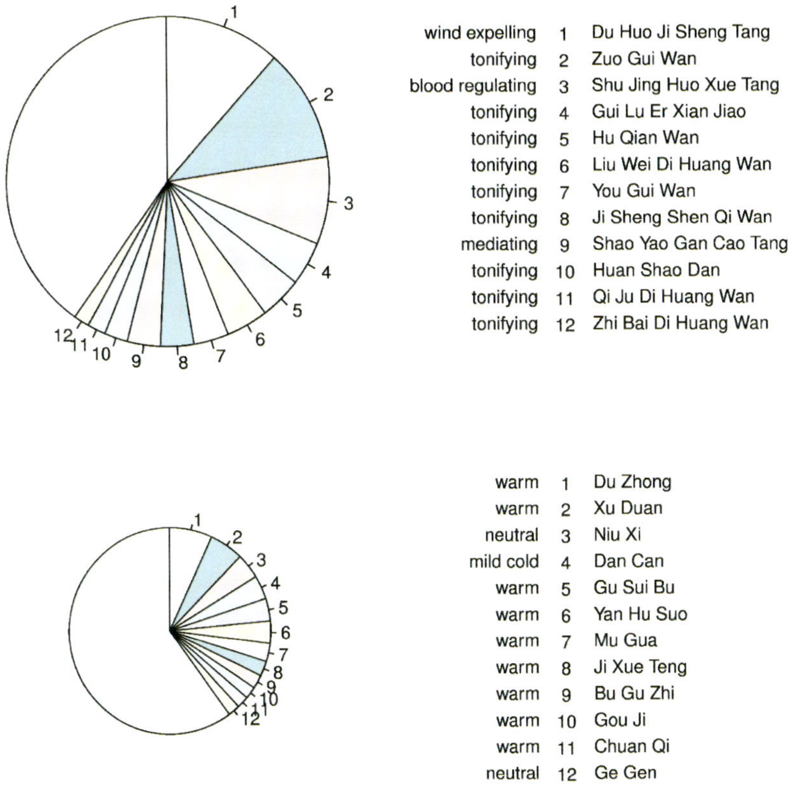

FIGURE 9.13a

Osteoporosis (ICD-9 = 7330) is treated by TCM tonifying formulas ($p = 0.000001$) and TCM warm herbs ($p = 0.0005$). The top 12 ingredients are shown. The areas of the pies indicate the relative weights of the formulas and herbs in the prescription for the condition. *P* values are from overrepresentation tests.

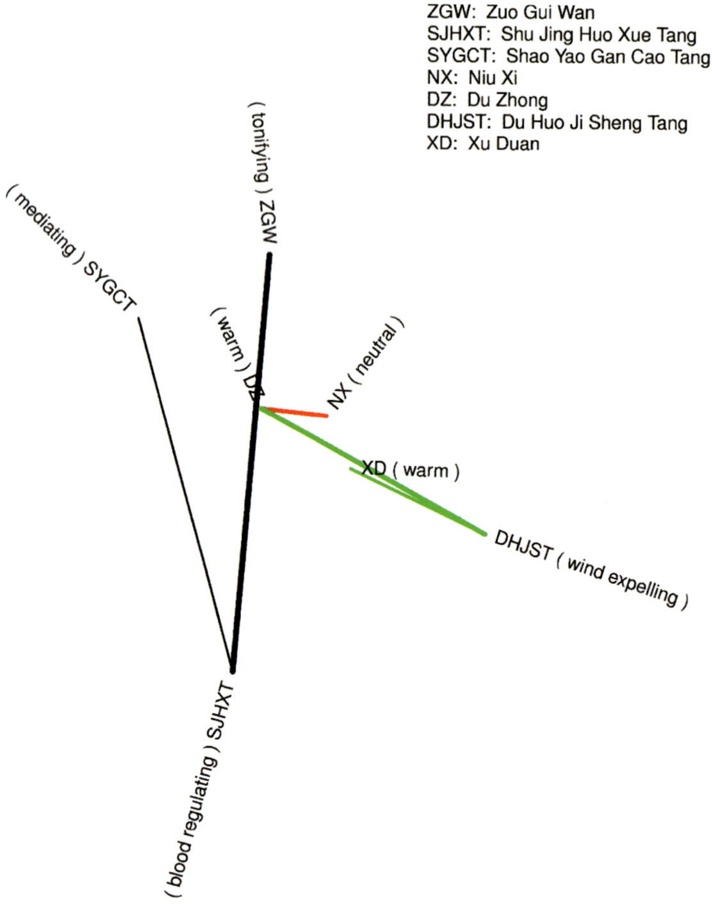

FIGURE 9.13b

The commonest TCM formula pair is SJHXT–ZGW, the commonest formula–herb pair is DHJST–DZ and the commonest herb pair is DZ–NX for the treatment of osteoporosis. The thickness of the line indicates the prevalence of the pair. Formula pairs are in black, formula–herb pairs in green and herb pairs in red. The TCM pharmacotherapeutic categories of the formulas and the TCM natures of the herbs are shown in parentheses.

9.15 Female Infertility (Unspecified Origin): *Shen Ling Bai Zhu San* and *Tu Si Zi*

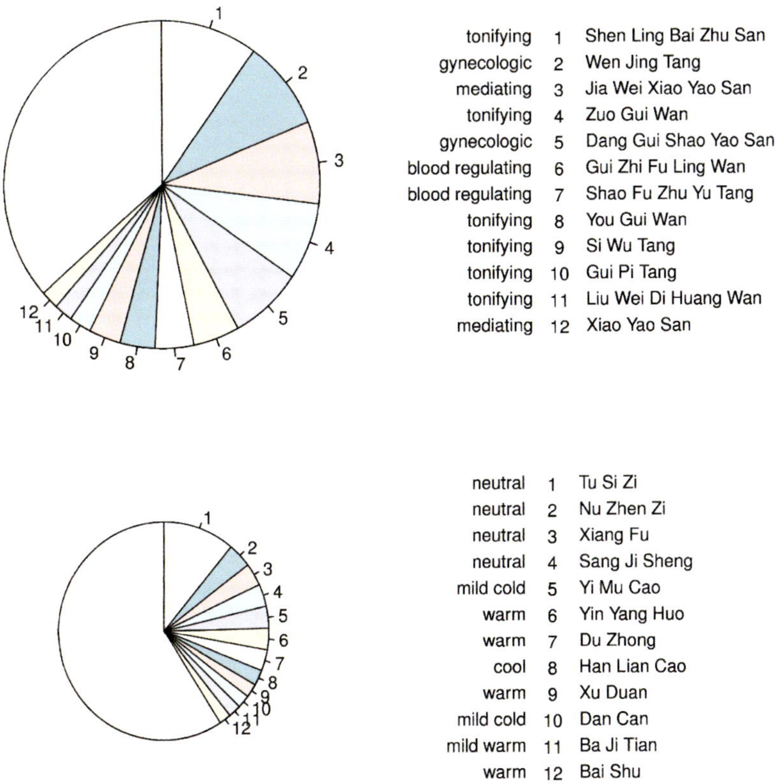

FIGURE 9.14a

Female infertility (ICD-9 = 6289) is treated by TCM tonifying formulas ($p = 0.002$). The top 12 ingredients are shown. The areas of the pies indicate the relative weights of the formulas and herbs in the prescription for the condition. *P* values are from overrepresentation tests.

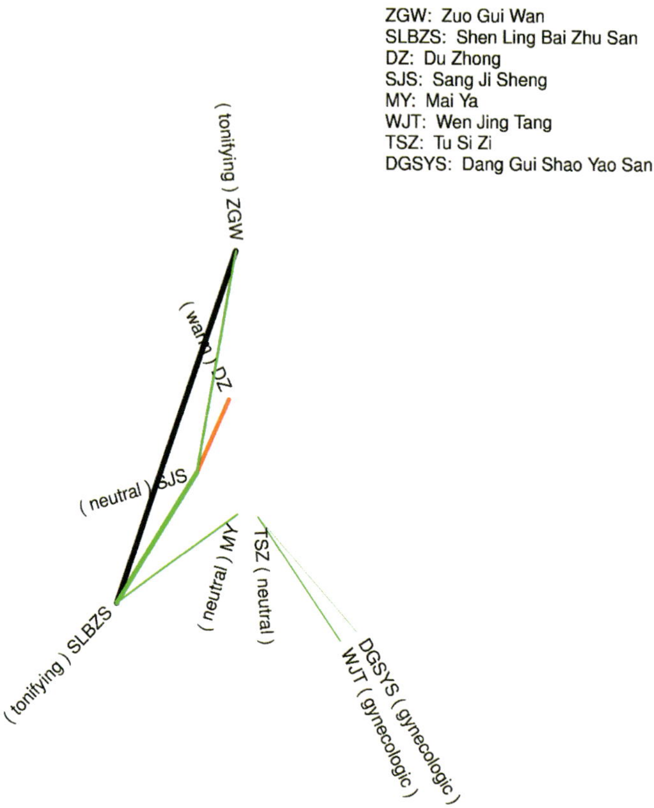

FIGURE 9.14b

The commonest TCM formula pair is SLBZS–ZGW, the commonest formula–herb pair is SLBZS–SJS, followed by ZGW–SJS and SLBZS–MY, and the commonest herb pair is SJS–DZ for the treatment of female infertility. The thickness of the line indicates the prevalence of the pair. Formula pairs are in black, formula–herb pairs in green and herb pairs in red. The TCM pharmacotherapeutic categories of the formulas and the TCM natures of the herbs are shown in parentheses.

9.16 Male Infertility (Unspecified Origin): *Huan Shao Dan* and *Yin Yang Huo*

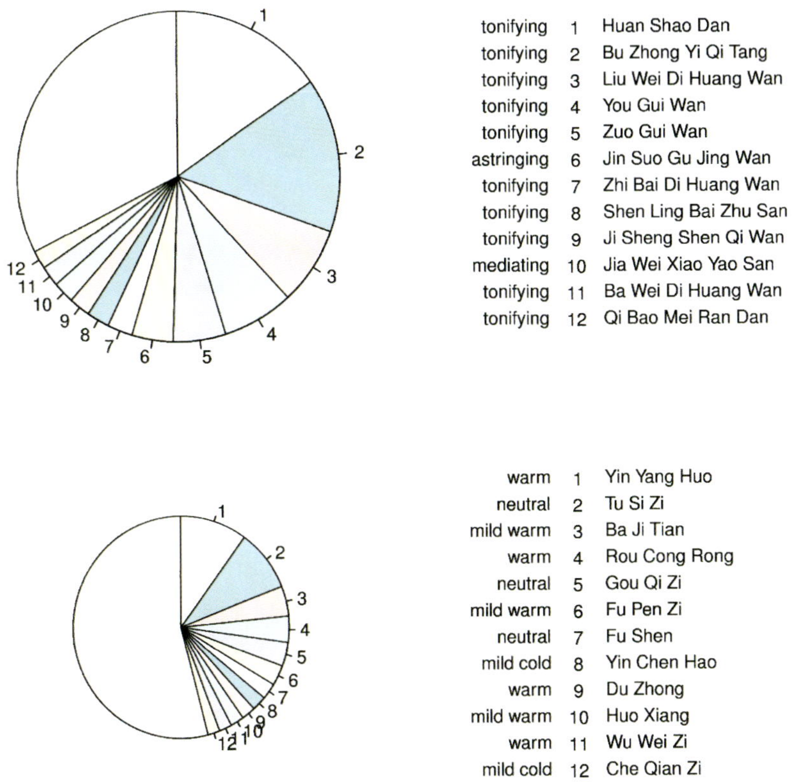

FIGURE 9.15a

Male infertility (ICD-9 = 6069) is treated by TCM tonifying formulas ($p = 0.00000004$). The top 12 ingredients are shown. The areas of the pies indicate the relative weights of the formulas and herbs in the prescription for the condition. *P* values are from overrepresentation tests.

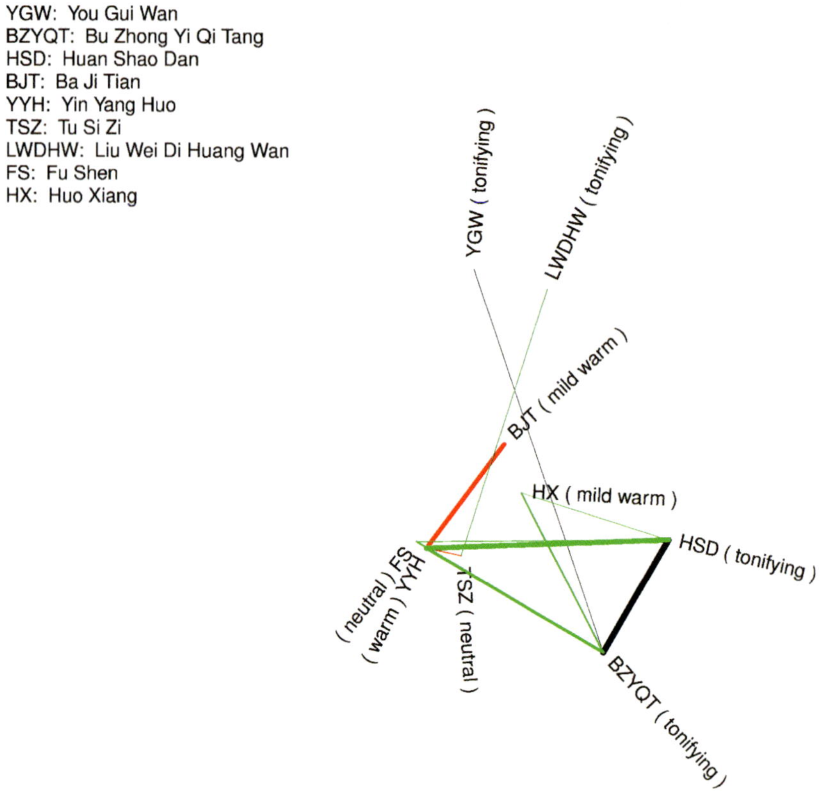

FIGURE 9.15b

The commonest TCM formula pair is HSD–BZYQT, the commonest formula–herb pair is HSD–YYH, followed by BZYQT–YYH, and the commonest herb pair is YYH–BJT for the treatment of male infertility. The thickness of the line indicates the prevalence of the pair. Formula pairs are in black, formula–herb pairs in green and herb pairs in red. The TCM pharmacotherapeutic categories of the formulas and the TCM natures of the herbs are shown in parentheses.

9.17 Impotence (Organic): *Huan Shao Dan* and *Yin Yang Huo*

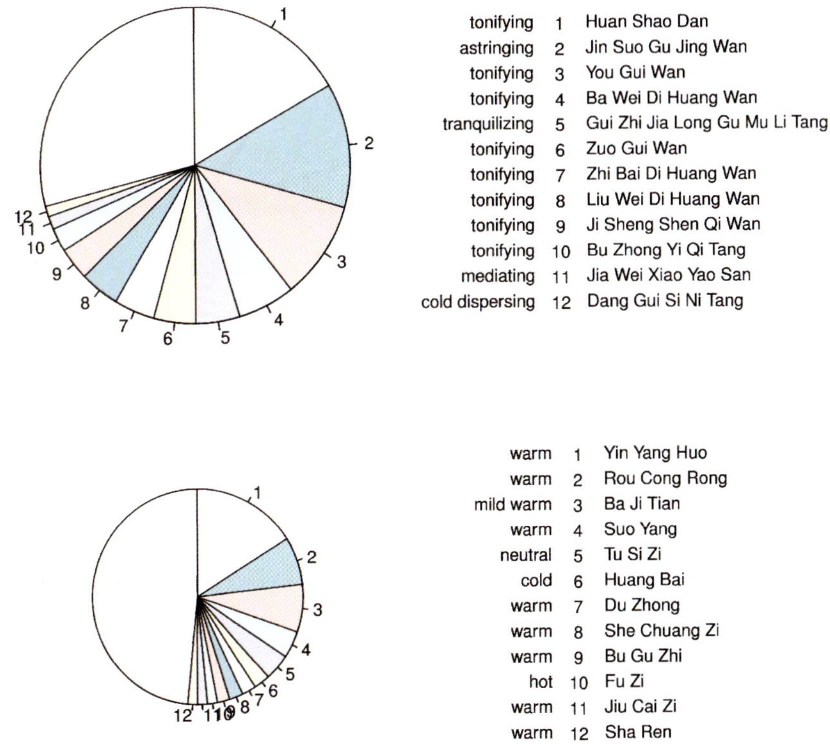

FIGURE 9.16a

Impotence (organic) (ICD-9 = 60784) is treated by TCM tonifying formulas ($p = 0.00002$) and TCM warm herbs ($p = 0.003$). The top 12 ingredients are shown. The areas of the pies indicate the relative weights of the formulas and herbs in the prescription for the condition. *P* values are from overrepresentation tests.

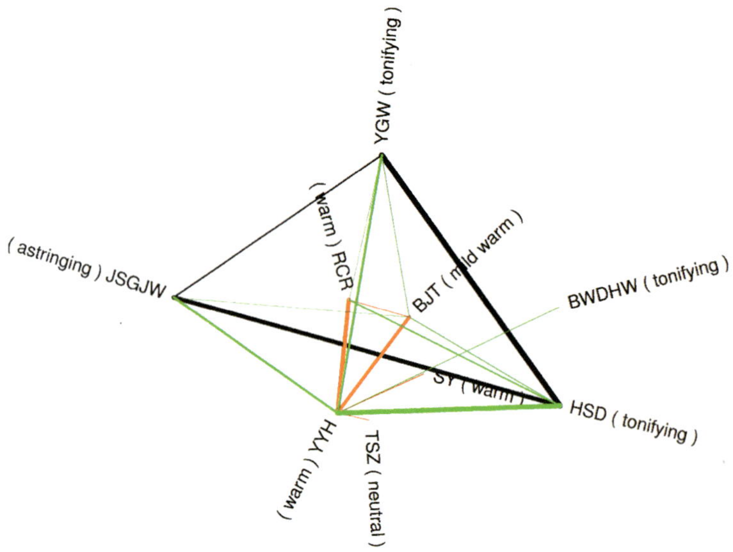

YGW: You Gui Wan
JSGJW: Jin Suo Gu Jing Wan
HSD: Huan Shao Dan
BJT: Ba Ji Tian
RCR: Rou Cong Rong
YYH: Yin Yang Huo
TSZ: Tu Si Zi
SY: Suo Yang
BWDHW: Ba Wei Di Huang Wan

FIGURE 9.16b

The commonest TCM formula pair is HSD–YGW, the commonest formula–herb pair is HSD–YYH, followed by YGW–YYH and JSGJW–YYH, and the commonest herb pair is YYH–RCR for the treatment of organic impotence. The thickness of the line indicates the prevalence of the pair. Formula pairs are in black, formula–herb pairs in green and herb pairs in red. The TCM pharmacotherapeutic categories of the formulas and the TCM natures of the herbs are shown in parentheses.

9.18 Impotence (Psychosexual Dysfunction): *Huan Shao Dan* and *Yin Yang Huo*

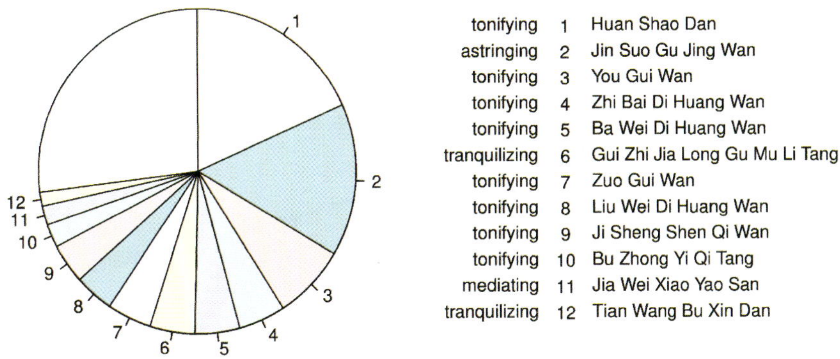

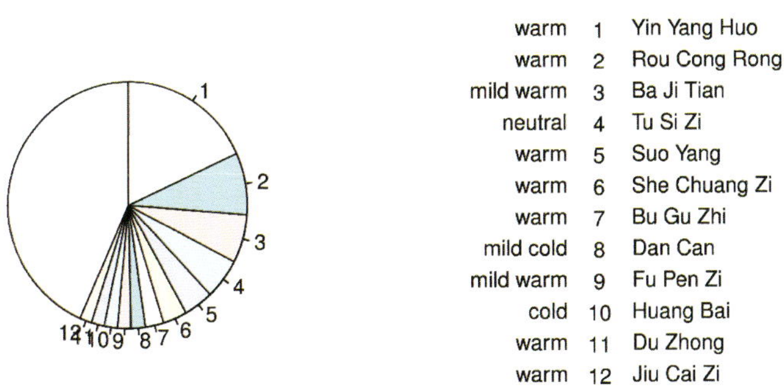

FIGURE 9.17a

Impotence (psychosexual dysfunction) (ICD-9 = 30272) is treated by TCM tonifying (p = 0.00002) and tranquilizing (p = 0.05) formulas and TCM warm (p = 0.02) herbs. The top 12 ingredients are shown. The areas of the pies indicate the relative weights of the formulas and herbs in the prescription for the condition. P values are from overrepresentation tests.

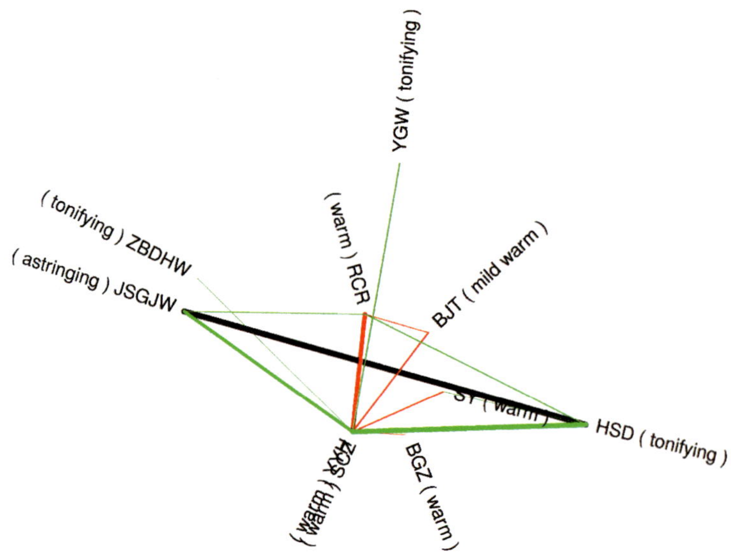

JSGJW: Jin Suo Gu Jing Wan
HSD: Huan Shao Dan
BJT: Ba Ji Tian
RCR: Rou Cong Rong
YYH: Yin Yang Huo
SCZ: She Chuang Zi
BGZ: Bu Gu Zhi
SY: Suo Yang
YGW: You Gui Wan
ZBDHW: Zhi Bai Di Huang Wan

FIGURE 9.17b

The commonest TCM formula pair is HSD–JSGJW, the commonest formula–herb pair is HSD–YYH, followed by JSGJW–YYH and YGW–YYH, and the commonest herb pair is YYH–RCR, followed by YYH–BJT, for the treatment of psychogenic impotence. The thickness of the line indicates the prevalence of the pair. Formula pairs are in black, formula–herb pairs in green and herb pairs in red. The TCM pharmacotherapeutic categories of the formulas and the TCM natures of the herbs are shown in parentheses.

Part III

Longevity

10

Theories of Aging

Dozens of aging theories exist in the western biomedical literature. They belong to one of two genres: (1) genetically programmed aging; (2) damage and error aging. Rats live many times shorter than birds of similar size. Genetics therefore plays a role in aging. Aging as a multifaceted complex phenomenon is, however, hardly believed to be influenced by a single factor. For example, cell cycle arrest for a longer time allows the cell to invest more in the repair of DNA damage, extending the species' maximum lifespan. Aging theories therefore are not necessarily mutually exclusive. A synthesis of the theories can hopefully help us better understand aging.

We start from modern western aging theories and proceed to traditional eastern aging theories, sweeping across molecular, systemic and suprasystemic (i.e. whole-person) aging hypotheses. As biochemical reactions underlie all living processes, the free radical or oxidative stress theory of aging applies not only to human cells but also primitive single-celled organisms. Oxygen-containing free radicals generated in aerobic respiration damage DNA, proteins and lipids, causing cellular senescence. Cellular-level theories of aging, albeit universal, fall short of organ- or system-specificity. The immune system can become overwhelmed over time by chronic stress. The neuroendocrine system and immunity are intimately correlated. An antagonistic pleiotropic theory of aging therefore involves a deregulated neuroendocrine system.

Pitta dosha in Ayurveda governs digestion, metabolism and energy production. The Ayurvedic theory of aging, that *pitta* aggravation drives premature aging is in concert with the oxidative stress theory of aging. The functions of the TCM kidney encompass those of the hypothalamus–pituitary–gonad axis. The functions of the TCM spleen/stomach include digestion and transformation. TCM *qi* aids body defense. The three TCM theories of aging therefore recapitulate the oxidative stress, immunosenescence and endocrine theories of aging. In summary, the theories of aging reviewed here suggest that antioxidant, anti-inflammatory and TCM kidney tonifying diets are potentially anti-aging. *Dosha*- or TCM-syndrome-specific regimens should further be prescribed for individualized prevention of aging.

10.1 Oxidative Stress Theory of Aging

In 1908, Max Rubner observed that the maximum lifespan of mammals and birds negatively correlates with the basal metabolic rate measured in kJ/day/kg. The observation implies that the *faster* a species lives, the more their bodies wear and the sooner they die. Since aerobic metabolism generates reactive oxygen species (ROS) that are tissue-damaging, it was proposed by Denham Harman in 1956 that aging *per se* or age-associated degenerative diseases were a result of endogenous free radical or oxidative damage [Harman, 1956].

The ROS superoxide O_2^-, generated as a byproduct of aerobic respiration in the electron transport chain (ETC) of mitochondria, damages DNA, proteins and lipids. For example, one of the major DNA oxidation products is 7,8-dihydro-8-oxo-deoxyguanosine (8-oxo-dG), which is known for its mutagenic potential resulting in G-to-T transversion in mitochondrial or nuclear DNA. Because of the ubiquity of oxidative reactions, defense mechanisms have evolved in cells to repair damaged DNA. Mechanisms that repair single-strand DNA damage using the undamaged strand as a template include base excision repair, nucleotide excision repair and mismatch repair. Mechanisms that repair double-strand breaks — which, if not repaired, can bring about genome rearrangements — include nonhomologous end joining. Unrepaired DNA damage can halt the cell cycle at the G1 phase indefinitely, giving rise to senescent cells. Tissues and organs stop growing. Further DNA damage triggers programmed cell death, leading to atrophy.

In the oxidative stress or somatic DNA damage theory of aging, increased oxidant resistance by overexpressing DNA repair genes and/or decreased ROS production by the use of antioxidants should extend the maximum lifespan. While experiments on lower organisms such as yeast, roundworms and fruit flies are generally supportive of the prediction, results from mammals such as rats have been inconclusive. ROS, although detrimental, are needed in redox homeostasis and signal transduction. Balance in ROS production and antioxidant defense is probably the key to health.

10.2 Telomere and Mitochondrial Theories of Aging

Leonard Hayflick in 1961 found that the number of times a normal cell divides is limited and that the limit correlates with telomere length [Hayflick and Moorhead, 1961]. Telomeres are repeated DNA at the tips of chromosomes. It is now known that vertebrate telomeres are TTAGGG tandem repeats, containing no genes. In DNA replication, DNA cannot be replicated all the way down to the ends of chromosomes. A telomeric section of about 20 bp is lost in each DNA replication. Telomeres function to maintain genome integrity by preventing chromosome fusion and rearrangement. When they become depleted after successive cell divisions over time, senescence or apoptosis can be induced to stop or destroy the aged cell. Telomeres are thus molecular clocks which count down the time to cellular demise.

Mitochondria are power generators in cells, producing more than 90% of all ATP made in the body. A cell contains dozens to

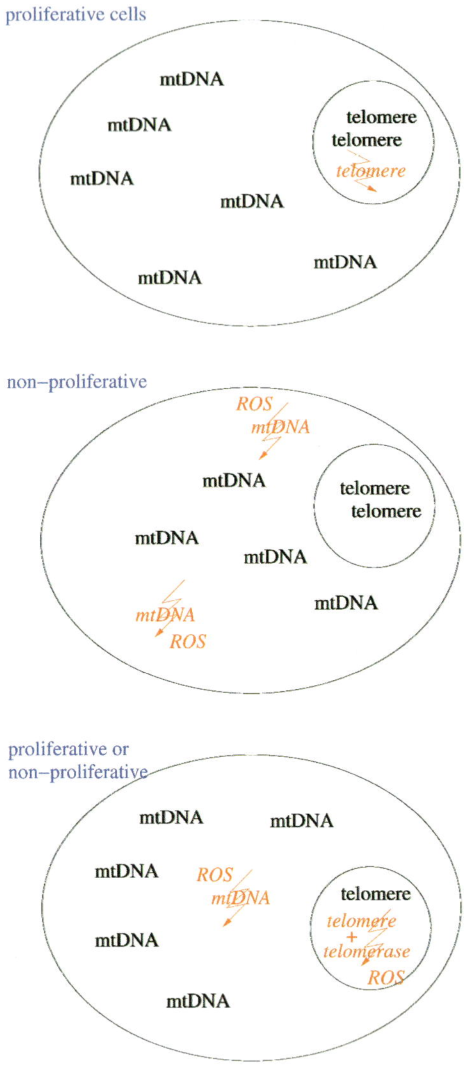

FIGURE 10.1

Telomere shortening in proliferative cells (*top*) and mtDNA mutation in nonproliferative cells (*middle*) can induce cell senescence or apoptosis. ROS damage not only mitochondrial but also telomeric DNA through telomerase damaging (*bottom*).

thousands of mitochondria, each of which has several copies of mitochondrial DNA (mtDNA) in the mitochondrial matrix close to the inner membrane where oxidation takes place through the process of ETC. Because of their proximity to the ETC, mtDNA molecules are susceptible to DNA damage by the leaking superoxide anion (O_2^-) and other secondary ROS, including hydrogen peroxide (H_2O_2) and hydroxyl radicals (OH). The 16 kb mtDNA contains 13 protein-coding genes, 8 of which encode the polypeptides of the energy-transducing enzymes complexes I and III of the ETC. Damage to mtDNA impairs the ETC, multiplying O_2^- leakage and aggravating mtDNA damage [Loeb *et al.*, 2005]. Defective mitochondria diminishes energy production, resulting in physical frailty a characteristic of aging.

Shortening of telomeres in nuclei accounts for aging of proliferative cells such as blood. On the other hand, oxidation of mtDNA in mitochondria explains aging of nonproliferative cells such as the brain, heart and liver. Aging, as a whole-organism, multifocal pathology, can result from damage to the DNA in both cellular compartments. For example, the enzyme telomerase is known to add a lost bit of DNA back to shortened telomeres. In adults, telomerase is expressed in regularly dividing cells such as germ, immune and stem cells. ROS from mitochondria can damage telomeric DNA and telomerase. Damaged telomeric DNA lowers the binding affinity between telomeric DNA and telomerase. Mitochondrial biogenesis and telomerase reactivation are potential interventions for rejuvenation. However, telomerase has also been found to be activated in many cancers. Before its role in cancerogenesis is better understood, one should remain cautious about telomerase therapy.

10.3 Immunosenescence Theory of Aging

ROS, originating in mitochondrial respiration, and which can damage nuclear and mtDNA, are an endogenous chemical stressor on cells. A myriad of other stressors also take a toll on organismal survival. They include physical stressors such as UV radiation and heat, biological stressors such as viruses and bacteria, and socio-psychological stressors on humans such as divorce and unemployment. As a consequence, species have evolved a battery of defense mechanisms against the challenges. Examples of the defense components are: superoxide dismutase (SOD) and catalase, which scavenge free radicals; heat shock proteins (HSPs), which refold heat-denatured proteins; poly[ADP-ribose] polymerase 1 (PARP1), which recovers DNA damage; and RAS and AP-1 genes, which are involved in UV response.

Along the evolution, invertebrates have first evolved an innate immune system which mounts an immediate and nonspecific response to pathogens. Major players in the innate immunity are the long-lived macrophages, which, besides engulfing and digesting cellular debris and pathogens, secrete proinflammatory cytokines such as IL-1, IL-6 and TNF-α. Jawed vertebrates have evolved an adaptive immune system which, together with the innate immunity, enables the host to respond to specific pathogens in a stronger manner. The strong and specific response is due to antigen-specific receptor binding of the clones of B and T lymphocytes that have developed in the host since the host first encountered the antigen. In higher vertebrates like humans, a highly integrated immuno-neuroendocrine suprasystem emerges to efficiently safeguard organismal integrity. The network of antistress systems consisting of the defense functions and immune responses altogether can be thought of as an anti-aging mechanism.

Cooperating macrophage- and lymphocyte-based immunities confer capability of adaptive and successful stress coping. However, over many years or decades, the cumulative impact of evolving antigens and chronic stress eventually tips the balance toward macrophage-based immunity. Such an immunosenescent phenotype, which has been observed in the aged, is characterized by an increase in the number of macrophages, expansion of memory cells, exhaustion of naïve cells and shrinkage of the T cell repertoire [Franceschi *et al.*, 2000]. An escalating proinflammatory status thus manifests as a common biological background of the aged. Furthermore, different individuals are more likely to be hit by different organ-specific diseases, depending on their genetic makeup.

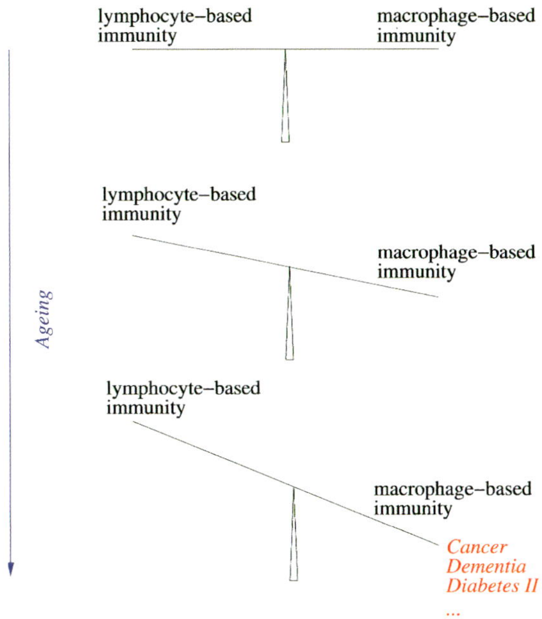

FIGURE 10.2

In aging, macrophage-related inflammation escalates, manifesting a low-grade inflammation which predisposes an individual to inflammatory diseases such as cancer, cardiovascular disease or dementia.

As a result, various chronic inflammatory disorders, including atherosclerosis, Alzheimer's disease, osteoarthritis and diabetes, are found to be most common among the elderly. Proinflammation which is beneficial for the young and adults turns out to be detrimental late in life, when the force of natural selection is weak. The rate of the inflammation surge can have a genetic component too. Nevertheless, anti-inflammatory regimens such as exercise should be favored to rein in inflammation.

10.4 Endocrine Theory of Aging

A communication network among neurotransmitters, hormones and immune cells began to be unraveled in 1975. An example of cooperative neuroendocrine systems is the HPG axis, which consists of the hypothalamus, anterior pituitary and gonads working together to regulate development, reproduction and aging. Gonadotropin-releasing hormone (GnRH) synthesized in the hypothalamus activates release of luteinizing hormone (LH) and follicle-stimulating hormone (FSH) from the pituitary gland into the blood circulation. LH and FSH bind to the receptors in ovaries and testes to stimulate secretion of sex hormones, i.e. estrogen and progesterone in females and testosterone in males, which in turn promote female ovulation and male spermatogenesis. Progesterone and testosterone inhibit production of GnRH, forming a negative feedback control of HPG axis activity. Interactions between HPG and immunity are through the estrogen and androgen receptors expressed in primary lymphoid organs and peripheral immune cells. Estrogen tends to have a stimulatory effect and testosterone/progesterone a suppressive effect on the immune system. On the other hand, cytokine IL-1 can inhibit GnRH release from the hypothalamus and LH from the pituitary, leading to reduced sex hormone release from the gonads.

Sustained and mature activity of the HPG axis kicks off puberty. In women, production of hormones in the ovaries does not decline until their midlife. In men, decline in testosterone production is believed to start in their early 30s, manifesting in progressive loss of muscle, libido and potency. A decrease in sex hormones results in an increase in LH, FSH and GnRH because of the negative feedback loop. Sex hormones are mitogenic, while LH, FSH and GnRH are differentiative. An imbalanced ratio of mitogenic to differentiative hormones disrupts cell cycle control and leads to aging-related diseases, including cancer, osteoporosis, Alzheimer's disease, dementia, coronary heart disease and cerebrovascular disease. Epidemiological studies have lent support to the reproductive hormone theory of aging [Atwood and Bowen, 2011]. For example, later menopause has been associated with a longer female lifespan, and earlier and later menarche have been associated with higher and lower mortality, respectively. However, a large-scale randomized controlled prevention trial found an increased risk of invasive breast

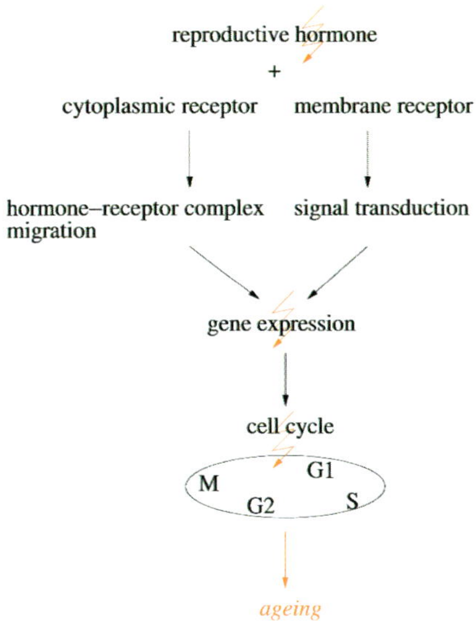

FIGURE 10.3

An imbalanced mixture of reproductive hormones disrupts the cell cycle, leading to aging.

cancer in healthy postmenopausal US women receiving estrogen and progestin [Rossouw *et al.*, 2002]. The benefit and risk profile of a sex-hormone-rejuvenating therapy (estrogen for women and testosterone for men) should therefore be carefully evaluated.

10.5 Ayurvedic Theory of Aging

According to the main Ayurvedic texts, i.e. *Charaka Samhita*, *Susruta Samhita*, *Ashtanga Sangraha*, *Ashtanga Hridaya* and commentaries, all creations, animate and inanimate, are made up of space, air, fire, water and earth. The total of the creations constitutes the universe, which is limited by time, called *kala* in Sanskrit. *Kala* as a factor interacts with the body from conception to death, in a time period called *ayu*. Through the interactions, changes, pleasant or not, occur naturally in the body and are divided into growth, achievement, maintenance and decay. Aging is a process of decay and degeneration, a process as natural as hunger, thirst and death. An age older than 60 or 70 is considered old age in Ayurveda. The degenerative signs and symptoms of old age include decay in anatomic tissues, perceptive power of the sensory and motor organs, strength, speech, potency, and mental and cognitive functions.

Although aging is natural, defective diet and/or defective lifestyle can bring forward the onset of aging through vitiation of *tridoshas*, causing premature, untimely or unnatural aging. Untimely aging, due to aggravated doshic imbalance, is a disease. Defective diets are those that are deficient or unplanned. Defective lifestyles include indulgence in day sleep, daily coitus without aphrodisiacs, daily alcohol drinking, excessive physical work, lack of exercise, mental and emotional fluctuations, and so forth [Devi *et al.*, 2010].

In Ayurveda, an individual comes with a predominant *dosha*, called *prakriti*. *Prakriti* is determined at conception and remains unchanged from fertilization till death. Because of the fundamental importance of doshic functions, *prakriti* determines not only one's psychophysiological traits but also prognosis and treatment of disease. According to *Charaka Samhita*, *pitta* aggravation, supported by *vata*, induces changes in related physiology, which in turn induce decay and degeneration of anatomic structure, leading to premature aging [Purvya and Meena, 2011]. In modern terms, since *pitta* is responsible for metabolism, biotransformation and energy

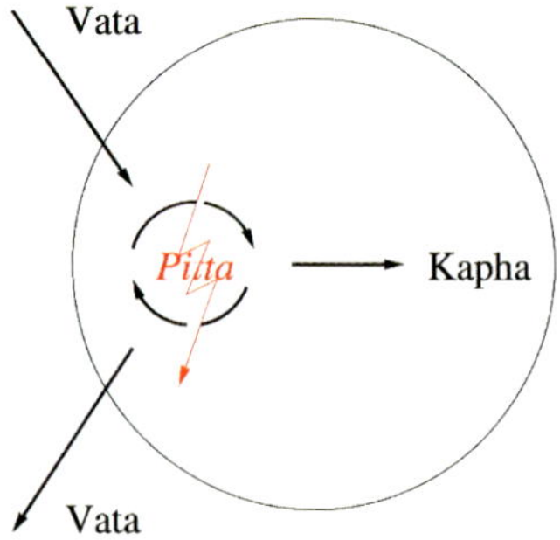

FIGURE 10.4

In Ayurveda, *pitta* aggravation, due for example to improper diet and lifestyle, causes untimely aging.

production, aggravated *pitta* functions raise basal metabolism and energy consumption and expedite tissue destruction through oxidized DNA, proteins and lipids. Health is achieved through balanced *tridoshas*. One is advised to design his or her diet/lifestyle opposite to the aggravated *dosha*(s).

10.6 TCM Theories of Aging

The Yellow Emperor's Inner Canon describes the progression of men's aging in the following way. Men start aging in their 40s, with the signs of gray hairs and slowing motion. Men at 50 experience decreased bile and blurred vision. Gloomy mind and wilting *qi*/ blood loom at 60. Atrophic skin develops at 70. Declining cognition

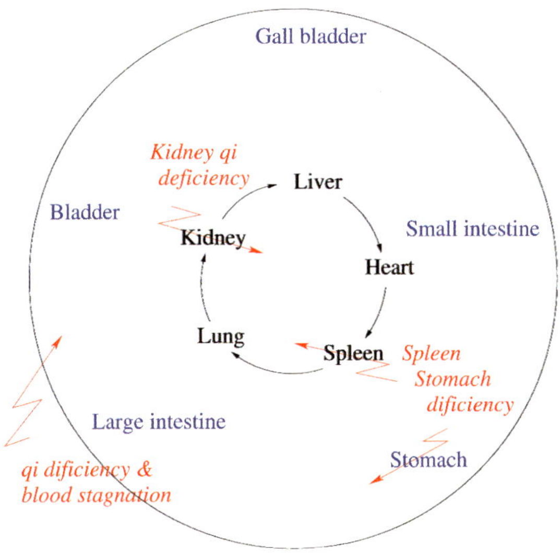

FIGURE 10.5

In TCM, three mechanisms are believed to be responsible for aging: (1) kidney *qi* deficiency; (2) spleen/stomach deficiency; (3) *qi* deficiency and blood stagnation. The first two mechanisms can exacerbate each other through the interrelated five viscera. Deteriorated viscera cause death. The third mechanism can perish viscera through the interconnected TCM meridians. The first two manifest interior TCM syndromes and the third an exterior TCM syndrome.

such as slips of the tongue strikes at 80. Debilitating viscera and meridians appear at 90. Death occurs at 100. Women age faster than men. For example, menarche starts at 14, aging at 35 and menopause at 49. The three prevailing TCM theories or syndromes of aging, based on *The Yellow Emperor's Inner Canon*, are: (1) kidney *qi* deficiency; (2) spleen and stomach deficiency; (3) *qi* deficiency and blood stagnation.

The kidney in TCM is regarded as the inborn root of an individual. The stronger the kidney, the longer one lives, and the speed of aging is determined by the functions of the kidney, i.e. kidney *qi*. The signs of kidney *qi* deficiency include depletion of blood, bodily fluids and bone marrow, decline in reproductivity, gray hairs, osteoporosis, fracture, loose teeth, weak waist/knees, insomnia, forgetfulness, obtuse reaction, falling intellect, impaired hearing, urination and defecation. The spleen in TCM is responsible for transformation, and its *yang* counterpart, the stomach, for digestion. The spleen in TCM is therefore regarded as the acquired root of an individual. The enfeebling spleen and stomach impair transformation of food and absorption of nutrition. As a result, decreased production of essence, *qi*, blood and bodily fluids withers visceral organs and peripheral meridians, causing aging. *Qi* in TCM energizes and also immunizes the body. Blood in TCM circulates substances, including nutrients and wastes, throughout the body. *Qi* and blood flow in meridians which interconnect viscera and peripherals. Deficiency in *qi* blunts one's response to climate changes or, in modern terms, weakens one's defense against infections and injuries. Blood flow can slow down due to deficient *qi*. Blood congestion can in turn block *qi* circulation. Deficient *qi* and stagnant blood, a mixture of depletive (i.e. *qi* deficiency) and excessive (i.e. blood stagnation) *zheng* in TCM, manifest disorders such as age pigmentation spots, cataract, atherosclerosis, hypertension, coronary heart disease, stroke, dementia, prostate enlargement and cancer.

The cause of an individual's aging will depend on his or her constitution — a concept akin to Ayurvedic *prakriti*. The TCM doctor will differentiate an individual's *zheng* before making a prescription. The three *zhengs* are interrelated. Kidney *qi* activates the functions of the spleen, whose products in turn nourish the kidney. Dysfunction in one imperils the other. Furthermore, the five TCM *zangs* regulate one another in the following sequence according to the five elements (or five phases) theory of TCM: kidney (water) → liver (wood) → heart (fire) → spleen (earth) → lung (metal). A defective kidney or spleen eventually compromises all the five visceral organs, which in turn impede *qi* and blood. Deficient *qi* and stagnant blood jeopardize viscera as these are interconnected through the flow of *qi* and blood in the intertwined meridians. The kidney *qi* deficiency, spleen and stomach deficiency and *qi* deficiency and blood stagnation perspectives on aging in TCM are, respectively, reminiscent of the endocrine, oxidative stress and immunosenescence theories of aging in modern western biomedicine.

11

Regenerative Medicine

The term "stem cell" was coined in 1908. The existence of adult stem cells was implicated in neurogenesis in the brain in the 1960s. Hematopoietic stem cells were discovered in human cord blood in the late 1970s. Stem cell research has received impetus since the successful reprogramming of human somatic cells into pluripotent stem cells by Shinya Yamanaka and coworkers in 2007. Although investment in scientific endeavor is continuous and linear, advancement in scientific knowledge is discrete and periodic. The singular events are called breakthroughs or revolutions. In evolutionary biology, new species periodically evolve in a pattern called punctuated equilibria. Stem cells have the potential to revolutionize therapeutics through their roles in tissue repair and regeneration.

Many modalities of complementary and alternative medicines, including Ayurveda and TCM, promote the concept of self-healing. Some of the classical yoga postures flex the spine, which accommodates a bulk of adult stem cells, including hematopoietic stem cells and multipotent stromal cells. Adequate mechanical stress on the axial skeleton in yoga exercise and TCM acupoint stimulation may retard aging through adult stem cell rejuvenation. Tonics in western healthcare refer to such supplements as vitamins C and E and the minerals selenium and zinc. Tonifying ingredients have, however, been part of TCM prescriptions and culinary preparations for thousands of years. TCM tonifying ingredients are commonly prescribed for chronically ill patients. It is speculated that TCM tonifying formulas and herbs work to activate adult stem cells.

11.1 Adult Stem Cells, Tissue Homeostasis

Life begins at the moment when a sperm fertilizes an egg. Within hours of conception, the fertilized egg, called a zygote, undergoes cleavage into two cells, which in turn cleave into four cells. Cycles of cell divisions continue throughout development till adulthood. An adult human body contains about 100 trillion cells of over 200 different cell types. Different cell types differ in morphology and specialize in distinct functions. Neuron cells look different and undertake different tasks from blood cells, for example. Specialized cells cooperate to efficiently meet the demand of the multicellular organism. Greater prowess is conferred on the multicellular organism as a consequence of subsystem (i.e. tissue) specialization within the organism during evolution.

The process of transformation from a zygote to a specialized cell is called cellular differentiation. All the different types of cells making up a human body originate from the fertilized egg. Zygotes are totipotent, in the sense that they are capable of differentiating into all kinds of cells. At the opposite extreme lie specialized, or somatic cells, which are terminally differentiated cells. Along the course of differentiation, the number of different cell types which a cell can differentiate into decreases. Cellular potencies, ranging from totipotency, pluripotency, multipotency, oligopotency to unipotency, are referred to in cell biology. Adult stem cells are cells that possess two properties, i.e. self-renewal and potency, and that are present in adult (and juvenile) tissues. Multi/oligopotent stem cells are sometimes called progenitor cells. Unipotent cells are also called precursor cells. As with the differentiation potential, the number of times a stem cell can self-renew decreases with its decreasing potency. Examples of better-characterized adult stem cells are hematopoietic stem cells in bone marrow, neural stem cells in some areas of the brain, intestinal stem cells in intestinal epithelium, satellite cells in muscle, melanocyte stem cells in hair follicles and dental pulp stem cells inside a tooth.

The process of self-renewal produces stem cells of the same undifferentiated state. Two mechanisms exist for stem cell self-renewal. In asymmetrical cell division, a stem cell divides, producing one stem cell and one differentiated cell. In symmetric cell division, two differentiated cells or two stem cells result after division. Like somatic cells, a stem cell can become dysfunctional — due, for example, to oxidative stress — and die with increasing age. The self-renewal process is meant to perpetuate the stem cell pool throughout the organismal lifetime. Moreover, in the event of normal cell turnover in, for example, blood, intestinal mucosa and the mammary gland, the stem cells differentiate into their respective cell types, replenishing lost cells. In response to tissue injury, resident adult stem cells differentiate into all the different cells of the damaged tissue, repairing the tissue. Adult stem cells thus play central roles in tissue homeostasis and organ regeneration. The mobilizing, proliferating and differentiating capabilities of adult stem cells depend, however, on tissue and decline with age [Pollina and Brunet, 2011].

11.2 De/Transdifferentiation, Reprogramming, *In Vivo* and *In Vitro* Regenerative Therapy

Many nonmammalian vertebrate species show extensive regenerative capability. For example, the salamander can regenerate a complete limb after amputation. The zebrafish can fully regenerate its heart after less than 20% of the organ's pumping chambers is amputated. In the regenerating process, the terminally differentiated cells (e.g. adult cardiomyocytes) that are still present regress cellular differentiation and dedifferentiate into less-differentiated cells (e.g. immature cardiomyocytes). The less-differentiated cells subsequently proliferate by entering the cell cycle. Finally, the less-differentiated cells differentiate into differentiated cells, replacing the missing ones. The gene expression profiles of the less-differentiated cells are usually characterized by downregulation of differentiation genes and upregulation of cell cycle activator genes. The detailed mechanisms responsible for initiating the switch between genomic programs are not known. Extracellular cues are believed to play decisive roles. Indeed, it was shown that regeneration-incompetent myotubes of mice started dedifferentiation and cell cycle re-entry after treatment with an extract isolated from the regenerating limbs of newts [McGann *et al.*, 2001].

Adult newts are capable of regenerating not only limbs but also eyes. In particular, it was shown that the iris' pigmented epithelium adjacent to their eye lens regenerated a new lens after lens removal [Tsonis *et al.*, 2004]. Pigmented epithelial cells and lens cells belong to different lineages of cellular differentiation. Lens regeneration of adult newts thus gives a classic example of transdifferentiation in nature. It has spurred experimental investigation of the transdifferentiation potential of mammalian systems. Successful examples in the lab include transdifferentiation of B cells into macrophages, hepatocyes into pancreatic cells, pancreatic exocrine cells into beta cells, fibroblasts into neurons, and fibroblasts into cardiomyocytes [Jopling *et al.*, 2011]. Induction of transdifferentiation often involves identification of transcription factors that are differentially expressed between the two lineages. The identified factors are then transfected into the differentiated cells, such as fibroblasts, in the hope that the exogenous factors will hijack the genomic program of the transfected cells. Should that work, the transfected cells are steered toward the cell fate, such as cardiomyocytes, dictated by the hijacking factors.

With the strategy, a minimal set of factors that reverted fibroblasts all the way back to embryonic stem cells (ESCs) were identified, they being Oct4, Sox2 and Nanog [Rodda *et al.*, 2005]. As ESCs are pluripotent, the reprogrammed cells are called induced pluripotent stem cells, or iPSCs for short. Oct4, Sox2 and Nanog, together with chromatin regulators, cooperate to upregulate pluripotency-associated genes and downregulate differentiation genes in iPSCs. As cellular differentiation is a continuous process, it can be expected that the less differentiated the cells are, the less effort is required for their reprogramming into iPSCs. It was indeed found that while fibroblasts required three factors, umbilical cord blood required only two, Oct4 and Sox2; and neural stem cells required only one, Oct4 [Jopling *et al.*, 2011].

Elucidation of *in vivo* dedifferentiation, *in vivo* transdifferentiation and *in vivo* reprogramming has tremendous implications for regenerative medicine. On the other hand, if genes are defective, *in vivo* regeneration will not help as the same defective genes will be expressed in the redifferentiated cells. If the defective genes can be fixed during *in vitro* reprogramming of cells, engraftment of the autologous, differentiated and repaired cells back to the patient can cure the disease. However, iPSCs by current techniques exhibit subtle epigenomic differences from ESCs. In addition, self-renewal is a precisely regulated process to maintain stem cell population. Dysregulated self-renewal can lead to overproliferative stem cells, explaining why iPSCs tend to be tumorigenic. Therefore, despite promising advances (illustrated below), before stem cell therapies are proven to be safe and effective, patients should remain cautious.

11.3 Hematopoietic Stem Cells, Multipotent Stromal Cells, Bone Marrow

More than seven billion new blood cells per kilogram of the body weight of a healthy adult have to be produced per day. Among the commonest debilitating conditions of the aged is immunosenescence. Hematopoiesis, which refers to blood cell production, is therefore of particular interest. In adult mammals, hematopoiesis is mostly accomplished by the hematopoietic stem cells (HSCs) in bone marrow. HSCs, being multipotent, can differentiate into all the cellular elements of blood, including: (1) oxygen-carrying red blood cells; (2) T and B white blood cells; and (3) granulocytes, macrophages and blood-clotting platelets. Blood vessels and capillaries are interwoven with bone marrow. Mature blood cells pass the endothelium of the blood vessels, called the bone marrow barrier, to reach the circulation. HSCs are also able to cross the bone marrow barrier. Circulating HSCs reach the thymus, where they differentiate into T cells. A small number of HSCs can proliferate into a whole HSC population. For example, the number of neutrophils, a major type of granulocytes, rapidly expands upon infection. Radiation and chemotherapy are known to damage the rapidly dividing cells in bone marrow. HSCs are sometimes extracted from cancer patients before radio/chemotherapy and injected back into them after radio/chemotherapy. The reinjected HSCs will repopulate the bone marrow to reconstitute the immunity.

The other abundant cells with multilineage differentiation potential are mesenchymal stem cells or multipotent stromal cells (MSCs). In contrast to the functional cells of a tissue or organ, stroma refers to the structural parts of it. Stroma is therefore the connective tissue and associated cells that surround and support the functional cells. MSC morphology is usually small, long, thin and adherent in comparison with the small, round and nonadherent HSCs. Prominent sources of MSCs include umbilical cord blood, amniotic fluid, tooth buds, adipose tissue and bone marrow. MSCs have been found to differentiate into a variety of cell types, including bone-forming cells, cartilage cells, fat cells, muscle cells, beta cells and neurons. More importantly, because MSCs are hypoimmunogenic, they have been found to avoid the immune rejection between mismatched allogeneic tissue in humans and animal models. Emerging MSC-related regenerative experiments show encouraging results. For example, infusion of human MSCs (hMSCs) raised the insulin and lowered the glucose of diabetic mice [Lee *et al.*, 2006]. Human Alu sequences were also detected in the pancreatic and renal DNA of the hMSC-treated diabetic mice, suggesting that hMSCs may enhance insulin secretion and improve renal lesions in diabetics. Neural implantation of hMSCs increased endogenous neural stem cell (NSC) proliferation and differentiation in the striatum of the hMSC-implanted Huntington's disease mice by upto to 30% [Snyder *et al.*, 2010]. In yet another study, hMSC administration attenuated inflammation in a rodent model of lipopolysaccharide-infected acute lung injury [Danchuk *et al.*, 2011]. Despite proof of principle, parameters such as dose, treatment schedule and route of administration have yet to be optimized. Again, before the risk-versus-benefit profile of the intervention in human subjects is better understood, patients should remain skeptical.

Bone marrow is the spongy tissue that fills the cavities of bones. It accounts for 4% of the total body weight of an adult, representing one of the primary sources of HSCs and MSCs. Bone marrow can be classified into two types: red marrow and yellow marrow. Red marrow consists of HSCs, MSCs, fibroblasts, osteoblasts, osteoclasts, macrophages and endothelial cells, and is hematopoietic. Yellow marrow contains fat cells and is nonhematopoietic. Bone marrow is thus also the major tissue of the lymphatic system in addition to the thymus. At birth, an individual's bone marrow is all red marrow. As one ages, red marrow turns into yellow. In adults, red marrow mainly resides in the axial skeleton and flat bones, including the cranium, sternum, ribs, vertebrae, ilium, scapulae, and rounded ends of the humerus and femur which are proximal to joints. The middle portion of long bones is lost to yellow marrow by the age of about six. Beef/lamb bone marrow has been used as a soup ingredient in several traditional cuisines, such as Italian, French, German, Hungarian, Iranian, Pakistani, Indian, Indonesian, Vietnamese, Filipino and Chinese.

11.4 Irreversible and Reversible Factors in Adult Stem Cell Aging

Just like any somatic cells, adult stem cells lose their functionality during aging. The declining plasticity of adult stem cells is evidenced by the increasing failure of HSC/MSC transplantation for recipients with increasing age of donor and time in culture. The number of cells in the stem cell pool can change in aging. Decreasing melanocyte stem cell numbers in hair follicles are an example, giving rise to gray hair. The potential of differentiation into specific cell fates can also change. Aged HSCs have been found to skew toward the myeloid lineage [Rossi *et al.*, 2007]. Aged NSCs and satellite cells (the resident stem cells of skeletal muscle) also showed astroglial and fibroblastic lineage bias, respectively [Liu and Rando, 2011]. Thus, adult stem cell aging has impact on the endogenous regenerating or self-healing power of the elderly. Understanding the factors that contribute to the altering quantity and quality of adult stem cells in aging, is therefore rewarding. From a practical point of view, we divide the factors into irreversible and reversible ones.

ROS, which are byproducts of cellular respiration, can damage DNA and proteins. If DNA impairment occurs in mitochondria, more ROS can be generated, causing more DNA damage. Each cycle of DNA replication shortens telomeres. Misfolded proteins form aggregates, becoming proteotoxic to cells. Such intracellular genomic and proteomic changes are irreversible. Compromised adult stem cells fail to repair tissue damage, contributing to organismal aging.

Undifferentiated ESC nuclei show elevated activities of nuclear proteins, including histones, lamins and chromatin modifiers, in comparison with differentiated cell nuclei. Over the course of cell fate acquisition, heterochromatic repeats and silent tissue-specific genes anchor and sequester on nuclear peripheral while active tissue-specific genes relocate and express toward nuclear internal. Such nuclear reorganization events are accompanied by chromatin compaction. Chromatin de/compactibility and mobility therefore correlate with the degree of stem cell plasticity. Chromatin conformation is determined by posttranslational modifications to the histones which make up chromatin. For example, histone acetyltransferases (HATs) open chromatin and histone deacetylases (HDACs) condense chromatin. As histone-modifying and histone-demodifying enzymes exist in mammalian cells, chromatin changes are reversible.

Apart from the above intracellular factors in stem cell aging, extracellular factors are as important or seem even more important in terms of their clinical relevance. In the so-called heterochronic parabiosis experiment, a young mouse is surgically joined to an old mouse so that the conjoined mice have a common circulation. It was found that the circulatory factors, such as WNT, NOTCH and TGF-beta inhibitors, from the young mouse blood restored the proliferative potential of the satellite cells from the old mouse [Conboy *et al.*, 2005]. Other examples of reversible systemic factors are inflammatory cytokines and stress hormones. Specifically, reduced corticosteroids induced neurogenesis; increased IGF-1 restored neurogenesis and muscle regeneration [Drummond-Barbosa, 2008]. Physical exercise was found to promote neurogenesis [Van Praag, 2008]. It is believed that circulating factors such as cytokines, IGF-1 and WNT ligand activate NF-kappa B, FOXO and beta-catenin through signal transduction pathways. Once inside the nucleus, these transcription factors, together with such histone modifiers as HATs and HDACs, alter the gene expression of the stem cells. Reversible factors behind the extrinsic and intrinsic cellular mechanisms are potential targets for stem cell rejuvenation.

11.5 Stem Cell Niche, Mechanotransduction, Axial-Skeletal Flexing Yoga Asanas, Acupressure

Somatic stem cells proliferate during development to populate the stem cell pool. In the event of tissue damage, adult stem cells migrate and differentiate to replace lost cells. They proliferate to replenish the drained stem cell pool and then stay dormant until the next tissue injury. The microenvironment that regulates stem cell fate is called the stem cell niche. A functional stem cell niche not only provides anatomic structural support but also maintains a balance between stem cell quiescence and activity. To meet the need for spatiotemporal regulation of stem cells, a niche can consist of a wide range of cellular and molecular elements, including differentiated cells, extracellular matrix (ECM) components, blood vessels, adhesion molecules, growth factors, cytokines, oxygen,

Ca^{2+}, metabolites/ATP, and so forth. Examples of adult stem cells and their niches are intestinal stem cells in the intestinal crypt base; satellite cells under basal lamina separating muscle fibers from interstitial space; epithelial stem cells in the hair follicle bulge; and neural stem cells in the dentate gyrus of the hippocampus. Stem cells and their niches interact reciprocally to maintain stemness. An aging adult stem cell niche contributes to stem cell aging. The best-studied niche is bone marrow. HSC niches in bone marrow are known to contain the following cell types: osteoblasts, osteoclasts, reticular cells, sympathetic nerve fibers, perivascular mesenchymal stem cells and macrophages. Bleeding and bacterial/viral infection impose constant stress on the hematopoietic system throughout the lifetime. It was found that the human bone marrow fat content increased with aging and that the increased fat content correlated with decreased HSC numbers in bone marrow [Tuljapurkar *et al.*, 2011].

Proliferation versus differentiation of stem cells in normal development and tissue homeostasis is subject to mechanical containment imposed by the rigid external boundaries. Stromal cells serve as anatomical support for functional cells, connecting the functional parts into a complete whole. Many studies of mechanical regulation of stem cells have thus been concerned with MSCs. Mechanical forces can be of three kinds: compressive pressure, tensile force and shear stress, manifesting through mechanical loading, mechanical stretching and laminar fluid flow, respectively. Compressive pressure constrains proliferating tissues such as the skeleton during bone remodeling. Tensile force is exerted on articulated tissues such as tendons, muscles and bones. Shear stress applies to endothelia such as myocardium, lung epithelium, the kidney and vascular remodeling. In adapting to mechanical stimuli over the microenvironment, MSCs change their gene expression via mechanotransduction, which converts mechanical force to biochemical signals. The mediators in mechanotransduction involve cadherins in cell–cell adhesions, integrins in cell–ECM junctions, fibronectin and collagen in ECM, microfilaments and microtubules in the cytoskeleton, ion channels and surface adhesion receptors in membranes, and FAK and ERK signaling. Mechanical forces have been shown to change MSC cell fate. For example, a study demonstrated that mechanical loading favored osteoblastogenic over adipogenic differentiation in rat bone marrow MSCs [David *et al.*, 2007]. Suppression of adipogenesis was through chromatin inactivation of PPAR gamma. An applied static 5% axial stretch (i.e. physiological level) was found to promote myogenic differentiation and antagonize adipogenic differentiation in mouse lung MSCs [Jakkaraju *et al.*, 2005]. The lineage preference was mediated via overexpression of TIPs, which are a HAT. Furthermore, fluid shear stress was shown to induce differentiation of human peripheral blood-derived endothelial progenitor cells into mature arterial (instead of venous) endothelial cells *in vitro* [Obi *et al.*, 2009]. Mechanical factors, in addition to chemical factors, are therefore likely to play critical roles in functional tissue engineering which requires differentiation of adult stem cells into multiple cell types *in situ*.

Given that stem cells are regulated by mechanical cues, yoga postures that stimulate stem cell niches should confer

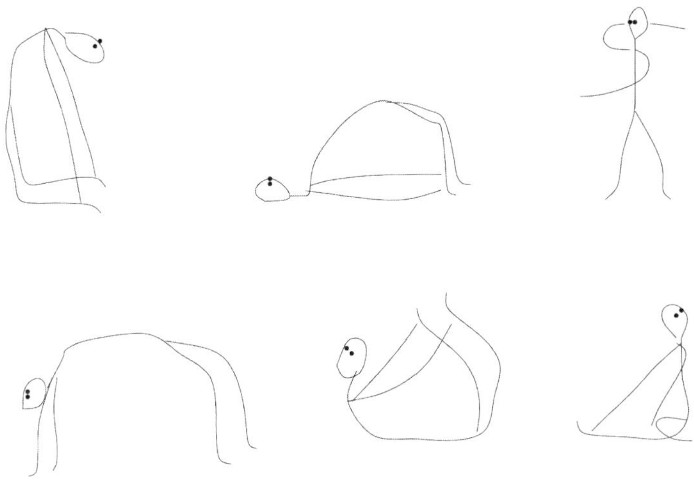

FIGURE 11.1

Examples of yoga *asanas* that stretch and twist the spine. The adult spine houses much of the red marrow, which contains hematopoietic stem cells and multipotent stromal cells.

physiological benefits. Among the various stem cell niches, bone marrow is of particular interest because of the ease of mechanical accessibility and its relevance to human aging. Examples of the yoga poses that manipulate the spine and pelvis, which house hematopoietic bone marrow, are: sun salutation backbend, standing forward bend, triangle pose (and its variants, such as revolved triangle), eight-limb pose, locust pose, half-fish, cobra pose (and its variants, such as frog cobra and revolved cobra), bow pose, camel pose, bridge pose, one leg revolved seated pose and one leg revolved belly pose. Specific breathing patterns usually accompany the pose, enhancing the mechanical force on the pulmonary and gastrointestinal tracts, e.g. backbend while inhaling and forward bend while exhaling. Note that yoga *asanas* are performed when one is in a healthy condition. Some postures are challenging and one should perform poses without feeling discomfort. By the same reasoning, the belly dance is beneficial to health through undulation of the spine and isolation and swiveling of the hips.

The network of interstitial connective tissue has been found to map to the network of acupuncture meridians in TCM. In particular, the connective tissue planes between and within muscles correspond to the sites of acupuncture points [Langevin and Yandow, 2002]. Needle lifting, thrusting and twirling introduce traction forces to the acupoint which harbors MSCs. Application of physical pressure by hand, elbow or devices to the acupoints in principle works the same way as needling. *hegu* (LI-4), *neiguan* (PC-6) and *zusanli* (ST-36) are among the best-investigated acupoints, relieving nervous, cardiac and gastrointestinal symptoms, respectively. The skull and scalp, below which reside red marrow and hair follicles, also teem with acupoints. Massaging the skull using the fingers' middle knuckles (or a wooden paddle hairbrush with ball-tipped bristles) stimulates scalp circulation. On the other hand, gently massaging the bony rims of eye sockets using the thumbs' top knuckles relaxes the eyes. Mechanical regulation of the MSCs in the connective tissue throughout the body may contribute to the cellular mechanisms of acupuncture.

11.6 Seasonal Tonifying Herbal Regimens, Personalized Preventive Medicine, Adult Stem Cell Rejuvenation

TCM formulas have commonly been classified into 22 categories according to their pharmacotherapeutic effects. A majority of the formulas are tonifying formulas under the classification. According to TCM theories, tonifying formulas (1) replenish to supplement deficiency and (2) nourish to sustain adequacy. TCM argues that individuals are rarely endowed with a balanced quality at birth. One can be congenitally deficient in *yin*, *yang*, blood or/and *qi*. TCM sages start treatment before diseases develop. Treating the disease after one is diseased is like digging wells only when one feels thirsty. Tonification is prevalent not only in Chinese medicine but also in Chinese cuisine. TCM predisease treatment heralds contemporary preventive medicine.

Prenatal deficiency varies from individual to individual. Postnatal deficiency acquired through injury, emotional disturbance, improper diet or lifestyle adds to the variation. Tonification therefore depends on the differentiated TCM syndrome of an individual. For instance, for lung impairment, one should invigorate *qi*, for heart impairment, one should regulate nutrition/defense, for spleen impairment, one should adjust diet, for liver impairment, one should nourish blood, and for kidney impairment, one should replenish essence, according to the *Canon of Difficult Questions* (*c.* 400 CE). TCM tonification aims to restore the *yin*/*yang*, *qi*, blood balance of any deficient *zang* and *fu*. As the innate and acquired deficiencies display interindividual variability, a view similar to Ayurvedic *prakriti*, TCM tonification is personalized.

In clinical practice, tonifying formulas appear across the TCM prescriptions for diseases of diverse origins, as evidenced by the prescriptions in Part II of this book. It is conceivable that TCM tonifying formulas, which show invariable presence in TCM prescriptions, function via adult stem cell activation. A carbuncle-treating formula together with a tonifying formula in a TCM prescription would provide a synergistic therapeutic effect of the prescription, via anti-inflammation and adult stem cell activation, to better address inflammation-associated disorders. Moreover, among the commonly used TCM single herbs, 212 of them also serve as culinary ingredients. Some well-known examples are ginger root, ginseng root, lotus seed, wild yam tuber and wolfberry. Other examples include red jujube fruit (*hong zao*), Astragalus root (*huang qi*), dong quai (*dang gui*), licorice root (*gan cao*), Rehmannia root (*di huang*), cnidium root (*chuan xiong*), poria/hoelen fungus (*fu ling*), white peony root (*bai shao*), white Atractylodes rhizome (*bai zhu*) and eucommia bark (*du zhong*). These herbs, when served at a limited quantity, are thought to provide long-term healthy effects for normal individuals. Tonification changes with seasons. For example, cooling and warming tonifying regimens are prescribed in summer and winter, respectively. We postulate that the tonifying herbal regimens, which have a long history in traditional Chinese recipes and medicine seeking health and longevity, work via adult stem cell rejuvenation.

12

Longevity

One's lifespan is largely determined by one's genetic makeup. What one can do, given the genome, is then to maximize the health-span. As there currently exist no prescription drugs for anti-aging, behavioral and nonpharmaceutical interventions that help maintain a healthy state are the choice. Among the drugless approaches, moderate exercise and dietary restriction are better studied and known in the West. As both interventions are concerned with energetics, a regular sleep–wake cycle which aligns activities, including resting and feeding, within and between days keeps one fit. Mind–body approaches that aim to enhance the mind's capability to positively affect bodily functions add to the arsenal against unhealthy aging. Yogic meditation and *tai chi* exercises are examples of the mind–body techniques popularly practiced in the East. Two recent long-term (>20 years) longevity studies of rhesus monkeys, by the US National Institute on Aging and the Wisconsin National Primate Research Center, indicate that food composition is as important as genetics in determining the survival of the monkeys. The Mediterranean diet has long been known for its beneficial effects on cardiovascular health. Chinese dietary therapy, which incorporates medicinal herbs in culinary recipes, is considered personalized regimens for healthy eating. Man, as a social species, lives with others in the environment. The sustainability of human health depends, through the food web, on the health of the soils, plants and animals. The holistic heritage of Ayurveda and TCM considers all parties in the ecosystem as an integral whole.

12.1 Moderate Physical Activity, Anti-Inflammation, Neural Plasticity

All modern humans stem from a single group of *Homo sapiens* who successfully emigrated from East Africa about 60,000 years ago and gradually spread throughout Eurasia, according to the Recent African Origin model of human evolution. The model was supported by analysis of large-scale, present-day mitochondrial DNA and Y chromosome sequences. In the cycles of exodus and settlement along human dispersion, our ancestors faced constant challenges of food scarcity, predator–prey interactions and climate extremes that threatened survival. To adapt, humans collaborate, as in the development of agriculture, which first appeared about 9000 years ago. The labor in farming has almost been replaced by machines since the beginning of the Second Industrial Revolution, about 150 years ago. Moreover, swift advances in the automotive industry and public transportation in the last 30 years have led to a physically inactive or sedentary lifestyle for the people in developed countries.

In 99.9% of human history, humans have been physically active. The transition to the sedentary lifestyle of the recent generations is considered too abrupt for the human genome to adapt to. Physical inactivity has therefore been found to be associated with a myriad of chronic disorders such as type II diabetes, cardiovascular disease and depression. For example, a landmark epidemiological study by Jeremy Noah Morris in the 1950s first showed that physically inactive double-decker bus drivers, postal clerks and telephonists had a higher rate of coronary heart disease than their physically active coworkers, bus conductors and postmen delivering the mail on foot. The specific conditions that have since been shown to be prevented by physical activity and voluntary exercise are pulmonary disease, cardiovascular disease, metabolic syndrome, musculoskeletal disorders, cancer (in particular, colon and breast cancer), depression and anxiety [Woods *et al.*, 2012].

In physical activity and exercise, contraction of skeletal muscle converts ATP into mechanical work. The major source of ATP is glucose coming from glycogen through glycogenolysis. In short-lasting (<2 min) and high-intensity bursts of exercise, glucose goes through glycolysis and ends up as lactic acid in anaerobic respiration for ATP production in the cytosol of muscle cells. In mild- and moderate-intensity exercise, glycolytic products go through aerobic respiration in mitochondria for more efficient ATP production. Exercise generally involves both anaerobic and aerobic respiration. Aerobic respiration kicks off later than anaerobic, because it takes time for oxygen to be transported to the contracting muscles. In exercise of prolonged duration, the glycogen in the liver undergoes glycogenolysis to supply glucose, via blood circulation, for muscle consumption. When carbohydrate storage starts running out, the plasma glucose level drops and fatigue sets in. Free fatty acids transported from remote adipose tissue are also an ATP source, through beta oxidation in the mitochondria of muscle cells. Fat metabolism is, however, a slow process and fuels the muscle for exercise of prolonged and mild-to-moderate intensity or in a fasting state. The heart and breathing rates rise to speed blood flow, which is rerouted from inactive viscera to active muscles. Body temperature climbs as a result of the buildup of metabolic waste heat. Sweat evaporates to bring down the body temperature. However, dehydration also leads to fatigue.

One of the beneficial effect of physical activity is anti-inflammation. In large-cohort studies of individuals over 60 years old, an inverse, dose-dependent relation between inflammation markers (serum CRP and IL-6) and physical activity was found [Woods *et al.*, 2012]. Obese adipose tissue, especially abdominal visceral fat, is known to be characterized by macrophage infiltration and pro-inflammatory adipocytokine overproduction. Loss of fat mass may underlie the anti-inflammatory effect of physical activity. A sense of psychological well-being, or so-called exercise-induced euphoria, can arise during and after exercise. Engagement of the nervous system is implicated. This should not be surprising, as exercise requires cerebral processing of sensory information for proper musculoskeletal coordination. The psychoactive effects of exercise were found to involve improved cognitive function via activation of hippocampal BDNF, the hippocampus being a region of the brain for memory and spatial navigation, and BDNF being a gene long known for its central role in synaptic plasticity and neurogenesis [Vaynman *et al.*, 2004].

Physical activity and exercise can therefore be prescribed as not only a behavioral prevention but also intervention against chronic disorders. Just like for any drug, the dose is a parameter that is of critical importance for efficacy. The latest and largest-scale epidemiological studies concluded that weekly moderate-intensity exercise gave an approximately 20% lower risk of dying from any cause [Wen *et al.*, 2011]. The suggested intensity and duration of exercise per week is, using jogging as an example, less than 20 miles of jogging at 10 min per mile, i.e. jogging at 10 km/h for up to 3 h per week. The studies also showed that a longer length or higher intensity of exercise did not necessarily offer extra benefits; prolonged and/or vigorous exercise could be counterproductive in some cases. Moderate-intensity exercises are those during which one can comfortably speak. Examples of moderate-intensity aerobic exercises are walking, cycling, jogging, swimming and stair-climbing.

12.2 Calorie Restriction, Alternate-Day Fasting, Mitochondrial Hormesis

Farmers have grown crops and raised animals for their own need. However, as with the Industrial Revolution, agriculture has undergone a revolution since about 100 years ago. Pesticides, herbicides, synthetic fertilizers, antibiotics, growth hormones, selective breeding, genetically modified organisms (GMOs) and government subsidies are common practices in modern farming and food industries.

Advances in the chemical, biotechnological and commercial developments result in a surplus of grains and meat and a plunge in food prices in the global marketplace. The fast-paced lifestyle of modern society leads to preference for foods of high-energy content. Our environment has become obesogenic.

Calorie restriction without malnutrition (CR) remains the most robust nongenetic dietary intervention to extend lifespan for a variety of species ranging from single-cell yeast, multicellular fruit flies, invertebrate nematodes, vertebrate fish to mammalian rats, mice and dogs. For example, in rodents, a 30%–60% reduction in calorie intake below *ad libitum* consumption initiated early in life has been shown to cause a proportionate extension of the maximal lifespan [Gonzalez *et al.*, 2012]. CR beginning in mouse adulthood increased the maximal lifespan by up to 20%. Specific rodent diseases onsets which were delayed by CR included cancer, nephropathies, cardiomyopathies, atherosclerosis, diabetes, autoimmune and respiratory diseases, Alzheimer's, Parkinson's, Huntington disease and stroke [Omodei and Fontana, 2011]. However, even though CR delayed age-dependent decline in IL-2 production and T-cell proliferation, severe CR seemed to impair monocyte- and macrophage-controlled microbial infections in rodents [Sun *et al.*, 2001]. Positive CR responses to age-associated diseases in rodents have prompted studies of CR effects on nonhuman primates. Two recent large-scale, long-term studies of rhesus monkeys on CR showed mixed results [Mattison *et al.*, 2012]. In humans, an epidemiological study involving 1.46 million white adults found the lowest all-cause mortality among individuals with a low body mass index between 20 and 24.9 [Berrington de Gonzalez *et al.*, 2010]. Further studies are needed to untangle the complex aging mechanisms in primates.

The amount of energy that is needed by an adult at rest is called the resting energy expenditure or basal metabolic rate (BMR). Rest here, is defined as no stimulation of the sympathetic nervous system. The BMR can be calculated from the energy required to sustain one's body temperature. It is usually measured in kcal/day, and depends on age, lean body mass, sex and temperature. Most of the BMR is spent by the liver, brain, skeletal muscle, kidney and heart. In particular, the liver, brain, kidney and heart account for 60%–70% of the BMR spent and the skeletal muscle for 20%–30%, although the combined mass of the liver, brain, kidney and heart is only <6% of the total body weight and the mass of the skeletal muscle is 40%–50%. The total amount of energy one needs per day is over the BMR by a factor of about 1.2–1.9, depending on the physical activity, stress and illness. At rest, 70% and 30% of ATP is derived from fats and carbohydrates, respectively. During aerobic exercise, ATP comes mainly from carbohydrates.

One mol of glucose generates 4 mol of ATP via glycolysis and 30 mol of ATP via aerobic respiration. Mouse cells under CR showed enhanced mitochondrial activity for efficient ATP production [Nisoli *et al.*, 2005]. Elevated ROS, a deleterious byproduct of aerobic respiration, induces endogenous defense against ROS. Such an adaptive response of the cell to CR, which serves as a low-dose stress, leads to functional improvement of cells and organisms. The phenomenon of the beneficial effects of mild stress is called hormesis, preconditioning or priming. As the ROS-related stress emanates from mitochondria, it is called mitochondrial hormesis or mitohormesis [Ristow and Zarse, 2010]. As the energy-devouring liver, brain, kidney and heart are all vital organs, mitohormesis in them is considered one of the mechanisms underlying the lifespan-extending and health-promoting effects of CR. Notably, the finding of the beneficial effects of regular exercise at moderate intensity can represent another example of oxidative-stress-related adaptation for healthy aging. As the CR-induced lifespan extension is an acquired phenotype, epigenetic regulation is also involved. Indeed, SIRT1, an NAD^+-dependent protein deacetylase, has been shown to mediate many of the CR longevity effects in mammals [Guarente, 2012]. For example, SIRT1 deacetylates and downregulates NF-kappa B, which is a master gene in proinflammatory response. The search for an SIRT1 activator, such as resveratrol, has been one of the hottest areas of research and development in CR mimetics.

In most of the dietary restriction studies, not only the quantity but also the timing of food intake was restricted. Feeding of animals took place in a restricted short period of time per day. The temporal factor of the restricted feeding could contribute to the beneficial effect. For example, in so-called alternate-day fasting (ADF) experiments, rodents were fed every other day. On a feasting day, the rodents could eat up to twice as much as the controls in order to compensate for zero intake on the next day. It was found that ADF retarded or prevented cardiovascular disease, kidney disease, diabetes and cancer in rodents [Varady and Hellerstein, 2007]. The cardiovascular and glucoregulatory effects of ADF were thought to mediate the benefits. On humans, the feasibility of maintaining ADF was established but the effectiveness has not yet been conclusively proven as most of the trials are still short (<20 weeks) [Trepanowski *et al.*, 2011]. Food delivers the energy for organism growth and reproduction. Availability of food is also constrained by the light–dark cycle within days.

12.3 Circadian Rhythms, Sleep–Wake Cycle, Energy Homeostasis

Rotation of the Earth on its axis creates a 24 h light–dark cycle. To adapt, plants and animals find their temporal niches within the circadian cycle for optimal energy harvesting and utilization. Many mammals, including humans, are active and feed in the day, and rest and fast in the night. The periodic patterns of mammalian behavior and physiology include the sleep–wake cycle, core body temperature, blood pressure, cardiovascular activity, endocrinal secretion, and renal, gastrointestinal and hepatic metabolism.

In humans, deep sleep, or slow-wave sleep (SWS), which lasts hours after sleep onset, is characterized by a decrease in the heart rate, blood pressure, cerebral glucose utilization and sympathetic nervous activity. In SWS, anabolic growth hormones are released and stress hormones are inhibited. Furthermore, proinflammatory molecules (IL-1beta, TNF alpha) are somnogenic while anti-inflammatory molecules inhibit sleep. Infection increases sleep via proinflammatory cytokine secretion. Immune cells, except natural killer cells, show peak proinflammatory activity at midnight. Sleep therefore improves the immune response and has a beneficial effect on infection. In the elderly, changes are found in the amplitude and timing of sleep rhythms that manifest in reduced hours of SWS and increased hours of wakefulness. In response to the sleep loss, the aged increase release of sleep regulatory proinflammatory molecules. The deregulated immunity resulting from the disrupted sleep rhythm can be one of the mechanisms underlying aging-associated debilitations. Acute effects of disrupted sleep–wake cycles are common in modern society, as transmeridian air travelers experience jet lag symptoms. Repeated sleep rhythm disruptions can be detrimental, as shift work has been found to be associated with an increased risk of obesity, cardiovascular morbidity, mood changes, gastrointestinal problems, breast cancer, workplace injuries, motor vehicle accidents and family problems. Workers in long-haul flight, emergency, healthcare, security, military, transportation and public utilities are therefore susceptible to shift work disorders.

The expression levels of many genes in most human cells, including brain neurons, retina, liver, intestines, heart and adipose tissues, exhibit circadian rhythms. In particular, the rhythm in hypothalamic suprachiasmatic nuclei (SCN) self-sustains even when the neurons are in isolation. An intracellular circadian oscillator therefore exists in SCN neurons. The period of oscillation is not exactly 24 h and can also vary from cell to cell. The endogenous circadian clocks are therefore subjected to synchronization or entrainment by external stimuli. Ambient sunlight has been the primary *zeitgeber* (German for "time-giver") for all living cells throughout evolution. The photic input received by the retinal ganglion cells, which are photosensitive, is projected to SCN, which contain about 100,000 neurons. The network of SCN neurons then synchronizes the intracellular clocks in other areas of the brain and the oscillators in peripheral tissues, e.g. the liver, via the autonomic nervous system and circulating humoral factors such as melatonin.

The clock apparatus inside the cell is known to consist of CLOCK, BMAL1 activators and PER, CRY repressors in a negative feedback loop of transcriptional regulation [Huang *et al.*, 2011]. CLOCK, the master gene in circadian rhythm, binds to activate a number of target genes involved in lipid metabolism, glucose metabolism, bile acid synthesis and adipogenesis. It is also a histone acetyltransferase. Chromatin remodeling therefore mediates circadian-rhythmic gene expression. The functions of the CLOCK-controlled genes reinstate the role of circadian rhythms in energy homeostasis.

The hierarchy of circadian-rhythmic synchronization is not one-way, as it was found that metabolic cues such as glucose, caffeine and glucocorticoids entrained peripheral and/or cerebral circadian oscillators. The NAD^+/NADH ratio and NAD^+-dependent SIRT1 can affect the binding of the CLOCK–BMAL1 complex to the target genes. As NAD^+ and NADH are key metabolic cofactors, feeding cues add to the light cue as a synchronizer of circadian clocks [Huang *et al.*, 2011].

The lifestyle in modern urban cities has become round-the-clock since the invention of the electric light bulb by Thomas A. Edison in 1879. The liquid crystal displays (LCDs) of personal electronic gadgets have joined the electric lamps to illuminate one's retina in the night in recent years. The light–dark cycle of the natural world has become polluted by the artificial lights, resulting in disrupted light–dark cycles. Interestingly, advanced age is associated with a reduced amplitude and period of body temperature rhythm. Timed CR in mice, where feeding was restricted to a fixed time of day, was found to not only increase the amplitude of body temperature rhythm but also align the rise of body temperature toward the feeding time [Challet, 2010]. The mechanism is unknown but a keener energy homeostasis under timed CR is supposed to help better reset and synchronize cerebral and peripheral circadian oscillators. The synchronized biochemical, hormonal and physiological functions lead to better tissue and body homeostasis, extending the healthspan. Given the association of sleep disturbance in aging, the development of modulators for sleep regulation, such as melatonin, is important. Nonpharmacological interventions that have minimal adverse side effects are most welcome and mindfulness meditation appears to be one of such nonpharmacological options for sleep improvement [Brand *et al.*, 2012].

12.4 Mindfulness Meditation: A Mental Workout for Reduction of Perceived Stress

The invention of the steam engine and of the electric lamp have liberated our muscle and time, respectively. The advent of the Internet has further shortened interindividual distances. The complexity of social interactions in modern societies, however, increases psychological stress. Examples of psychological stressors are finances, relationships, work and caregiving. To deal with the stress, the body reacts, via sympathetic nervous system activation and adrenal hormone release, to dilate the pupil, increase the heart and respiration rates, tense the muscles, raise the blood pressure, reduce sensitivity to pain and shut down digestion. The elevated physiological arousal is an adaption of the human body to quickly resolve the stressful stimuli. Chronic stress prolongs physiological arousal and causes health issues.

Mindfulness meditation is a stress reduction program developed by Jon Kabat-Zinn in 1979. Although meditation has roots in yoga, Taoism and Buddhism, mindfulness meditation is taught and practiced independently of religious and cultural connotations. Mindfulness meditation is a psychotherapeutic technique, and a session of it consists of the following: (1) sit in a comfortable position with eyes closed and back upright and unsupported; (2) relax and take note of body sensations, including sounds and moods; (3) settle the mind to the rhythm of the breath; (4) redirect the attention back to the breath if the mind wanders; (5) notice the passing thoughts without judgment; and (6) stay with it for at least 10 min.

According to the "stress, appraisal and coping" theory (proposed by Richard S. Lazarus and Susan Folkman in 1984), which is one of the prevailing models of understanding what makes a situation stressful, one feels stressed when a situation is perceived to harm highly valued important goals. That is to say, a threat appraisal comes from the perception that demands of the situation outweigh one's coping resources. Threat appraisals drive such negative emotions as fear, anxiety, worry, anger and guilt. Coping then follows appraisal to resolve the situation. The opposite of threat appraisal is challenge appraisal, where situations are perceived to be controllable and one sees opportunities during coping and after resolution. Challenge appraisals drive positive emotions such as eagerness, confidence, hope, energization and elation. Humans exhibit interindividual variations in perception and reaction to stressful events. Threat appraisals amplify stressors. Rumination further prolongs negative emotional responses. Lack of control over a stressor breeds a sense of unpredictability and uncertainty, which over time disrupts the neuroendocrinal balance of catabolic and anabolic hormones, leading to, for example, a hypercatabolic and hypoanabolic profile of hormones and blunted diurnal rhythm of cortisol. Chronic stress can also reorganize one's outlook on life. Mind–body interaction has played roles in TCM diagnosis and treatment. For example, *The Yellow Emperor's Inner Canon* states that anger harms the liver, thrill harms the heart, grief harms the lung, worry harms the spleen and fear harms the kidney.

In the training of mindfulness meditation, when a stray thought or emotion enters the mind, let it pass and return the attention to the breath. Mindfulness meditation focuses the awareness on what is happening from moment to moment without judgment. It is thus a decentering, reperceiving and perspective-shifting process, in that what was a subject becomes an object. The letting-go and more objective perspective on mental content prevent one from lapsing into ruminative thinking. Thoughts are self-generating, passing events in the mind rather than accurate reflections of reality. The cognitive shift of conscious identification to conscious awareness of emotion inhibits automatic affective response. Mindfulness meditation, through nonjudgmental observation of the ongoing stream of inner experiences as they arise, helps one to endure floods of flashing emotions during meditation. The training ripples to alter one's reaction to daily experience in mundane life. A mindfulness meditation program usually lasts for eight weeks, with a two-hour course per week.

Mindfulness meditation is not to get rid of thoughts toward a blank mind. Attentional training is an intense mental workout. Indeed, meditation practice was found to correlate with the thickness of the cerebral cortex in areas involved in attention, interoception and sensory processing [Lazar *et al.*, 2005]. The finding suggests meditation to offset age-related cortical thinning. Furthermore, participants in intensive meditation retreats were found to show an increased telomerase activity in the peripheral blood mononuclear cells at the end of the retreat in comparison with waitlist controls [Jacobs *et al.*, 2011]. It was reported that the ratio of challenge appraisals to threat appraisals correlated with telomere length. It was thus proposed that mindfulness meditation confers a salutary effect on telomere length via: (1) decreased stress hormones and oxidative stress; (2) increased anabolic hormones (testosterone/vagal tone) which protect telomeres [Epel *et al.*, 2009].

12.5 Tai Chi: A Combination of Aerobic Exercise, Resistance Training and Mindfulness Meditation

Taijiquan, tai chi chuan, or tai chi, as it is being practiced worldwide now, is an exercise stereotyped by linked sequences of predetermined smooth-flowing movements. A tai chi master maintains an upright posture with a low center of mass. Locomotion then involves continuous maneuvers between single-legged and double-legged weight-bearing stances. The movements require various amounts of concentric and eccentric contractions of the musculature of the lower extremities. Physical exercises can generally be grouped into flexibility, aerobic and anaerobic, depending on whether they increase muscle/joint range of motion, cardiorespiratory endurance or muscle strength. Tai chi is one of the few exercises that improve the three aspects of physical fitness. The intensity of present-day tai chi exercise is between 2.3 and 2.6 MET; MET (metabolic equivalent of task), the energy cost of sitting quietly, is equal to 1 kcal per kg of body mass per hour. In comparison, desk work such as writing and typing costs 1.8 MET; walking at 2.7 km/h, 2.3 MET; cycling at 16 km/h, 4.0 MET; and jogging at 8 km/h, 8.0 MET. Tai chi is therefore considered a light-intensity, low-impact physical exercise most suitable for compromised, rehabilitating or aged individuals.

Tai chi is said to be traced to a breathing dance in ancient China called *tao yin*, which literally means "guiding and pulling." The phrase first appeared in the classic text *Zhuangzi*, authored by the influential Taoist philosopher Zhou Zhuang (*c*. 400 BCE). A routine of 72-move tai chi is said to have been inspired and created by Sanfeng Zhang, a legendary Taoist monk and Chinese martial artist, about 700 years ago. Tai chi has also been attributed to Wangting Chen, a Ming dynasty general who lived about 400 years ago, as documented in the Chen family's chronicles. Underlying tai chi movements is the flow of *qi* and *yin–yang* dynamics. Tai chi therefore has roots in Taoism, martial arts and TCM. There have evolved at least five major types or schools of tai chi over the course of its development: *chen*, *yang*, *hao*, *wu* and *sun*. They share much of the basic concepts, differing in approaches and training.

Belonging to Chinese internal martial arts, tai chi features self-defense and counteroffense, in that it emphasizes redirecting the attacker's force against the attacker or away from the defender, instead of meeting the force with an opposing block. Tai chi turns the attacker's force into his or her disadvantage with minimum exertion by the defender. The yielding to an incoming attack is then followed by the initiation of a counterattack via pivoting of the body, twisting of the trunk and leverage/flexibility through joints of the defender. Tai chi kinematics is therefore circular. The training of tai chi employs exercise sets or forms, which are series of choreographed movements coordinated with breathing and awareness. Two tai chi forms exist: solo forms and sparring forms. The slow tempo and even transition of the movements facilitate an increased sensory awareness of speed, force and relaxation throughout the exercise. Tai chi breathing aids the flow of *qi* (a vital energy or life force) to enhance internal strength. Focusing of the mind on movements and breathing engages one in a state of heightened awareness or a state of meditation. As maintenance of mind–body homeostasis has been recognized to be more important than development of martial arts skills, tai chi is now undertaken for health promotion rather than self-defense. Most contemporary tai chi training involves only solo forms. Nevertheless, tai chi that combines intense mental concentration with deliberate, graceful movements is considered meditation in motion.

The mind–body approach of tai chi intervention is believed to benefit health through improved balance ability, postural stability, musculoskeletal strength/flexibility, cardiorespiratory fitness, immune function and stress management. For example, the relatively frequent shifting of the center of mass in three dimensions helps postural control and balance. A wide range of motions of the joints improves muscular strength and endurance. Slow action facilitates muscle coordination [Hong and Li, 2007]. Scientific evidence of effectiveness has been assessed by randomized controlled trials (RCTs) in modern western medicine. However, RCTs on tai chi, which is characterized by a multicomponent whole-system approach, can be inadequate or inefficient, as traditional RCTs are designed for single active ingredient verification and optimization. Variability in tai chi forms and schedule also contribute to the inadequacy. Despite the limitations, growing evidence from systematic reviews and meta-analyses has emerged, suggesting that tai chi is a relatively safe and cost-effective intervention for coronary heart disease [Dalusung-Angosta, 2011], balance and balance confidence [Rand *et al.*, 2011], psychological well-being [Wang *et al.*, 2010], blood pressure [Yeh *et al.*, 2008] and bone mineral density [Wayne *et al.*, 2007]. Besides the behavioral interventions that have been elaborated on so far, diets are an indispensible part of the holistic approach to health promotion and disease prevention.

12.6 The Mediterranean Diet, Herbs and Spices, Organic Foods

The Mediterranean diet refers to the traditional style of diet and cooking of the areas bordering the Mediterranean Sea, including Greece, southern Italy, southern France, Spain and Morocco. It is characterized by (1) high consumption of fresh fruits, vegetables, whole grains, legumes, beans, seeds, spices and olive oil; (2) moderate consumption of seafood, cheese, yogurt, poultry and eggs; and (3) low consumption of red wine, red meat and meat products. The Mediterranean diet is therefore plant-based, minimizing dairy products and red meat. It has been associated with lowered risks of death from heart disease, diabetes, cancer, Parkinson's disease, Alzheimer's disease and depression in various large-scale epidemiological studies. Higher adherence to the diet was also shown to be correlated with lower risk of mortality. Olive oil and cashews are known to be rich in monounsaturated fat. Fish and walnuts contain abundant omega-3 fatty acids, a polyunsaturated fat. Replacement of saturated and trans fats, such as butter and lard, with unsaturated fats, such as olive oil and canola oil, helps lower the total, low-density lipoprotein (LDL; "bad") cholesterol and triglycerides in the blood. The fat composition of the Mediterranean diet is thought to contribute to its beneficial effect on cardiovascular disease. The high content of dietary fiber in the plant foods and unrefined cereals in this diet is believed to help prevent colon cancer. The antioxidant effect of the natural phenols in berries, olive oil, colored fruits, vegetables, nuts, herbs and spices is also believed to be contributing factors. The beneficial effect of moderate alcohol consumption has been debated. Physiological response to alcohol consumption may show hormesis. Use of alcohol in any case requires the doctor's guidance.

Mediterranean diet cooking methods include grilling, broiling, baking, sautéing, roasting and braising. By contrast, deep frying is heavily employed in the preparation of fast food. Oils can be maintained at temperatures well above 100 °C. Preprocessed ingredients are usually preserved with salt. The immersion of raw ingredients in hot oil and/or reheating of preprocessed ingredients is frequently done in order to rapidly serve foods. The prevalence of low-priced, high-calorie greasy foods and sugary drinks has recently been linked to the epidemics of childhood obesity, colon cancer and hypertension in both developed and developing countries. The Mediterranean diet, instead, makes heavy use of fresh fruits and vegetables that are purchased when they are in season. Herbs and spices, such as allspice, basil, cardamom, caraway, cinnamon, clove, coriander, cumin, dill, fennel, garlic, ginger, lemongrass, licorice, marjoram, mustard, nutmeg, onion, oregano, paprika, parsley, black/red pepper, peppermint, rosemary, saffron, sage, tarragon, thyme and turmeric, impart aromas and flavors to the dishes. In a study of the use frequency of 43 spices in meat-based cuisines in 36 countries, it was found that use of spices positively correlated with the annual mean temperatures of the countries, suggesting the role of spices in inhibiting food spoilage micro-organisms [Billing and Sherman, 1998]. The antimicrobial and antifungal functions of spices were important for the control of food-borne illness before the invention of refrigerators. Spices are therefore beneficial for alleviating gastrointestinal disturbances such as dyspepsia and gastritis. Most spices are pungent/warm in TCM flavor/nature. Section 8.6 and Figure 8.1 indeed find that digestive disorders are treated with herbs warm in TCM nature. As about 15% of cancers are of bacterial or viral origins, spices are potentially preventative against gastric and colon cancers [Kaefer and Milner, 2008]. As an example of one of the antitumorigenic mechanisms of spices, adding Asian spices to meat was found to reduce the formation and absorption of potentially carcinogenic components during high-temperature cooking of the meat [Puangsombat *et al.*, 2011]. Ayurveda also considers spices as part of every meal towards a balanced *dosha*. Replacing salt and sugar with culinary herbs and spices in dish seasoning is therefore recommended.

Developments and advances in industrialized production of crops, livestock, poultry and fish by the use of agriculture machinery, selective breeding and genetic technology have helped boost agricultural productivity. Concerns have, however, been raised about the impact on the environment. As humans are an integral part of the ecosystem, an unsustainable environment will in the long run scourge human health. For example, residues of synthetic growth hormones in the waste of livestock animals can contaminate the soil and waterway of the feedlot. The local terrestrial and aquatic wildlife exposed to escalating levels of hormones could show abnormal sex characteristics. Organic farming, which treats the farm as an organism, has therefore been on the rise, relative to the conventional chemical farming, which is not self-sustainable. Organic farming is a holistic and ecological approach to farming, centering on the concepts of resource recycling, ecological balance and biodiversity conservation. Animal manure, instead of synthetic fertilizers is used to fertilize soils. Biological pesticides rather than synthetic pesticides are used to control pests. Genetically modified organisms are prohibited. Foods free of synthetic pesticides and chemical fertilizers in production and free of extraction solvents, artificial food additives and nanomaterials in processing are labeled organic. As to animal husbandry, food-producing animals' feeds have to be organic. Synthetic hormones are not allowed, nor are antibiotics unless for bacterial control in the case of infection. High-density confinement of poultry and livestock increases the physiological stress of the confined and mistreated animals, which overwhelms the immune function and increases the risk of infection. Free-range poultry and pasture-raised livestock, if certified, are labeled in marketing.

Although the residual levels of synthetic pesticides, synthetic growth hormones and antibiotics in conventional farming are regulated, potential detrimental effects, direct or indirect, over time on human health should not be overlooked. The recent discovery — by the Human Microbiome Project on 242 healthy individuals — of a complex microbial ecosystem coevolving with us in and on the human body (i.e. ears, nose, mouth, skin, gut, vagina and stool) reminds us of the delicate symbiotics between humans and nonhuman species [Human Microbiome Project Consortium, 2012]. An adult carries 1–2 kg of microbiomes. The number of the microbes is, however, ten times the number of human cells. Humans share

99.9% of the human genome but no two human microbiomes overlap. Human microbiomes help shape what we are. For example, a viral flora was detected in the human body, attacking both bacteria and human cells. Our immune system has been trained to tolerate the good viruses while counteracting the bad ones. Disruptions in the microbiomic balance, by antibiotic abuse which kills off a spectrum of bad and good bacteria, are implicated in causing obesity and autoimmune disorders such as irritable bowel syndrome and asthma. Humans, including doctors, whether as consumers or food producers, should think like ecologists, as has been advocated in the movement of organic agriculture.

12.7 Self-Assembly Principle, TCM Fire-Purging Diet, Personalized Anti-Inflammatory Regimens

The *yin*-nourishing school of TCM, founded by Danxi Zhu (1281–1358 CE), is one of the seven important TCM schools throughout TCM development. Summarizing his clinical experiences, Zhu concluded that human morbidities often resulted from a depleted *yin*. In TCM, *yin* refers to the material and structural aspects of human physiology, and *yang* to the activity and functional aspects. *Yin* has the qualities of tangibility, statics and coolness, and *yang* those of intangibility, dynamics and warmth. *Yin* is considered the collection of metabolites (e.g. ATP), biopolymers (e.g. proteins, carbohydrates, lipids, DNA/RNA), cells, humoral factors, blood, organs/tissues and pathogens of a biological system. *Yang* represents the bioenergetics that maintains the vitality (or self-assembly) of the biological system in an open environment. The principle of self-assembly requires: (1) a blueprint for the ultimate form; (2) forces of interaction that bring together parts of the system; (3) error correction which can fix the pieces when they assemble in the wrong way; and (4) an external force that activates the (re)assembling. For a biological system, the genome is the blueprint. DNA, proteins, ligands and so on are the parts and van der Waals attraction brings them together. DNA repair pathways, heat shock proteins and apoptosis support error correction. Heat and ATP from catabolism of digested foods are the energy sources facilitating biopolymer interactions and fueling error correction. For the system and environment that meet the requirements, parts self-assemble, defying the second law of thermodynamics. *Yin* represents the physical parts and *yang* the heat/ATP production and associated activities.

Yin and *yang* nourish each other in a living organism. The *yin* and *yang* of an individual grows from birth until adulthood. The level of *yang* is delicately maintained. In the self-assembly model of living systems, excessive heat undoes van der Waals attraction, disintegrating protein complexes. Deficient heat/ATP disables error correction, accumulating misfolded proteins and unrepaired DNA. *Yin* and *yang* levels are thus balanced to sustain one's health. *Yang* at the normal level of the *yin–yang* balance is called *qi*. Otherwise, it is called fire. When *yang* exceeds its normal level, it is called real fire or real heat. When *yin* goes below its normal level, the residual *yang* is called virtual fire or virtual heat. Physiologically, real fire manifests fever, a strong and quick pulse, and a red tongue with a yellow coating. Virtual fire displays fever, a thin and quick pulse, and a red tongue with no coating. Both real fire and virtual fire manifest fever because of an ostensible *yang* surplus. The treatment, however, is different in TCM. For the white-collar workers in modern societies, *yang* surplus is caused by psychological stress and/or hypercaloric intake, both of which are proinflammatory through elevated levels of free radicals. Excessive *yang* overtaxes *yin*, leading to *yin* depletion, which mirrors Danxi Zhu's proposition. Correlation between maternal caregiving and telomere shortening is an example. TCM *yin*-nourishing or fire-purging regimens for people over their middle age therefore prevent disease and promote longevity.

According to TCM, fire-setting ingredients are those which are warm in TCM nature. The warm ingredients are, in decreasing order, beef, lamb, pork, chicken, duck, fish, pungent spices (e.g. ginger, onion, garlic and pepper) and nuts (e.g. peanuts and cashews). Oil frying increases the warmness of the ingredients. Warm fruits include custard apple or sugar apple, durian, litchi (or lychee), mango and longan. Sweet desserts and drinks which contain starch, fats and sugar are fire-setting.

Fire-purging ingredients are those which are cool in TCM. Fresh juicy fruits are effective in fire-purging. They include watermelon, banana, sugarcane, pear, tomato, kiwi, mulberry, pitaya, cantaloupe melon, honeydew melon, lemon, orange, papaya and wax apple. In particular, watermelon is helpful for real fire and banana for virtual fire.

Most vegetables are fire-purging. They include water spinach (*Ipomoea aquatica Forsk*), spinach, cabbage, bean sprouts, wax gourd, white radish, white gourd, balsam pear, cucumber, loofah, lotus root, celery, asparagus, winter bamboo shoots, edible tree fungus, lentils and water chestnut.

A fire-purging soup would mix mung beans, Job's tears, lotus seeds and white edible tree fungus in the preparation. Mint tea,

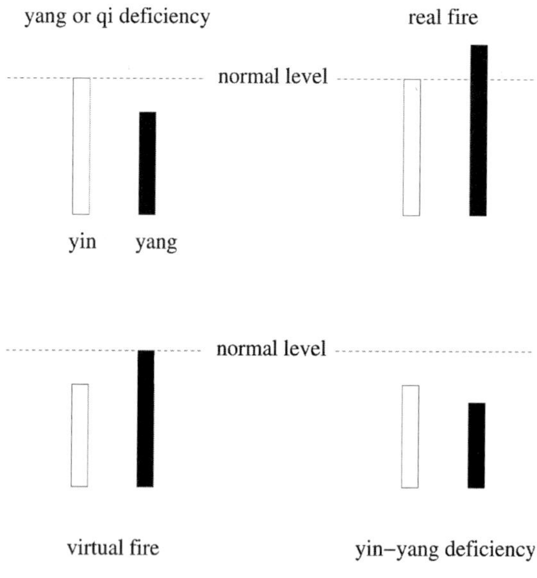

FIGURE 12.1
Imbalance of *yin* and *yang*. Real fire reflects acute symptoms such as infection and inflammation. Virtual fire reflects chronic conditions such as obesity and diabetes. An example of *qi* deficiency is constipation. Deficiency in both *yin* and *yang indicates* terminal illness. The dashed lines show the adequate level of *yin* and *yang*.

rose tea, roselle tea, jasmine tea, chrysanthemum tea and American ginseng tea are all fire-purging green teas. A herbal tea constituting Chinese brake herb (*Pteris multifida*), Asiatic plantain, mint and beggar ticks is a potent fire-purging drink.

The TCM herbs to antagonize virtual fire syndromes would nourish *yin*, including *mai dong* (dwarf lilyturf root), *tian dong* (wild asparagus root), *shen di* (raw Rehmannia root), *yu zhu* (fragrant Solomon seal rhizome), *huang jing* (King Solomon's seal), *shan yao* (Chinese yam), *sha can* (root of straight ladybell) and *xi yang can* (American ginseng). On the other hand, the TCM herbs against real fire syndromes would clear heat, including *huang lian* (Chinese goldthread), *huang qin* (baikal skullcap root), *huang bai* (Amur cork-tree bark), *zhi zi* (cape jasmine fruit) and *long dan cao* (Chinese gentian root). One should differentiate one's TCM syndrome before fire-purging TCM herbs are taken. More detailed TCM diagnosis would differentiate the *yin–yang* homeostasis of individual viscera/meridians. For example, diabetics are associated with deficiency in kidney *yin*. A viscera-specific *yin*-nourishing or fire-purging regimen, together with such lifestyle interventions as tai chi, can be thought of as a personalized holistic approach to anti-aging.

12.8 Social Integration, Brain Aging Reversal, Longevity

Social animals live in groups. Theories exist to explain the evolutionary origin of sociality. An animal in a group of 100 has one hundredth the chance of becoming prey than a lone animal does. An animal in a group of 100 has a hundred times the defense and knowledge (that are shared within the group) compared to a solitary animal. Animals in a group have also a better chance of finding mates. Coordination and cooperation within groups is essential for groups to outcompete individuals and for large groups to outcompete small groups. A dominance hierarchy therefore usually develops in a group to resolve conflict and competition among the members, establishing order. Hierarchy builds up class tension and psychosocial stress. Gregariousness spreads infectious diseases. Nevertheless, if group-living increases overall survival in a population, as more social members reproduce, social members displace asocial ones in the population. Primates, including humans, are social beings.

Honeybees, being an eusocial species with a complex societal structure and dynamic social environment, have been a model organism for the study of the neurobiological underpinnings of mammalian behavior, including human behavior. For example, comparison of the gene expression profiles between scout and nonscout bees has recently led to the identification of genes responsible for the scouting trait [Liang *et al.*, 2012]. The identified genes were found to relate to dopamine, glutamate and gamma-aminobutyric acid (GABA) signaling between neurons. The same neurotransmitters are known to regulate novelty-seeking behavior in humans. Honeybees nurse larvae in the nest when they are young. They leave the nest to scout for nectar when they get old. The scouting bees age quickly; owing to wearing of wings or body hairs and loss of brain functions during the long duration of food foraging. Cognition was measured as the ability to learn new things. Old scouts can revert to their social role as nurses when young nurse bees in the colony are in shortage. Role reversal showed recovery of learning ability. Gene expression profiling identified increased levels of stress response and antioxidant proteins in old reverters in comparison with old nonreverters. One of the identified genes homologous to mammals' is PRX6, which in humans has been associated with anti-inflammation against Alzheimer's and Huntington disease. The findings suggest that cognitive decline is an effect of the social role, not of the chronological age, at least in honeybees [Baker *et al.*, 2012]. In the fight against dementia in our rapidly aging society, in addition to drug treatment, social interventions involving active social (re)engagement such as a second career after retirement, cross-cultural immersion, volunteer jobs and amateur activities are potentially effective in slowing or treating age-related dementia.

Isolation of the social determinants for healthy aging is challenging given the continual nature of psychological development throughout one's life, although insightful results from primates are emerging [Silk *et al.*, 2010]. The study involved a group of 44 free-ranging, adult female baboons in a reserve in southern Africa. Rates of approaches and grooming were used to measure the relationship between each female dyad. The top three partners of each female in a year were also identified. The strength and consistency of the relationships were quantified and found to correlate with each other. They were thus lumped together into a single factor called relationship quality. Analysis then showed that relationship quality and dominance rank both positively correlated with female longevity. Relationship quality had a stronger effect than dominance rank on longevity. Since strong and stable bonds were also equitable (i.e. reciprocal grooming) bonds, the result suggested that a strong and stable relationship offsets the fitness loss due to low dominance rank. In humans, marriage represents a form of strong, equitable and stable relationship. Epidemiological studies across a range of human cultures have indeed found that married men or women have a longer life expectancy, higher quality of life and higher rate of survival from such medical interventions as coronary artery bypass and chemotherapy than their single counterparts [Gallacher and Gallacher, 2011]. Social connectedness seems to enhance the anabolic processes involved in somatic maintenance and repair, buffering the stress-activated adrenocortical activities. Although epidemiological studies are correlative in nature, cross-species results suggest the adaptive value of social bonds in reproduction and longevity.

Bibliography

Adams, C.P., Brantner, V.V. (2006). Estimating the cost of new drug development: is it really 802 million dollars? *Health Aff (Millwood)*, 25, pp. 420–428.

Atwood, C.S., Bowen, R.L. (2011). The reproductive-cell cycle theory of aging: an update, *Exp Gerontol*, 46, pp. 100–107.

Audette, J.F., Ryan, A.H. (2004). The role of acupuncture in pain management, *Phys Med Rehabil Clin N Am*, 15, pp. 749–772.

Auyeung, T.W., Lee, J.S., Leung, J., Kwok, T., Leung, P.C., Woo, J., Wing, Y.K. (2012). Cognitive deficit is associated with phase advance of sleep–wake rhythm, daily napping, and prolong sleep duration — a cross-sectional study in 2,947 community-dwelling older adults, *Age (Dordr)*, doi: 10.1007/s11357-011-9366-6.

Baccarelli, A., Wright, R.O., Bollati, V., Tarantini, L., Litonjua, A.A., Suh, H.H., Zanobetti, A., Sparrow, D., Vokonas, P.S., Schwartz, J. (2009). Rapid DNA methylation changes after exposure to traffic particles, *Am J Respir Crit Care Med*, 179, pp. 572–578.

Baker, N., Wolschin, F., Amdam, G.V. (2012). Age-related learning deficits can be reversible in honeybees *Apis mellifera*, *Exp Gerontol*, 47, pp. 764–772.

Berrington de Gonzalez, A., Hartge, P., Cerhan, J.R., Flint, A.J., Hannan, L., Maclnnis, R.J., Moore, S.C., Tobias, G.S., Anton-Culver, H., Freeman, L.B., Beeson, W.L., Clipp, S.L., English, D.R., Folsom, A.R., Freedman, D.M., Giles, G., Hakansson, N., Henderson, K.D., Hoffman-Bolton, J., Hoppin, J.A., Koenig, K.L., Lee, I.M., Linet, M.S., Park, Y., Pocobelli, G., Schatzkin, A., Sesso,

H.D., Weiderpass, E., Willcox, B.J., Wolk, A., Zeleniuch-Jacquotte, A., Willett, W.C., Thun, M.J. (2010). Body-mass index and mortality among 1.46 million white adults, *N Engl J Med*, 363, pp. 2211–2219.

Billing, J., Sherman, P.W. (1998). Antimicrobial functions of spices: why some like it hot, *Q Rev Biol*, 73, pp. 3–49.

Bornstein, S.R., Licinio, J. (2011). Improving the efficacy of translational medicine by optimally integrating health care, academia and industry, *Nat Med*, 17, pp. 1567–1569.

Brand, S., Holsboer-Trachsler, E., Naranjo, J.R., Schmidt, S. (2012). Influence of mindfulness practice on cortisol and sleep in long-term and short-term meditators, *Neuropsychobiology*, 65, pp. 109–118.

Cao, C.F., Sun, X.P. (1998). Herbal medicine for periodontal diseases, *Int Dent J*, 48, pp. 316–322.

Carlson, L.E., Speca, M., Faris, P., Patel, K.D. (2007). One year pre-post intervention follow-up of psychological, immune, endocrine and blood pressure outcomes of mindfulness-based stress reduction (MBSR) in breast and prostate cancer outpatients, *Brain Behav Immun*, 21, pp. 1038–1049.

Challet, E. (2010). Interactions between light, mealtime and calorie restriction to control daily timing in mammals, *J Comp Physiol B*, 180, pp. 631–644.

Champagne, F.A., Curley, J.P. (2009). Epigenetic mechanisms mediating the long-term effects of maternal care on development, *Neurosci Biobehav Rev*, 33, pp. 593–600.

Chen, Y.S., Torroni, A., Excoffier, L., Santachiara-Benerecetti, A.S., Wallace, D.C. (1995). Analysis of mtDNA variation in African populations reveals the most ancient of all human continent-specific haplogroups, *Am J Hum Genet*, 57, pp. 133–149.

Chiu, P.H., Hsieh, H.Y., Wang, S.C. (2012). Prescriptions of traditional Chinese medicine are specific to cancer types and adjustable to temperature changes, *PLoS One*, 7: e31648.

Coller, B.S., Califf, R.M. (2009). Traversing the valley of death: a guide to assessing prospects for translational success, *Sci Transl Med*, 1, 10cm9.

Colloca, L., Miller, F.G. (2011). Harnessing the placebo effect: the need for translational research, *Philos Trans R Soc Lond B Biol Sci*, 366, pp. 1922–1930.

Conboy, I.M., Conboy, M.J., Wagers, A.J., Girma, E.R., Weissman, I.L., Rando, T.A. (2005) Rejuvenation of aged progenitor cells by exposure to a young systemic environment, *Nature*, 433, pp. 760–764.

Dalusung-Angosta, A. (2011). The impact of Tai Chi exercise on coronary heart disease: a systematic review, *J Am Acad Nurse Pract*, 23, pp. 376–381.

Danchuk, S., Ylostalo, J.H., Hossain, F., Sorge, R., Ramsey, A., Bonvillain, R.W., Lasky, J.A., Bunnell, B.A., Welsh, D.A., Prockop, D.J. Sullivan, D.E. (2011). Human multipotent stromal cells attenuate lipopolysaccharide-induced acute lung injury in mice via secretion of tumor necrosis factor-alpha–induced protein 6, *Stem Cell Res Ther*, 2, p. 27.

David, V., Martin, A., Lafage-Proust, M.H., Malaval, L., Peyroche, S., Jones, D.B., Vico, L., Guignandon, A. (2007). Mechanical loading down-regulates peroxisome proliferator–activated receptor gamma in bone marrow stromal cells and favors osteoblastogenesis at the expense of adipogenesis, *Endocrinology*, 148, pp. 2553–2563.

Devi, D., Srivastava, R., Dwivedi, B.K. (2010). A critical review of concept of aging in Ayurveda, *Ayu*, 31, pp. 516–519.

DiMasi, J.A., Feldman, L., Seckler, A., Wilson, A. (2010). Trends in risks associated with new drug development: success rates for investigational drugs, *Clin Pharmacol Ther*, 87, pp. 272–277.

Drummond-Barbosa, D. (2008). Stem cells, their niches and the systemic environment: an aging network, *Genetics*, 180, pp. 1787–1797.

Egger, M., Smith, G.D., Phillips, A.N. (1997). Meta-analysis: principles and procedures, *BMJ*, 315, pp. 1533–1537.

Epel, E., Daubenmier, J., Moskowitz, J.T., Folkman, S., Blackburn, E. (2009). Can meditation slow rate of cellular aging? Cognitive stress, mindfulness, and telomeres, *Ann NY Acad Sci*, 1172, pp. 34–53.

Fan, T.P., Deal, G., Koo, H.L., Rees, D., Sun, H., Chen, S., Dou, J.H., Makarov, V.G., Pozharitskaya, O.N., Shikov, A.N., Kim, Y.S., Huang, Y.T., Chang, Y.S., Jia, W., Dias, A., Wong, V.C., Chan, K. (2012). Future development of global regulations of Chinese herbal products, *J Ethnopharmacol*, 140, pp. 568–586.

Fasinu, P.S., Bouic P.J., Rosenkranz, B. (2012). An overview of the evidence and mechanisms of herb–drug interactions, *Front Pharmacol*, 3, p. 69.

Franceschi, C., Bonafe, M., Valensin, S., Olivieri, F., De Luca, M., Ottaviani, E., De Benedictis, G. (2000). Inflamm-aging: an evolutionary perspective on immunosenescence, *Ann NY Acad Sci*, 908, pp. 244–254.

Galkina, E., Ley, K. (2009). Immune and inflammatory mechanisms of atherosclerosis, *Annu Rev Immunol*, 27, pp. 165–197.

Gallacher, D., Gallacher, J. (2011). Are relationships good for your health? *Student BMJ*, 19: d404, doi: 10.1136/sbmj.d404.

Gonzalez, O.A., Tobia, C., Ebersole, J.L., Novak, M.J. (2012). Calorie restriction and chronic inflammatory diseases, *Oral Dis*, 18, pp. 16-31.

Gonzalez-Coloma, A., Martin-Benito, D., Mohamed, N., Garcia-Vallejo, M.C., Soria, A.C. (2006). Antifeedant effects and chemical composition of essential oils from different populations of *Lavandula luisieri L.*, *Biochem Syst Ecol*, 34, pp. 609–616.

Gronniger, E., Weber, B., Heil, O., Peters, N., Stab, F., Wenck, H., Korn, B., Winnefeld, M., Lyko, F. (2010). Aging and chronic sun exposure cause distinct epigenetic changes in human skin, *PLoS Genet*, 6: e1000971.

Guarente, L. (2012). Sirtuins and calorie restriction, *Nat Rev Mol Cell Biol*, 13, doi: 10.1038/nrm3308.

Hanahan, D., Weinberg, R.A. (2011). Hallmarks of cancer: the next generation, *Cell*, 144, pp. 646–674.

Harman, D. (1956). Aging: a theory based on free radical and radiation chemistry, *J Gerontol*, 11, pp. 298–300.

Hayflick, L., Moorhead P.S. (1961). The serial cultivation of human diploid cell strains, *Exp Cell Res*, pp. 585–621.

Hong, Y., Li, J.X. (2007). Biomechanics of Tai Chi: a review, *Sports Biomechanics*, 6, pp. 453–464.

Huang, W., Ramsey, K.M., Marcheva, B., Bass, J. (2011). Circadian rhythms, sleep, and metabolism, *J Clin Invest*, 121, pp. 2133–2141.

Human Microbiome Project Consortium (2012). Structure, function and diversity of the healthy human microbiome, *Nature*, 486, pp. 207–214.

Hsieh, H.Y., Chiu, P.H., Wang, S.C. (2011). Epigenetics in traditional Chinese pharmacy: a bioinformatic study at pharmacopoeia scale, *Evid-Based Compl Alternat Med*, 2011: 816714.

Ito, S. (2012). Cardiorenal connection in chronic kidney disease, *Clin Exp Nephrol*, 16, pp. 8–16.

Jacobs, T.L., Epel, E.S., Lin, J., Blackburn, E.H., Wolkowitz, O.M., Bridwell, D.A., Zanesco, A.P., Aichele, S.R., Sahdra, B.K., MacLean, K.A., King, B.G., Shaver, P.R., Rosenberg, E.L., Ferrer, E., Wallace, B.A., Saron C.D. (2011). Intensive meditation training, immune cell telomerase activity, and psychological mediators, *Psychoneuroendocrinology*, 36, pp. 664–681.

Jakkaraju, S., Zhe, X., Pan, D., Choudhury, R., Schuger, L. (2005). TIPs are tension-responsive proteins involved in myogenic versus adipogenic differentiation, *Dev Cell*, 9, pp. 39–49.

Jopling, C., Boue, S., Belmonte, J.C.I. (2011). Dedifferentiation, transdifferentiation and reprogramming: three routes to regeneration, *Nat Rev Mol Cell Biol*, 12, pp. 79–89.

Kaefer, C.M., Milner, J.A. (2008). The role of herbs and spices in cancer prevention, *J Nutr Biochem*, 19, pp. 347–361.

Kennedy, D.O., Wightman, E.L. (2011). Herbal extracts and phytochemicals: plant secondary metabolites and the enhancement of human brain function, *Adv Nutr*, 2, pp. 32–50.

Khatib, F., DiMaio, F., Foldit Contenders Group, Foldit Void Crushers Group, Cooper, S., Kazmierczyk, M., Gilski, M., Krzywda, S., Zabranska, H., Pichova, I., Thompson, J., Popovic, Z., Jaskolski, M., Baker, D. (2011). Crystal structure of a monomeric retroviral protease solved by protein folding game players, *Nat Struct Mol Biol*, 18, pp. 1175–1177.

Klinger, R., Soost, S., Flor, H., Worm, M. (2007). Classical conditioning and expectancy in placebo hypoalgesia: a randomized controlled study in patients with atopic dermatitis and persons with healthy skin, *Pain*, 128, pp. 31–39.

Langevin, H.M., Yandow, J.A. (2002). Relationship of acupuncture points and meridians to connective tissue planes, *Anat Rec*, 269, pp. 257–265.

Lansing, J.S. (2003). Complex adaptive systems, *Annu Rev Anthropol*, 32, pp. 183–204.

Lazar, S.W., Kerr, C.E., Wasserman, R.H., Gray, J.R., Greve, D.N., Treadway, M.T., McGarvey, M., Quinn, B.T., Dusek, J.A., Benson, H., Rauch, S.L., Moore, C.I., Fischl, B. (2005). Meditation experience is associated with increased cortical thickness, *Neuroreport*, 16, pp. 1893–1897.

Lee, R.H., Seo, M.J., Reger, R.L., Spees, J.L., Pulin, A.A., Olson, S.D., Prockop, D.J. (2006). Multipotent stromal cells from human marrow home to and promote repair of pancreatic islets and renal glomeruli in diabetic NOD/*scid* mice, *Proc Natl Acad Sci USA*, 103, pp. 17438–17443.

Liang, Z.S., Nguyen, T., Mattila, H.R., Rodriguez-Zas, S.L., Seeley, T.D., Robinson, G.E. (2012). Molecular determinants of scouting behavior in honey bees, *Science*, 335, pp. 1225–1228.

Liu, L., Rando, T.A. (2011). Manifestations and mechanisms of stem cell aging, *J Cell Biol*, 193, pp. 257–266.

Loeb, L.A., Wallace, D.C., Martin, G.M. (2005). The mitochondrial theory of aging and its relationship to reactive oxygen species damage and somatic mtDNA mutations, *Proc Natl Acad Sci USA*, 102, pp. 18769–18770.

Manheimer, E., Wieland, S., Kimbrough, E., Cheng, K., Berman, B.M. (2009). Evidence from the Cochrane Collaboration for traditional Chinese medicine therapies, *J Alternat Compl Med*, 15, pp. 1001–1014.

Mattison, J.A., Roth, G.S., Beasley, M., Tilmont, E.M., Handy, A.M., Herbert, R.L., Longo, D.L., Allison, D.B., Young, J.E., Bryant, M., Barnard, D., Ward, W.F., Qi, W., Ingram, D.K., de Cabo, R. (2012). Impact of caloric restriction on health and survival in rhesus monkeys from the NIA study, *Nature*, doi: 10.1038/nature11432.

McGann, C.J., Odelberg, S.J., Keating, M.T. (2001). Mammalian myotube dedifferentiation induced by newt regeneration extract, *Proc Natl Acad Sci USA*, 98, pp. 13699–13704.

Melzack, R., Wall, P.D. (1965). Pain mechanisms: a new theory, *Science*, 150, pp. 971–979.

Montezano, A.C., Touyz, R.M. (2012). Oxidative stress, Noxs, and hypertension: experimental evidence and clinical controversies, *Ann Med*, 44, pp. S2–S16.

Nerio, L.S., Olivero-Verbel, J., Stashenko, E. (2010). Repellent activity of essential oils: a review, *Bioresour Technol*, 101, pp. 372–378.

Newman, D.J., Cragg, G.M. (2007). Natural products as sources of new drugs over the last 25 years, *J Nat Prod*, 70, pp. 461–477.

Nisoli, E., Tonello, C., Cardile, A., Cozzi, V., Bracale, R., Tedesco, L., Falcone, S., Valerio, A., Cantoni, O., Clementi, E., Moncada, S., Carruba, M.O. (2005). Calorie restriction promotes mitochondrial biogenesis by inducing the expression of eNOS, *Science*, 310, pp. 314–317.

Norden, A.D., Drappatz, J., Wen, P.Y. (2009). Antiangiogenic therapies for high-grade glioma, *Nat Rev Neurol*, 5, pp. 610–620.

Nortier J.L, Martinez, M.C., Schmeiser, H.H., Arlt, V.M., Bieler, C.A., Petein, M., Depierreux, M.F., De Pauw, L., Abramowicz, D., Vereerstraeten, P., Vanherweghem, J.L. (2000) Urothelial carcinoma associated with the use of a Chinese herb (*Aristolochia fangchi*), *N Eng J Med*, 342, pp. 1686–1692.

Obi, S., Yamamoto, K., Shimizu, N., Kumagaya, S., Masumura, T., Sokabe, T., Asahara, T., Ando, J. (2009). Fluid shear stress induces arterial differentiation of endothelial progenitor cells, *J Appl Physiol*, 106, pp. 203–211.

Omodei, D., Fontana, L. (2011). Calorie restriction and prevention of age-associated chronic disease, *FEBS Lett*, 585, pp. 1537–1542.

Pollina, E.A., Brunet, A. (2011) Epigenetic regulation of aging stem cells, *Oncogene*, 30, pp. 3105–3122.

Puangsombat, K., Jirapakkul, W., Smith, J.S. (2011). Inhibitory activity of Asian spices on heterocyclic amines formation in cooked beef patties, *J Food Sci*, 76, pp. T174–T180.

Purvya, M.C., Meena, M.S. (2011). A review on role of prakriti in aging, *Ayu*, 32, pp. 20–24.

Pyne, D., Shenker, N.G. (2008). Demystifying acupuncture, *Rheumatology (Oxford)*, 47, pp. 1132–1136.

Rand, D., Miller, W.C., Yiu, J., Eng, J.J. (2011). Interventions for addressing low balance confidence in older adults: a systematic review and meta-analysis, *Age Aging*, 40, pp. 297–306.

Ristow, M., Zarse, K. (2010). How increased oxidative stress promotes longevity and metabolic health: the concept of mitochondrial hormesis (mitohormesis), *Exp Gerontol*, 45, pp. 410–418.

Rodda, D.J., Chew, J.L., Lim, L.H., Loh, Y.H., Wang, B., Ng, H.H., Robson, P. (2005). Transcriptional regulation of nanog by OCT4 and SOX2, *J Biol Chem*, 280, pp. 24731–24737.

Rossi, D.J., Bryder, D., Weissman, I.L. (2007). Hematopoietic stem cell aging: mechanism and consequence, *Exp Gerontol*, 42, pp. 385–390.

Rossouw, J.E., Anderson, G.L., Prentice, R.L., LaCroix, A.Z., Kooperberg, C., Stefanick, M.L., Jackson, R.D., Beresford, S.A., Howard, B.V., Johnson, K.C., Kotchen, J.M., Ockene, J., Writing Group for the Women's Health Initiative Investigators (2002). Risks and benefits of estrogen plus progestin in healthy postmenopausal women: principal results form the Women's Health Initiative randomized controlled trial. *JAMA*, 288, pp. 321–333.

Shang, A., Huwiler, K., Nartey, L., Juni, P., Egger, M. (2007). Placebo-controlled trials of Chinese herbal medicine and conventional medicine comparative study, *Int J Epidemiol*, 36, pp. 1086–1092.

Silk, J.B., Beehner, J.C., Bergman, T.J., Crockford, C., Engh, A.L., Moscovice, L.R. Wittig, R.M., Seyfarth, R.M., Cheney, D.L. (2010). Strong and consistent social bonds enhance the longevity of female baboons, *Curr Biol*, 20, pp. 1359–1361.

Staud, R. (2007). Mechanisms of acupuncture analgesia: effective therapy for musculoskeletal pain? *Curr Rheumatol Rep*, 9, pp. 473–481.

Strauss, J., Reyes-Dominguez, Y. (2011). Regulation of secondary metabolism by chromatin structure and epigenetic codes, *Fungal Genet Biol*, 48, pp. 62–69.

Sun, D., Muthukumar, A.R., Lawrence, R.A., Fernandes, G. (2001). Effects of calorie restriction on polymicrobial peritonitis induced by cecum ligation and puncture in young C57BL/6 mice, *Clin Diagn Lab Immunol*, 8, pp. 1003–1011.

Surathu, N., Kurumathur, A.V. (2011). Traditional therapies in the management of periodontal disease in India and China, *Periodontol 2000*, 56, pp. 14–24.

Synder, B.R., Chiu, A.M., Prockop, D.J., Chan, A.W.S. (2010). Human multipotent stromal cells (MSCs) increase neurogenesis and decrease atrophy of the striatum in a transgenic mouse model for Huntington's disease, *PLoS ONE*, 5: e9347.

The Cancer Genome Atlas Research Network (2012). Comprehensive genome characterization of squamous cell lung cancers, *Nature*, doi: 10.1038/nature11404.

Trepanowski, J.F., Canale, R.E., Marshall, K.E., Kabir, M.M., Bloomer, R.J. (2011). Impact of caloric and dietary restriction regimens on markers of health and longevity in humans and animals: a summary of available findings, *Nutr J*, 10, p. 107.

Tsonis, P.A., Madhavan, M., Tancous, E.E., Rio-Tsonis, K.D. (2004). A newt's eye view of lens regeneration, *Int J Dev Biol*, 48, pp. 975–980.

Tuljapurkar, S.R., McGuire, T.R., Brusnahan, S.K., Jackson, J.D., Garvin, K.L., Kessinger, M.A., Lane, J.T., O'Kane, B.J., Sharp, J.G. (2011). Changes in human bone marrow fat content associated with changes in hematopoietic stem cell numbers and cytokine levels with aging, *J Anat*, 219, pp. 574–581.

Van Praag, H. (2008). Neurogenesis and exercise: past and future directions, *Neuromol Med*, 10, pp. 128–140.

Varady, K.A., Hellerstein, M.K. (2007). Alternate-day fasting and chronic disease prevention: a review of human and animal trials, *Am J Clin Nutr*, 86, pp. 7–13.

Vaynman, S., Ying, Z., Gomez-Pinilla, F. (2004). Hippocampal BDNF mediates the efficacy of exercise on synaptic plasticity and cognition, *Eur J Neurosci*, 20, pp. 2580–2590.

Vickers, A.J., Cronin, A.M., Maschino, A.C., Lweith, G., MacPherson, H., Foster, N.E., Sherman, K.J., Witt, C.M., Linde, K., for the Acupuncture Trialists' Collaboration (2012). Acupuncture for chronic pain individual patient data meta-analysis, *Arch Intern Med*, doi: 10.1001/archinternmed.2012.3654.

Wallace, D.C. (2010). Bioenergetics, the origins of complexity, and the ascent of man, *Proc Natl Acad Sci USA*, 107, pp. 8947–8953.

Wang, C., Bannuru, R., Ramel, J., Kupelnick, B., Scott, T. Schmid, C.H. (2010). Tai Chi on psychological well-being: systematic review and meta-analysis, *BMC Compl Alternat Med*, 10, p. 23.

Warburg, O. (1956). On the origin of cancer cells, *Science*, 133, pp. 309–314.

Wayne, P.M., Kiel, D.P., Krebs, D.E., Davis, R.B., Savetsky-German, J., Connelly, M., Buring, J.E. (2007). The effects of Tai Chi on bone mineral density in postmenopausal women: a systematic review, *Arch Phys Med Rehabil*, 88, pp. 673–680.

Wen, C.P., Wai, J.P., Tsai, M.K., Yang, Y.C., Cheng, T.Y., Lee, M.C., Chan, H.T., Tsao, C.K., Tsai, S.P., Wu, X. (2011). Minimum amount of physical activity for reduced mortality and extended life expectancy: a prospective cohort study, *Lancet*, 378, pp. 1244–1253.

Woods, J.A., Wilund, K.R., Martin, S.A., Kistler, B.M. (2012). Exercise, inflammation and aging, *Aging Dis*, 3, pp. 130–140.

Yeh, G.Y., Wang, C., Wayne, P.M., Phillips, R.S. (2008). The effect of tai chi exercise on blood pressure: a systematic review, *Prev Cardiol*, 11, pp. 82–89.

Yildirim, M.A., Goh, K.I., Cusick, M.E., Barabasi, A.L., Vidal, M. (2007). Drug-target network, *Nat Biotechnol*, 25, pp. 1119–1126.

Zlokovic, B.V. (2011). Neurovascular pathways to neurodegeneration in Alzheimer's disease and other disorders, *Nat Rev Neurosci*, 12, pp. 723–738.

Index